HANDBOOK OF
MEDICAL AND PROFESSIONAL
STAFF MANAGEMENT

Second Edition

Contributors

Morgan Brown, MA, CMSC, CPHQ
Senior Consultant
HealthCare Resource Group
Whittier, California

Wendy R. Crimp, RN, MBA
Director, Operations Consulting
BDO Seidman, LLP
Costa Mesa, California

Merialice (Mimi) Cruse, BA, CMSC
Former Director, Medical Staff Services
St. John and St. John West Shore
    Hospital
Westlake, Ohio

Cindy A. Gassiot, CMSC, CPCS
Director, Medical Staff Services
Cook Children's Medical Center
Fort Worth, Texas

Joanne P. Hopkins, Esq.
Partner
Haynes and Boone, LLP
Austin, Texas

Janet Reagan, PhD
Professor and Director
Health Administration Programs
California State Univesity
Northridge, California

Opal Reinbold
Director, Accrediation Services
BDO Seidman, LLP
Costa Mesa, California

Jodi Schirling, CMSC
Director, Quality Assurance, Utilization
    Management & Medical Staff
    Services
Alfred I. Dupont Institute
Wilmington, Delaware

Madeline Schneikart, CMSC
Director, CheckPoint Credentials
    Management Services
COHR
Chatsworth, California

Vicki L. Searcy
Principal
Healthcare Advisory Services
BDO Seidman, LLP
Costa Mesa, CA

Carla D. Thompson, Esq.
Attorney
Guest Lecturer, Chemeketa Community
    College
Salem, Oregon

Richard E. Thompson, MD
President
Thompson, Mohr and Associates
Dunedin, Florida

HANDBOOK OF MEDICAL AND PROFESSIONAL STAFF MANAGEMENT

Second Edition

Edited by

Cindy A. Gassiot, CMSC, CPCS

Director, Medical Staff Services
Cook Children's Medical Center

Fort Worth, TX

Vicki L. Searcy

Principal, Healthcare Advisory Services
BDO Seidman, LLP
Costa Mesa, CA

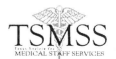

A Texas Society for Medical Staff Services Publication
Austin, Texas • 1998

Texas Society for Medical Staff Services grants permission for
photocopying for limited personal or internal use. This consent does
not extend to other kinds of copying, such as copying for general
distribution, for advertising or promotional purposes, for creating
new collective works, or for resale. For information, address Texas
Society for Medical Staff Services, Permissions Department, 1033
La Posada Drive, Suite 220, Austin, Texas 78752-3880.
Editorial Services: Tracie Harris

Library of Congress Catalog Card Number: 98-61267
ISBN: 0-9666564-0-7

Printed in the United States of America

Acknowledgments

This book could not have been written without the work of the contributors, whom the editors sincerely thank.

Our thanks also to the Board of Directors of the Texas Society for Medical Staff Services for recognizing the need for an updated text.

The editors gratefully acknowledge Tracie Harris and Roy Bohrer of Association and Society Management, Inc., Austin, Texas, whose assistance in producing this book was invaluable. Caroline Leyva of BDO Seidman, LLP, Costa Mesa, California, was also a great help in compiling the manuscript.

The editors also acknowledge F.C. Dimond, Jr., MD (now deceased) and Charles Matthews, MD, whose chapters from the first edition were used in part in this edition. We are indebted to these physicians for their initial contributions.

And to Sharon Lindsey, who co-edited the first edition of this book, best wishes with your new interests.

Cindy A. Gassiot
Vicki L. Searcy
July, 1998

Table of Contents

Chapter   9 — Credentials Verification Organizations 165
Madeline Schneikart, CMSC

**Chapter 10 — The Role of the Medical Staff in the Assessment
         and Improvement of Patient Care 183**
Opal Reinbold

Chapter 11 — Program-specific Accreditation 213
Cindy A. Gassiot, CMSC, CPCS

Preface

I began my career in health care in the early 1980s. My first job in health care was working for Sister John, the administrator of a community hospital. I had a variety of responsibilities but the most interesting for me from the very beginning was coordinating some of the medical staff committees and participating in the credentialing process. This was also the most frustrating of my responsibilities, because no one at the hospital could explain to me why committees were meeting, what was supposed to be documented in the minutes, who would be reading the minutes, or the purpose (and procedures) involved in the credentialing process. The physician leaders certainly didn't know and everyone else seemed to be doing things that "had always been done this way." I asked "why" so many times that I knew if I asked one more time, Sister John was likely to banish me from the administrative wing.

Fortunately, Sister John's secretary went on vacation shortly after I began asking all these questions. One day I was searching at her desk for a document and came upon a red manual called *Medical Staff Services Manual* written by Cindy Orsund (Gassiot) and Patricia Starr. I found the answers I was searching for in that manual. More importantly, however, that red manual gave me the vision for a career in medical staff services that has been enormously exciting and fulfilling.

Many medical staff services professionals have similar stories about how they stumbled into medical staff organization management. Many of these individuals still have copies of the "red manual" which helped so many of us understand how to support a medical staff organization.

Since those early days, I have had the opportunity to work with Cindy Gassiot on a variety of projects and am always in awe of Cindy's commitment to the medical staff services profession. She is a tireless advocate for providing education and resource materials to individuals who are new to the profession.

Thanks, Cindy, for inspiring me, writing the original manual that helped me find my career, and for asking me to work with you on this book. I hope the *Handbook of Medical and Professional Staff Management* will prove to be a valuable resource to those who work with medical and professional staffs.

Vicki L. Searcy
Costa Mesa, California

The Handbook of Medical and Professional Staff Management is a revised and updated edition of the *Handbook of Medical Staff Management.* The second edition of this work has new and revised chapters addressing the significant changes that have occurred, mainly due to the role that managed care now plays in the health care delivery system, since the first edition was published eight years ago. Most chapters have been extensively rewritten. New chapters have been written addressing managed care credentialing and the many accreditation programs that influence and drive the operation of medical and professional staff services and credentials verification organizations. The Current Legal Issues chapter has been updated to include information on managed care credentialing and emerging case law in that area. The Credentialing and Peer Review Issues chapter addresses some newer issues such as telemedicine and fast-track credentialing as well as provides information about credentialing and peer review in academic hospitals. A new chapter deals with the changes occurring in many medical staff services departments that now serve integrated health care delivery systems and have had to tailor operations to meet these needs.

This book is a definitive text and resource for medical staff services practitioners, managed care credentialing managers and specialists, students, and those preparing to earn their credentials in the fields. Physician leaders of professional staff organizations should also find the book to be of value. Credentialing specialists in managed care organizations should find the book especially helpful. The editors hope that this work will assist medical staff services and managed care credentialing professionals to understand and appreciate the other's roles to a greater degree.

It is also my wish that others, like Vicki Searcy, will come across this book on someone else's desk and be inspired to enter this challenging and rewarding field.

Thank you, Vicki, for collaborating with me on this book, for finding time to work on this project in spite of a very demanding schedule, for your unfailing good humor and positive attitude, and for providing a brief respite from the heat of a Texas summer.

Cindy A. Gassiot
Grapevine, Texas
July 1998

Chapter 1

Health Care Delivery Systems

Janet Thompson Reagan, Ph.D.

A BRIEF HISTORY

Health care is one of the largest industries in the United States, both in size of expenditures and number of persons employed. In 1995 expenditures on health care totaled $988.5 billion, or 13.6 percent of the gross national product (GNP). Expenditures for hospital care totaled $350.1 billion, followed by expenditures for physician services, ($201.6 billion).[1] In 1996 hospitals employed 5,041,000 people while over 11 million were employed in health services delivery.[2] The industry is rapidly changing in response to legal, cultural, technological, and economic changes in its environment. Terms commonly used to describe the environment are turbulent, unstable, and complex.

What began as a cottage industry of individual providers has evolved into a complex array of providers, service delivery mechanisms, payment mechanisms, and regulatory agencies. Torrens described the development of the health care system according to the predominant health problem of the period, the technology available, and the social organization for the application of the technology.[3] The development of the industry was divided into four periods, 1850-1900, 1900 to World War II, World War II to roughly 1980, and the future. Other authors have used similar approaches in tracing the development of the health care system. For example, Odin W. Anderson discussed the periods from 1875 to 1930, 1930 to 1965, and 1965 to 1985.[4] This brief overview of the industry will begin at an earlier point, the pre-1750 era, and then will follow the periods of development described by Torrens. The primary emphasis of this chapter will be on the private sector, and within that sector, on the hospital and managed care industries.

Pre-1750

During the pre-industrial revolution years (pre-1750), the practice of medicine was relatively primitive.[5] The scientific viewpoint was undeveloped and medical practice was often based on speculation, trial and error, and even superstition. Medical education was neither standardized nor regulated. Hospitals in their current form did not exist. Institutions for care were essentially pesthouses or almshouses established and run by religious organizations, or, in some cases, by local governments. Medical technology and the kind of social organization required for its application were largely nonexistent.

During this period, activities focused on attempts to control epidemics, prevent the entry of new diseases, and ensure a safe water supply. For example in 1647, the Massachusetts Bay Colony passed a regulation to prevent pollution of the Boston Harbor, and in 1701, the Commonwealth of Massachusetts passed a law requiring isolation of persons with smallpox.[6]

Industrial Revolution 1750-1850

During the Industrial Revolution, developments occurred largely in the area of public health. Local and state health agencies were established in response to epidemics and the need to ensure safe water supplies and adequate sanitation. Medical science advanced as a result of an increasing emphasis on logical experimentation and controlled observation. Medical training improved, beginning with the establishment of the first American medical school at the College of Philadelphia in 1765.[7] The American Medical Association was founded in 1847 and had as one of its primary goals the improvement of medical education. Yet, rigorous training was still rare. "In 1800 there were only four functioning medical colleges; in 1825 there were eighteen."[8]

Hospitals were still primarily almshouses serving the indigent. Yet toward the end of this period, hospitals began to emerge as legitimate providers of care, and not only for individuals with communicable diseases who had to be isolated and for the indigent who had no other options for care but also for individuals in the larger community who had resources to pay.

The Shattuck Report of 1850 can be viewed as the culmination of advances in public health during this period. Although the report did not initially stimulate dramatic changes in the provision of public health services, it set out far-reaching recommendations that not only held true for that time, but continue to hold true today. For example, Shattuck included recommendations regarding the control of alcoholism, smoke nuisances, routine physical examinations, and family records of illness, to name only a few.[9]

1850-1900

The period from 1850 to 1900 was characterized by only moderate progress in the medical field. Diagnostic and therapeutic techniques were improved and anesthesia and antisepsis were developed.[10,11] Medical education and practice, however, were still poorly developed. Although many medical schools existed, over 450 at times, many of the new schools were proprietary and curricula and programs varied widely.[12] Schools were not held accountable for the ability or the quality of the physicians produced. At the end of this period, licensure of physicians emerged as medical practice acts began to be enacted by the states in the 1870s.

Nursing emerged as the first allied health profession, and hospital-based training programs for nurses were established. Although Florence Nightingale is credited with the "transformation of nursing into a profession," it was Dorothea Dix who recruited and encouraged nursing training programs in this country during the Civil War.[13] Permanent schools of nursing were established in the post-Civil War years. The health care team now consisted of the physician and the nurse.

Hospitals became legitimate providers of care. As surgery developed, the affluent sought the services of surgeons, who in turn sought to practice in hospitals. "By 1900 there were 4,000 general hospitals in the United States."[14]

1901-1945

The period from 1901 to roughly 1945 included remarkable medical advances, the expansion of state and federal subsidies for health services, the revamping of medical education, and the emergence of the framework for the health care system as it currently exists. During this period, the focus of health care shifted from epidemics to individual episodes of acute disease.[15] Support for medical research was greatly expanded, and advances were made in diagnosis, treatment, and prevention of disease. The period of antibiotics began with the discovery of penicillin in 1941. With the advances in medical science, health care professionals began to combat successfully individual episodes of acute disease.

Medical education was revolutionized as a result of the efforts of the American Medical Association, the advances in medical science, and the publication of the Flexner Report in 1910.[16] Although the number of medical schools declined as a result of the closure of substandard schools (down to 85 in 1920), those that remained built their curricula on a sound scientific base, and the four-year program of preparation became standard. Additionally, "by 1925 forty-nine boards (for medical licensure) required candidates for their examinations to be graduates of a medical college...".[17] During this period, many of the medical specialties developed. Only one specialty existed in 1920; by 1940 there were 16.[18]

Government involvement at both the state and federal level increased. At the federal level, the Pure Food and Drug Act was passed in 1906. The Sheppard-Towner Act of 1921 made small federal grants available to state and local governments for maternal and child health programs and for the development and strengthening of local health departments.[19] Other federal action included the 1935 Social Security Act. Title V of this act increased federal assistance to maternal and child health programs and greatly expanded assistance to state and local health departments. Another outcome of this legislation was the growth in proprietary nursing homes. Guaranteed monthly incomes through the old age survivors insurance and the old age assistance programs enabled the elderly to pay for boarding home or nursing home care. Payments were not made to the elderly in almshouses or government facilities. Finally, the 1944 Public Health Service Act brought all the federal public health programs together under one agency.

The Committee on the Costs of Medical Care was created in 1927 through the support of private foundations.[20] A series of 27 field studies were conducted, and a total of 28 reports published. The last report, published in 1932, recommended that health services be delivered through organized groups and that the costs of medical care should be financed on a group basis. This restructuring of the health care system was proposed as a means of addressing economic inefficiency and reducing preventable pain and needless deaths.

It was during this period that the third-party pay system emerged as an important source of financing for health services. During the Depression, the Blue Cross and Blue Shield plans were developed to ensure that individuals would have access to hospital and physician services. The first commercial insurers also entered the marketplace, and the first prepaid group, the Ross-Loos Plan, was established.

Any attempt to summarize the medical advances during this period would be futile. Progress was made on all fronts. New diagnostic procedures developed; treatment, especially surgical procedures, were improved; and prevention of diseases, especially infectious diseases became more successful.

1946-1965

The period from 1946 to 1965 was one of rapid advancement in the medical sciences, expansion of federal effort in the health care field, and the continued growth of third-party payers. "From 1947 to 1963 federal support of medical research increased at an average annual rate of 26 percent."[21] The National Institutes of Health increased in prestige and set the agenda for medical research during this period.

The role of the federal government in health services was greatly expanded. With the passage of the Hill-Burton Act (Hospital Survey and Construction Act) in 1946, the federal government began to subsidize the construction of hospitals. Between 1947 and 1971, Hill-Burton funds helped to build 345,000 hospital beds.[22] Through amendments to the original legislation, funds were later used for hospital renovations and for the construction of ambulatory clinics and nursing homes. Mental health services were supported through the 1946 Mental Health Act and later through the 1963 Mental Retardation Facilities and Community Mental Health Centers Construction Act.[23]

The federal government also subsidized the development of human resources through a variety of programs, including the Vocational Education Act of 1946, the Grants-in-Aid to Schools of Public Health in 1958, and the Health Professions Education Assistance Act of 1963. New occupations emerged in response to the introduction of new technology and advances in medical practice. The practice of medicine became increasingly specialized.

1966-Present

The mid-sixties are considered by many to be a turning point in the health care industry. The predominant health care focus shifted from individual episodes of acute disease to chronic health conditions, partly as a result of our aging population and partly as a result of medicine's success in preventing and treating acute disease.[24]

The federal government began to play an ever larger role in health services. Lawrence Brown identified the main function of the federal government from 1966 to the mid-seventies as the provision of financing.[25] With the implementation of Medicare and Medicaid in 1966, the federal government became a major source for financing of health services. Medicare is a federal insurance program for those qualifying for Social Security benefits, and Medicaid is a federal-state assistance program for the indigent.

Although a description of these programs is beyond the scope of this chapter, an indication of their impact on the health care system is essential. Expenditures for both programs soon far exceeded projected levels. Since both were entitlement programs, expenditures were difficult to project and control. Federal expenditures for Medicare alone went from $4.5 billion in 1967 to $15.6 billion in 1976.[26] For Medicaid, federal response was to allow states to reduce covered services, restrict the eligible population, and modify reimbursement methods to control expenditures. For Medicare, the federal government sought to control expenditures through regulation and reimbursement, for example, through the introduction of Professional Standards Review Organizations (PSROs) in 1972 and the Prospective Payment System (PPS) in 1982.

Brown characterizes federal policy in the 1970s as one of reorganization and regulation.[27] Reorganization was seen as a way of increasing system efficiency and controlling expenditures. The Health Maintenance Organization Act (HMO) of 1973 is an example of action in this area. Additionally, Title XIX of the Social Security Act was amended to encourage the enrollment of persons covered by Medicaid in alternative delivery systems, usually prepaid groups.

The federal government sought to regulate the system through the new health planning legislation passed in 1974 (P.L. 41-93), replacing the planning system authorized in 1966. The Social Security Amendments of 1972 authorized PSROs, whose function was to monitor the appropriateness and quality of care rendered under the Medicaid and Medicare programs. PSROs were replaced by the Professional Review Organizations (PROs) in 1982 with the passage of the Tax Equity and Fiscal Responsibility Act (TEFRA). TEFRA also modified the method of reimbursement under Medicare. A prospective payment system based on diagnosis related groups (DRGs) replaced the retrospective cost-based system.

In the 1980s the health care industry continued to evolve. Innovations included the development of new alternative delivery systems, the introduction of new financing mechanisms, and the first attempts by states (Hawaii and Massachusetts) to provide universal health insurance coverage.

For a summary of the history, see Table 1-1.

THE HOSPITAL SECTOR

The preceding discussion of the evolution of the health care system traced the development of hospitals as one component of the larger service delivery

Table 1-1. Overview of the Development of the U.S. Health Care System (1776-present).

	Pre-1776	1776-1876
Major health issues	Plagues Epidemics Sanitation Dietary deficiencies	Infections Sanitation Epidemics
Health care policy/laws	1602 Massachusetts Bay Colony regulation to prevent pollution of Boston Harbor 1701 Massachusetts - Law to require isolation of persons with small pox	Health of the people is the responsibility of the states: sporadic attempts to legislate public health; spirit of laissez-faire 1850 Shattuck Report
Federal government's role		1798 Congress created the Marine Hospital Svc. 1875 Surgeon General appointed
Professional growth - medicine	In colonies, clergy were doctors 1765 College of Philadelphia - first medical school in U.S.	1783 Harvard Medical School opens 1812 New England Journal of Medicine 1848 American Medical Association 1873 First state board of medical examiners
Professional growth - allied health	Nursing performed by religious orders; midwives delivered babies	1861 Dorothea Dix establishes Army Nurses Corps 1862 Nightingale opens nurses' training school in London 1882 Clara Barton establishes American Red Cross
Delivery of care	Pts. treated in home; MDs treated by letter written to pts. far away; hospitals established to treat poor 1750 Pennsylvania Hospital	MDs had to practice surgery, obstetrics as well as internal medicine; all treatment, even surgery, performed at home. 1810 Mass. General Hospital became model for others 1872 American Public Health Association
Financial trends	Wealthy landowners paid MDs a yearly fee to provide care for family and slaves Others paid out of pocket	Cost of medical school approx. $150/yr. for 2-3 yrs. 1840 MDs office visit: $.05-10 Natural delivery: $4-30 1860 Natural delivery: $5-50

Table 1-1. Overview of the Development of the U.S. Health Care System (1776-present). *(continued)*

	1876-1946	1946-present
Major health issues	Acute infections and illnesses	Acute illnesses Chronic diseases AIDS Addiction Aging population
Health care policy/laws	Spirit of responsible concern; NY State requires reporting TB 1906 Food and Drug Act 1912 US Pubic Health Service 1914 Harrison Anti-narcotic Act 1921 Sheppard-Towner Act 1925 Social Security Act 1944 Public Health Service Act 1946 Hill-Burton Act National Mental Health Act 1946 Vocational Education Act	1958 Grants-in-Aid to Schools of Public Health 1963 Health Professions Assistance Act 1965 Community Mental Health Center Act 1966 Comprehensive Health Planning Act 1968 Health Manpower Act 1970 Occupational Safety and Health Act 1971 National Cancer Act 1972 PSROs established 1973 Health Maintenance Organization Act 1974 National Health Planning & Resources Development Act 1982 TEFRA (established DRGs and replaced PSROs with PROs) 1983 PL 98-21 created Prospective Payment System using DRGs for reimbursement 1986 Health Care Quality Improvement Act 1990 Americans with Disabilities Act
Federal government's role	Concern for public health 1876 Marine Hospital Service given power to cooperate with state boards of health 1879 National Board of Health Increased federal involvement after the Great Depression 1946 CDC established	Increasing amount of federal regulation, especially after Medicaid and Medicare Late 60s Blank check attitude to improving nation's health Early 70s Cost containment 1972 Intern salary: $9778 1974 Cost of medical school: $12,650/yr. 1980 Quality assurance; cost containment 1989 Agency for Health Care Policy & Research established
Professional growth - medicine	1863 Journal of the American Medical Assn. 1910 Flexner report on medical education 1936 American Cancer Institute	1949 National Institute of Mental Health Increased specialization; more MDs become board certified 1976 Health Professions Educational Assistance Act - focus on primary care New health professions 1995 Commission calls for 20% of medical schools to be closed by 2005 1996 Institute of Medicine's report: "The Nation's Physician Workforce: Options for Balancing Supply and Requirements"
Professional growth - allied health	1885 First visiting nurse service 1910 Public Health Nursing program at Columbia 1911 American Nurses' Association	Rapid increase in a wide variety of allied health professions 1966 Allied Health Professions Personnel Act
Delivery of care	As surgery became more complex, pts. had to go to hospitals; increased need for skilled nursing care; increased need to centralize expensive X-ray and lab equipment in hospitals 1899 American Hospital Association 1916 American College of Surgeons started hospital surveys 1927 Committee on the Costs of Medical Care 1929 Ross-Loos - first HMO founded 1933 First Blue Cross plan organized 1945 Kaiser Permanente started	Community outpatient mental health clinics 1952 Formation of JCAH Increase in large multihospital corporations; formation of PPOs, IPAs; increase in salaried MDs 1973 HMO Act 1980s Horizontal and vertical integration of health care organizations 1990s Period of consolidations and mergers of health care organizations 1991 National Committee for Quality Assurance begins accreditation of managed care organizations
Financial trends	1902 $4/day hospital stay $40/month nursing salary 1933 First Blue Cross plan organized By 1935 all but 4 states had workmen's compensation	1972 Cost of medical education:$9700/year 1974 $80-187/day for hospital stay Increased involvement by business in health care finances; decreased cost shifting

Note: Revised and updated data from *Two Centuries of American Medicine* by J. Bordley and A. McGehee Harvey, W.B. Saunders Company, 1976.

system. Hospitals have evolved from simple institutions to organizations that provide a wide array of health services, utilize sophisticated technology and numerous health professions and allied health personnel, and exist under a variety of organizational and ownership arrangements. The free-standing hospital is increasingly rare as multi-hospital or multi-institutional systems emerge. Hospitals are expanding services to include not only inpatient care but also a broad array of services such as ambulatory clinics, membership programs for the elderly, psychiatric services, and substance abuse programs.

Hospital Size

Hospitals can be categorized in a number of ways, including size, ownership, and services provided. Of the 6,201 hospitals in the United States in 1996, 2,854 (46 percent) had 99 or fewer beds; 2,339 (38 percent) had 100 to 299 beds; 654 (10 percent) had 300-499 beds; and 354 (6 percent) had 500 or more beds.[28] Although a fairly large number (2,854 hospitals) are small (99 or fewer beds), these hospitals account for only 14 percent of the total beds.

Hospital Ownership

The categories of hospital ownership are voluntary (non-profit, including religious control), government (local, state, and federal), and proprietary. Most hospitals are non-profit followed by government and proprietary.[29] However, if one excludes government facilities, the percentage of proprietary hospitals has been relatively stable (20 percent in 1995, up from 18.4 percent in 1976).

Hospitals can also be described according to specialty. In 1996 most non-federal hospitals were classified as short-term general and other specialty (87 percent), followed by psychiatric facilities (11 percent); long term general and other specialty (2 percent); and tuberculosis and other respiratory disease (less than 1 percent).[30]

Hospitals are integrating vertically and horizontally in response to changes in the environment which have threatened their survival.[31] Horizontal integration refers to the addition of organizations of the same type (e.g., one hospital acquiring another hospital). Vertical integration occurs when the organization decides to engage in a new enterprise or new type of program. For example, as mentioned earlier, many hospitals are adding new services such as substance abuse clinics, long term care units, and psychiatric programs.

As a result of these organizational shifts, hospital systems grew rapidly in the late 1970s and early 1980s. In 1978, 1,455 hospitals were owned by multi-hospital systems; 628, by investor-owner systems; and 727, by non-profit systems.[32] In 1982, 1,740 hospitals were owned by multi-hospital systems, an increase of 19.6 percent.[33] The number of multihospital systems increased rapidly and controlled 2,058 hospitals in 1996.[34] In addition, 1,343 hospitals were in some type of health care network.

Hospital Reimbursement

Hospitals are reimbursed for services rendered through a variety of mechanisms. Most of their revenues are from third-party payers, including local, state, and federal governments; managed care organizations such as health maintenance organizations (HMOs) and preferred provider organizations (PPOs); Blue Cross and Blue Shield Plans; and indemnity insurance plans. Because of the large number of third-party payers and the variety of payment mechanisms, sound financial planning and information systems for financial management are essential to hospital survival.

To control costs many third-party payers are implementing new payment mechanisms and requiring utilization review and second opinions. For example, in California hospitals must contract with the state if they wish to serve Medicaid patients. Payment is a pre-negotiated flat per diem rate. Other payers who contract with hospitals are HMOs and PPOs. With the passage of the 1982 Tax Equity and Fiscal Responsibility Act (TEFRA) and the Social Security Amendments of 1983, Medicare replaced the cost-based retrospective payment system with a PPS based on DRGs. Medicare patients are assigned to a DRG and payment is based on the amount allowed for that DRG. The PPS provides incentives for efficient service delivery, since reimbursement is predetermined based on the DRG assignment and not on resource utilization.

There was some concern that hospitals might be tempted to reduce the number and quality of services to save money. Although the average length of stay (ALOS) declined for individuals aged 65 to 74 (from 8.3 days in 1985 to 6.5 days in 1995) it also declined for those aged 45–64 (from 7.1 days to 5.5 days).[35] This decline in ALOS means that hospitals are serving more acute patients and providing more intensive services during the short hospital stay. Patients are discharged earlier, many requiring a stay in a sub-acute or skilled nursing facility or services provided in the home, fueling the growth of these industries. Evidence to date does not indicate that the PPS has resulted in reduced quality of care.[36]

Hospitals are heavily regulated organizations. Not only must they comply with all relevant state, local, and federal requirements for businesses, but they must meet additional requirements because of the nature of their business—health care. Non-federal hospitals in each state are licensed and exist by the authority of the state under general statutes regarding corporations or under specific statutes or charters. Federal facilities (e.g., Veterans Administration hospitals) are an exception, since they are not regulated by the states. Hospitals also must meet Medicare and Medicaid conditions of participation if they wish to provide services to enrollees of those programs. In addition, most hospitals seek accreditation through the Joint Commission on Accreditation of Healthcare Organizations (JCAHO) or the American Osteopathic Association (AOA).

THE HEALTH CARE TEAM

Hospitals employ a bewildering array of health professionals and allied and ancillary health personnel. Over 200 different occupational groups exist, and in some hospitals the number of job titles approaches the number of employees. Staffing patterns and levels in hospitals and other health facilities have changed in recent years. The driving forces behind these changes include the introduction of new technology, advances in medical practice, and, in some cases, new requirements by state and federal governments (e.g., the conditions of participation under Medicare and Medicaid).

The large number of distinct professional and occupational groups complicates human resource management and requires skill in developing and maintaining productive health care teams. In contrast to the days when medical care was provided by the physician, possibly with the aid of a nurse, the provision of medical services today requires a team made up of diverse professionals. Often the members of the health care team come from disparate educational backgrounds and have been socialized into roles that do not easily mesh. Professionals have been characterized as desiring and expecting autonomy in the workplace, further complicating the development of cooperative and productive health care teams.

For the purpose of this discussion, human resources in the health care industry will be categorized as (1) management and administrative personnel, (2) professional and technical personnel, and (3) support personnel.[37] Occupations in the first two categories usually require the completion of special educational programs and licensure or certification.

Management and Administrative Personnel

Education for professional managers of health services emerged relatively recently. The first master's program was developed in 1934 at the University of Chicago. Graduate programs are found in various settings: schools of public health, business schools and schools of allied health. Programs of study are typically two years in length and prepare the graduate to enter middle-management positions in a wide variety of health care settings. In 1996, 69 programs were accredited by the Accrediting Commission on Education in Health Services Administration (ACEHSA) and were full members of the University Program in Health Administration (AUPHA).[38]

Undergraduate programs in health care management emerged in the 1960s in response to system expansion and an increased need for individuals trained to assume entry-level management positions. The AUPHA has established standards for baccalaureate programs and applies these standards to programs seeking full AUPHA membership. In 1996, 28 programs were approved for full AUPHA membership. Five programs were associate members preparing for full membership.[39]

Recent trends in health care management are the increasing number of women entering both the baccalaureate and graduate programs (from 8.1 percent in 1968-69 to 72.7 percent in 1984-85 for baccalaureate programs.)[40] Executive and non-traditional programs have been developed for physicians and allied health professionals seeking to move from clinical to management roles.

Professional and Technical Personnel

As mentioned earlier a large number of occupational groups contribute to the delivery of health care. Although it is beyond the scope of this chapter to discuss all or even most of these groups, the key ones will be described in terms of education, number in practice, and trends in the field. For the purpose of this discussion, a distinction will be made between independent practitioners and dependent practitioners. The former are allowed by law to provide a delimited set of services without the supervision or authorization by others; the latter provide services under supervision or after authorization by an independent practitioner.

Independent Practitioners

As discussed earlier in this chapter, medical education and the medical profession underwent major changes in the early twentieth century. The practice of medicine is now highly specialized, with over 80 specialties and subspecialties. Training programs are long, often requiring over seven years of postbaccalaureate study.

The number of active physicians increased from 380,500 in 1975 to 533,000 in 1985, and to 681,694 in 1995, and is projected to be 740,900 in 2000.[41] The practitioner per 100,000 population increased from 174 in 1975 to 220 in 1985, to 259 in 1995, and is projected to be 268 in 2000. Whether these figures represent a surplus, shortage, or supply-demand equilibrium is subject to debate.[42,43] Several factors complicate the supply and demand analysis of physicians. Geographic distribution, distribution across specialties, utilization patterns, and medical care practice are just a few of these.[44] For example, in 1994 the non-federal physician to population ratio varied from 323 per 100,000 population in the Northeast to 210.5 per 100,000 population in the South.

Podiatrists, dentists, psychologists and optometrists are also independent practitioners. Although the supply and practitioner-to-population ratio are expected to increase for all these groups, the percentage change will vary considerably. For example, the physician-to-population ratio is projected to change 21.8 percent from 1985 to 2000, yet the change for dentists is projected to be only 3.4 percent. Additionally, admissions to dental schools are declining, from 22,842 in 1980-81 to 16,178 in 1994-95.[45]

Dependent Practitioners

Professional nurses constitute the largest group of health personnel. In 1980 there were 1,272,000 active registered nurses (RNs), in 1990 there were 1,715,600, and in 1994 there were 2,044,000.[46] This represents an increase in the RNs from 560 in 1980 to 785 in 1984. Yet, hospitals and other health delivery sites are having difficulty filling vacant RN positions.[47]

Nurses may prepare to enter the field by completing any one of three educational programs. Diploma programs were the first ones developed and are usually two to three years in length and hospital based. The first year students enrolled in these programs dropped from 16,905 in 1980 to 7,717 in 1995.[48]

Baccalaureate programs typically are four to five years and are offered by colleges and universities. The number of first year students enrolled in these programs increased from 35,414 in 1980 to 43,451 in 1995.[49]

Associate degree programs developed in the fifties with the support of the federal government. Since the establishment of the first program in 1952, the growth of these programs has been rapid. The number of first year students enrolled in these programs increased from 53,334 in 1980 to 76,016 in 1995.[50]

Nurse training programs are accredited by the National League of Nursing. The key professional association is the American Nurses' Association. Registered nurses are licensed in all states. The first licensure act was passed in 1903, and by 1923 all states and the District of Columbia licensed nurses under nurse practice acts.[51]

Nursing practice, like medical practice, has become increasingly specialized. Among the specialty groups are nurse anesthetists, psychiatric nurses, and nurse practitioners. Specialties require training beyond the initial program of study and in some cases require a master's degree.

Current issues in nursing are the appropriate roles and tasks for professional nurses, the preferred educational program (diploma, associate degree, or baccalaureate degree), and the shortage of professional nurses. The full-time equivalent RN vacancy rate in hospitals increased from 4.4% in 1983 to 13.6% in 1986.[52]

Several factors may be responsible for the shortage of RNs, including increasing opportunities for women to enter other professions (e.g., law and medicine), the changing utilization of RNs, job stress, and limited salary progression.

Quite simply, women are seeking career opportunities in other fields, perhaps reducing the number entering nursing and the number remaining in nursing.

Practical nurses (licensed practical nurses or licensed vocational nurses) complete 9 to 12 months of training, usually in a vocational school or a community college. The first programs were established in 1917 as a result of the Vocational Education Act.[53]

Support Personnel

Other allied health personnel include workers in the medical laboratory, radiologic service workers, physical therapists, speech pathologists, occupational therapists, dental hygienists, and pharmacists, to list only a few. Although the educational and licensure requirements for individual occupations vary considerably, the general trend is for education requirements to increase over time and licensure and certification requirements to become more restrictive. For example, physical therapy is attempting to move the degree required for entry-level practice from the baccalaureate level to the master's. Another trend is for occupational groups to seek more autonomy in practice. For example, dental hygienists in California are seeking to change licensure laws so that they can engage in a mode of independent practice[54] and pharmacists in Florida are seeking changes that would allow them to prescribe drugs in delimited circumstances.

As the health care industry evolves, new specialties develop. The field of medical records management, developed in the mid-1900s, has become increasingly important as reimbursement mechanisms change (for example, the move by Medicare to form cost-based reimbursement to reimbursement based on DRGs and the advances in sophistication of clinical information systems). Similarly, in response to the need for improved quality assurance mechanisms and the implementation of quality improvement programs, the field of quality assurance or improvement has developed. A final example is that of the medical staff services professional. Health care organizations of all types need staff to oversee the management of the medical staff organization, including credentialing and related activities. The National Association Medical Staff Services, with over 4000 members provides opportunities for education and certification in this field.[55]

PAYING FOR CARE

Payment mechanisms within the health care sector are complex and constantly changing. At the beginning of the twentieth century, payment was usually made out of pocket by the individual receiving the service. In some cases government and religious organizations would directly provide services through hospitals and clinics.

During the Depression, the Blue Shield and Blue Cross Plans were developed and the government began to subsidize health services for some indigent groups. For example, Title V of the Social Security Act provided support for maternal and child health programs. The importance of third-party payers increased steadily in the following decades. A third-party payer is a party—a government agency, insurance company, or employer—that reimburses providers for services delivered to others. In 1940 only 18.7 percent of the payments for personal health services were by third-party payers. In 1960, it was 44.1 percent, and by 1981, it was 67.9 percent. For hospitals it is now over 80 percent.[56,57]

MANAGED CARE

Health Maintenance Organizations

As Russell Coile points out in his book, *The New Governance*, the hospital is no longer the center of the health care system[58] and HMOs are no longer considered to be alternative delivery systems. Managed care organizations including HMOs, PPOs, managed indemnity plans, Medicare, and others, dominate. For example, in 1976 only 2.8 percent (6 million) of the population was enrolled in HMOs. By 1995, that percentage was 19.4 percent (53.4 million). The growth of PPOs has been even faster from 37.1 million enrollees in 1991 to 117.1 million enrollees in 1995.[59]

HMOs provide an alternative to traditional delivery financing mechanisms. An HMO is an organization that provides a comprehensive set of health services to a voluntarily enrolled population for a fixed monthly or annual fee. Although the first HMO, the Ross-Loos Health Plan, was organized in 1929 and the Kaiser Permanente Medical Program was established in northern and southern California in 1945, few HMOs existed until their growth was stimulated by the passage in 1973 of the Health Maintenance Organization Act.[60] The federal government supported the development of HMOs through a program of grants and loans. HMOs were considered to be an efficient means of providing and financing health services. The federal government hoped the growth of HMOs would help contain health care expenditures by reducing the use of costly health services and by competing with the commercial insurers and the Blue Cross and Blue Shield Plans.

Organizational Models

The predominant models for HMOs are the staff, group practice and the independent practice association (IPA). Common to all three models are (1) a component responsible for plan management, including the development of the service and payment structure and the acquisition of service providers, service delivery sites, and plan enrollees; (2) service providers, including physicians and other health care personnel; (3) service delivery sites, including hospitals and ambulatory clinics; and (4) enrollees.

In the staff model HMO the plan employs the providers and owns and operates the facilities. Physicians and other providers are generally salaried and provide services only to HMO enrollees.

In the group practice model, the HMO contracts with a multispecialty group and other facilities (e.g., hospitals) for the provision of services. The HMO reimburses the group on a capitation basis, and the group then reimburses the physicians and other providers. In some cases, a distinction is made between a group model in which plan management contracts with a single medical group and a group model in which the plan contracts with several medical groups or providers. The former mode is referred to as a group model and the latter as a network model.

In the IPA model, the plan contracts with multiple providers who maintain their own offices and may treat patients other than HMO enrollees. The plan reimburses the physicians directly, usually at a percentage of their usual and customary fees. In 1996 there were 122 (19.4 percent) group model HMOs (including networks and staff models), 366 (58.2 percent) IPAs, and 140 (22.3 percent) mixed model HMOs.[61]

The growth of HMOs was rapid. In 1976 there were only 174 HMOs serving 6 million enrollees. By 1990 there were 572 HMOs serving 33 million enrollees, and in 1996 there were 628 HMOs serving 55.7 million.[62]

Preferred Provider Organizations

PPOs contract with employers or other groups of enrollees to provide coverage for a comprehensive set of health services. A panel of health care providers is established through contracts based on negotiated discounted rates or a fixed fee schedule. Unlike HMOs, PPOs do not require prepayment. Also PPO enrollees have a broader choice of providers. A PPO usually contracts with a large panel of providers, but the enrollees may seek services from providers other than those contracting with the PPO. To encourage enrollees to use services of contracting providers, the PPO usually has a larger co-payment for services received from non-contracting providers. Providers enroll in PPOs because service costs are lower when contracting providers are used. Providers contract with a PPO in order to secure a larger patient base. Finally, the PPO seeks to contract with providers at favorable rates or discounts in order to keep premiums low and thus ensure their position in the insurance marketplace.

PPOs are growing rapidly. From 1984 to 1986 the number of people covered by PPOs increased from 1.4 million to 16.5 million.[63] Growth of PPOs was especially rapid in California with the passage of Assembly Bill 3480 in 1982, which allowed private insurers to negotiate rates with institutional providers and offer benefits of such rates to the insureds who select those providers. The sponsoring agency of a PPO is usually a hospital (27.7%) or a Blue Cross or Blue Shield Plan (27.7%).[64] Physicians, commercial insurers, and investor groups also sponsor PPOs. Because most PPOs were developed in the past ten years and because they vary so widely in structure, it is impossible to predict what their course of development will be in the coming decade.

Other Delivery Systems

As hospital care increased in cost and as patients sought convenient service delivery options, new service delivery sites and approaches emerged. Outpatient surgical centers began to appear (the first was established in Phoenix in 1970). Urgent care centers, free-standing diagnostic clinics, birthing centers, and renal dialysis clinics were developed to provide service options that were affordable and convenient. Hospitals have responded by adding some of these services. The net effect has been greater response to consumer desires by many health care providers.

THE FUTURE

Predictions regarding the future of the health care industry are risky. The industry is complex, rapidly evolving, and constantly impacted by changes in the larger environment. Yet, a few predictions can be safely made. Health care expenditures will continue to increase; it is the rate of increase that is subject to debate. If effective cost controls are implemented, the rate of increase may slow. If they are not, then expenditures will continue to account for an ever-larger percent of the gross national product. In the next decade, hospitals and other health care providers will continue to adjust to an increasingly competitive marketplace. Less successful providers will fail or be acquired by their competitors.

Financing

Financing of health service has undergone dramatic changes in the past two decades and even more dramatic changes have occurred in the 1990s. Factors related to anticipated changes in financing include (1) the need to provide coverage for the indigent, unemployed, and employed uninsured; (2) the need to develop financing methods that encourage efficient, high quality service delivery; and (3) the need to develop an easily understood unified approach to financing, thereby reducing the burden on both the patient and the provider.

Some states (e.g., Hawaii) have enacted programs to expand health care coverage for their populations. Other states may take similar action if these programs are effective and affordable. At the federal level, the idea of national insurance is still promoted by some, although how to structure and finance such a program is the subject of much debate.

Technology

Although the role of technology was addressed earlier, technological advances will continue to be a driving force in the industry. Unfortunately, these advances may not always lead to positive results. In health care, in contrast to other industries, new technologies often increase rather than decrease cost of care. Thus, careful cost-benefit analyses are necessary in determining which technologies should be adopted. Additionally, careful evaluation of new technologies will remain a problem as groups which might benefit from it press for adoption before adequate testing is completed.

New technologies also impact human resources. As new equipment and new methods of prevention, diagnosis, and treatment are developed, health care providers will need to acquire new skills and knowledge. New specialties may develop and new occupations emerge. The health care team will continue to evolve as technological advances impact the field of practice.

Ethical Issues

A consideration of issues related to bioethics and managerial ethics is essential in contemplating the future of the health care industry. The rapid expansion of medical technology virtually guarantees that new issues in bioethics will emerge while the system is still grappling with current ones. Questions related to organ transplants, genetic engineering, surrogate parenting, the definition of death, wrongful life, and rationing of health care, to name only a few issues, must be addressed through forums that consider economic, legal, and ethical ramifications of different courses of action.

Because of the unique nature of health services, managerial ethics assumes greater importance than for many other industries. Managers have to balance the responsibility that their organizations have to deliver services to those who need them against the need to remain financially sound. Should hospitals be expected to maintain trauma centers or emergency rooms that drain resources needed to maintain other services? No easy answers are available. One can only predict that issues in bioethics and managerial ethics will continue to be debated.

NOTES

1. "Key Industry Facts," *Healthcare Executive* (September/October 1997).

2. U.S. Department of Health and Human Services, Public Health Service, Bureau of Health Professions, *Health United States 1996-97* and *Injury Chartbook*, 1997, DHHS Pub. no. (PHS) 97-1232 (Washington, D.C.: Government Printing Office, 1997).

3. P.R. Torrens, *The American Health Care System: Issues and Problems* (St. Louis: C.V. Mosby, 1978), 3-15.

4. O.W. Anderson, *Health Services in the Unites States: Growth Enterprise Since 1875* (Ann Arbor, Mich: Health Administration Press, 1985).

5. J.J. Hanlon and G.E. Pickett, *Public Health: Administration and Practice*, 7th ed. (St. Louis: C.V. Mosby, 1979).

6. Ibid.

7. R. Stevens, *American Medicine and The Public Interest* (New Haven: Yale University Press, 1971), 7.

8. Ibid., 24.

9. Hanlon and Pickett, *Public Health*, 22.

10. Torrens, *American Health Care System*.

11. Anderson, *Health Services in the United States*.

12. Stevens, *American Medicine and the Public Interest*.

13. C.L. Haglund and W.L. Dowling, "The Hospital," in *Introduction to Health Services*, 3rd ed., ed. S.J. Williams and P.R. Torrens. (New York: Wiley, 1988).

14. Anderson, *Health Services in the United States*.

15. Torrens, *American Health Care System*.

16. Stevens, *American Medicine and the Public Interest*, 68.

17. Ibid.

18. R.W. Scott and J.C. Lammers, "Trends in Occupations and Organizations Health Care and Mental Health in Sectors," *Medical Care Review* 42 no. 1 (1985): 37-76.

19. Torrens, *American Health Care System*.

20. Anderson, *Health Services in the United States*.

21. A.R. Somers and H.M. Somers, *Health and Health Care: Policies in Perspective* (Rockville, Md.: Aspen Publishers, 1977): 8.

22. L.D. Brown, *Health Policy in the United States: Issues and Options* (New York: Ford Foundation, 1988).

23. F.A. Wilson and D. Neuhauser, *Health Services in the United States*, 2nd ed. (Cambridge, Mass.: Ballinger, 1985).

24. Torrens, *American Health Care System*.

25. Brown, *Health Policy in the United States*.

26. U.S. Department of Health and Human Services, Public Health Service, *Health United States*, 1996. DHHS Pub. No. (PHS) 87-1232(Washington, D.C.: Government Printing Office, 1997), Tables 106 and 107.

27. Brown, *Health Policy in the United States*.

28. American Hospital Association, *Hospital Statistics*, 1998 ed. (Chicago: American Hospital Association, 1998).

29. Ibid.

30. Ibid.

31. J.P. Clement, "Vertical Integration and Diversification of Acute Care Hospitals: Conceptual Definitions," *Hospital and Health Services Administration* 33 (1988): 99-110.

32. D. Ermann and J. Gabel, "Multi-hospital Systems: Issues and Empirical Findings," *Health Affairs* 3 no.1 (1984): 51-64.

33. American Hospital Association, *AHA Guide* (Chicago: American Hospital Association, 1988).

34. American Hospital Association, *Hospital Statistics* (Chicago: Health Care Info Source, Inc., 1998).

35. U.S. Department of Health and Human Services, *Health United States.*

36. J.R. Lave, "The Effect of the Medicare Prospective Payment System," *Annual Review of Public Health* 10 (1989): 141-61.

37. R.S. Hanft, "Health Manpower" in *Health Care Delivery in the United States*, 2nd ed, ed. Steven Jonas (New York: Springer, 1981): 61-95.

38. Association of University Programs in Health Administration, *Annual Report*, 1997 (Washington, D.C.: Association of University Programs in Health Administration, 1998).

39. Ibid.

40. U.S. Department of Health and Human Services, Public Health Service, Bureau of Health Professions, *Minorities and Women in the Health Fields*, DHHS Publication no. (HRSA) HRS-DV 171 (Washington, D.C.: Government Printing Office ,1987).

41. U.S. Department of Health and Human Services, Public Health Service, Bureau of Health Professions, *Fifth Report to the President and Congress on the Status of Health Personnel* (Washington, D.C.: Government Printing Office, March, 1986).

42. W.B. Schwartz, F.A. Sloan and B.A. Mendelson, "Why There Will Be Little or No Physician Surplus Between Now and the Year 2000," *New England Journal of Medicine*, 318 (1988): 892-896.

43. Graduate Medical Advisory Committee, *Report of the Graduate Medical Education Advisory Committee to the Secretary of DHHS*, vol. 1, Summary Report (Washington, D.C.: GPO, 1981).

44. R.D. Thomas, "Projecting Physician Demand and Supply: The Importance of Nonmedical Factors," *Journal of Health and Human Resources* (1988): 388-392.

45. U.S. Department of Health and Human Services, *Fifth Report to the President and Congress on the Status of Health Personnel.*

46. Ibid.

47. Ibid.

48. F.A. Wilson and Neuhauser, *Health Services in the United States*, 1985.

49. P.I. Berhaus, "Not Just Another Nursing Shortage," *Nursing Economics* 5, no.6 (1987): 267-79.

50. F.A. Wilson and Neuhauser, *Health Services in the United States*, 1985.

51. W. Frey and R. Gottschalle, "Round 3: California Dentists, Hygienists Still Skirmishing," *Healthweek*, July 17, 1989, 12.

52. National Association Medical Staff Services, "Application Packet," Lombard, Ill., 1998.

53. J. V. Vicenzino, "Trends in Medical Care - Update," *Statistical Bulletin*, Metropolitan Insurance Companies, January - March, 1989, 26-34.

54. "Key Industry Facts," *Healthcare Executive*, 1997.

55. R.C. Coile, Jr., *The New Grievance Strategies for an Era of Health Reform* (Ann Arbor, Mich.: American College of Healthcare Executives, 1994).

56. U.S. Department of Health and Human Service, *Health United States*, 1997.

57. Anderson, *Health Services in the United States.*

58. U.S. Department of Health and Human Service, *Health United States*, 1997.

59. Ibid.

60. G. deLissovoy, et al., "Preferred Provider Organizations - One Year Later," *Inquiry* 24 (Summer 1987): 127-34.

61. U.S. Department of Health and Human Service, *Health United States*, 1997.

62. Ibid.

Chapter 2

Health Care Organization Accreditation

Cindy A. Gassiot, CMSC, CPCS

Health care organizations strive to achieve and maintain accreditation that is awarded by a plethora of organizations. Fifteen major organizations in the United States survey and accredit health care organizations ranging from hospitals and ambulatory care centers to managed care organizations and blood banks.[1] The Joint Commission on Accreditation of Healthcare Organizations (JCAHO) and the National Committee for Quality Assurance (NCQA) are the organizations medical staff services professionals and managed care credentialing specialists are exposed to most frequently. While the focus of this chapter will be on those organizations, other accrediting bodies these professionals may encounter will be addressed as well. Later chapters will address meeting credentialing and performance improvement standards of these organizations.

HOSPITAL ACCREDITATION

The Joint Commission on Accreditation of Healthcare Organizations (JCAHO)

The JCAHO accredits hospitals, including acute, rehabilitation, long term care, children's, and behavioral health facilities as well as health care networks or systems, ambulatory care facilities, and home care programs. Standards have been developed for each accreditation program. The Board of Directors of JCAHO consists of representatives of the American Medical Association, the American Hospital Association, the American College of Physicians, the American College of Surgeons, the American Dental Association, nursing representatives and members of the business community. In 1965, the JCAHO received deemed status from the Health Care Financing Administration (HCFA) to survey and accredit hospitals as having met HCFA's Conditions of Participation for Medicare reimbursement. Forty-four states recognize JCAHO accreditation of hospitals in lieu of state certification for Medicare/Medicaid.

A History of the Joint Commission on Accreditation of Hospitals*

The history of the Joint Commission on Accreditation of Hospitals [now Joint Commission on Accreditation of Healthcare Organizations] is a story of the health professions' commitment to patient care of high quality in the 20th century. The story began on a summer day in England in 1910. While riding back to London from a visit to a tuberculosis sanitarium, Dr. Ernest Codman was explaining his end-result system of hospital organization to Dr. Edward Martin. According to Dr. Codman, his system would enable a hospital to track every patient it treated long enough to determine whether or not the treatment was effective. If the treatment was not effective, the hospital would then try to find out how to prevent similar failures in the future. Dr. Martin responded that he thought Dr. Codman's system was one of the important reasons why an American college of surgeons should be established:

> An American College would be a fine thing if it could be the instrument with which to introduce the End Result Idea into hospitals; in other words to standardize them on the basis of service to the individual patient, as demonstrated by available records.[2]

Beyond establishing the concept of a linkage between an American college of surgeons and hospital standardization, this conversation was also the first expression of the principle that was eventually to guide the standardization program: service to the patient.

Dr. Martin's interest in improving conditions in hospitals was shared by other physicians and by hospital administrators in the United States and Canada. Conditions in hospitals were embarrassing to the professions. Most hospitals were little more than boardinghouses for poor and sick persons. Patients were not examined when they were admitted, and because histories and diagnoses were seldom recorded, medical records were useless. Most hospitals also lacked the equipment and services necessary for conducting proper preoperative and postoperative evaluation of surgical patients. Furthermore, few efforts were made to determine the results of patient care and treatment. Leading physicians believed that the basis of the most serious problems was the lack of organized medical staffs. Certainly, no efforts were made to determine a physician's competence to practice in a hospital, and no one was held responsible for the quality of care provided to patients.[3]

While conditions in hospitals were viewed as grim, many involved in medicine and hospital administration were optimistic about the future. The

*The section, "A History of the Joint Commission on Accreditation of Hospitals," is reprinted with permission of the American Medical Association from *Journal of the American Medical Association*, 258(August 21, 1987):936–940, by James S. Roberts, MD; Jack G. Coale, MA; Robert R. Redman, MA. Copyright 1987, American Medical Association.

source of their optimism was the convergence of significant advances in the science of medicine and in management concepts, as well as the recognition of the value of hygiene in health care. Technological progress in the practice of medicine, particularly in the performance of surgery in hospitals, offered considerably safer care for patients. Management principles developed during the industrial revolution were also being applied successfully in all types of businesses, including hospitals. Interest in formulating standards of care and in developing systems to produce better products more efficiently began to spread. Dr. Codman's end-result system was just one example of the application of management principles to hospital care.

These several factors were the background against which the Third Clinical Congress of Surgeons of North America met in November 1912. At this historic meeting, Dr. Franklin Martin made a proposal that was to lead to the founding of the American College of Surgeons. Immediately following that proposal, Dr. Allen Kanavel set forth the following resolution at the request of Dr. Edward Martin:

> Be It Resolved by the Clinical Congress of Surgeons of North America here assembled, that some system of standardization of hospital equipment and hospital work should be developed, to the end that those institutions having the highest ideals may have proper recognition before the profession, and that those of inferior equipment and standards should be stimulated to raise the quality of their work. In this way patients will receive the best type of treatment, and the public will have some means of recognizing those institutions devoted to the highest ideals of medicine.[4]

It is a tribute to Dr. Martin's foresight that he managed to associate this first official expression of the need for hospital standardization so closely with the proposal that would result in the creation of the American College of Surgeons. There appeared to be a clear realization that the hospital standardization program must have the backing of a national organization if it were ever going to have a chance to succeed. Largely because of his efforts, hospital standardization became one of the stated purposes of the College when it was founded in 1913.

During the first few years of its existence, the College focused its energies on solving problems of vital concern to its survival and success. Hospital standardization quickly and unexpectedly became one of these problems. During the first three years of its existence, the College found it necessary to reject 60% of the applicants for fellowship because the 50 case records required from each fellowship applicant provided the college with an insufficient basis to determine clinical competence.[5] Shortly thereafter, John Bowman, PhD, the director of the College, used his influence with the Carnegie Foundation, New York, to obtain a gift of $30,000 to launch a hospital standardization program.

From October 19 to 20, 1917, 300 fellows from the Committees on Standards from every state in the union and every province in Canada, as well as

60 leading hospital superintendents, met in Chicago to discuss hospital standardization. During the conference, the participants described existing conditions in hospitals and discussed the kinds of improvements that would be necessary to ensure the proper care and treatment of patients. This conference, the papers and some of the discussions of which are published in the first issue of volume 3 of the 1917 *Bulletin of the American College of Surgeons*,[6] is of interest not only because it established the foundation for hospital standardization, but also because it created the concept that knowledgeable and experienced health care professionals should assess conditions in the hospital environment and work to achieve consensus on standards that would have the greatest positive effect on the quality of care provided to patients. That concept continues to underlie the accreditation process today.

On December 20, 1917, two months after the Conference on Hospital Standardization, the American College of Surgeons formally established the Hospital Standardization Program, and in March 1918, the College published a "Standard on Efficiency" in the *Bulletin*. Expecting to approve at least 1000 hospitals during the first year, the College staff began testing the program in April 1918.

The results of the field trials were announced by Bowman at a conference on hospital standardization in New York on October 24, 1919. Bowman told the audience that 692 hospitals of 100 beds or more had been surveyed and that only 89 hospitals had met the standards.[7] While these results are not surprising when one considers conditions in hospitals at the time, the results were nevertheless shocking.

Although the College made the numbers public, it burned the list of hospitals at midnight in the furnace of the Waldorf Astoria Hotel, New York, to keep it from the press. Some of the most prestigious hospitals in the country had failed to meet the most basic standards. However, 109 hospitals corrected deficiencies after their initial surveys and were subsequently approved. Although the field trials were disappointing, they dramatically demonstrated the need for a national hospital accreditation program, and they solidified national support for the program. Consequently, the College's Board of Regents adopted five official standards for the program at its December 1919 meeting (Table 2-1).[8] These standards, which are collectively known as the *Minimum Standard*, said it was intended to

> safeguard the care of every patient within a hospital by insisting upon competence on the part of the doctors, and upon adequate clinical and pathological laboratory facilities to insure correct diagnosis; by a thorough study and diagnosis in writing for each case; by a monthly audit of the medical and surgical work conducted in the hospital during the preceding interval; and by prohibiting the practice of the division of fees under any guise whatsoever.[9]

That these standards are as essential to the provision of quality care in hospitals today as they were in 1919 is no small tribute to the men who contributed to their development. In 1924, Dr. Franklin Martin said that the *Minimum Standard*, had "become to hospital betterment what the Sermon on the Mount is to great religion."[10]

With the adoption of the *Minimum Standard*, the accreditation process that continues today was set in motion. The following steps are included in

---

Table 2-1. The Minimum Standard*

---

1. That physicians and surgeons privileged to practice in the hospital be organized as a definite group or staff. Such organization has nothing to do with the question as to whether the hospital is "open" or "closed," nor need it affect the various existing types of staff organization. The word STAFF is here defined as the group of doctors who practice in the hospital inclusive of all groups such as the "regular staff," "the visiting staff," and the "associate staff."

2. That membership upon the staff be restricted to physicians and surgeons who are (a) full graduates of medicine in good standing and legally licensed to practice in their respective states or provinces, (b) competent in their respective fields, and (c) worthy in character and in matters of professional ethics, that in this latter connection in the practice of the division of fees, under any guise whatever, be prohibited.

3. That the staff initiate and, with the approval of the governing board of the hospital, adopt rules, regulations, and policies governing the professional work of the hospital; that these rules, regulations, and policies specifically provide:

   (a) That staff meetings be held at least once each month. (In large hospitals the departments may choose to meet separately.)

   (b) That the staff review and analyze at regular intervals their clinical experience in the various departments of the hospital, such as medicine, surgery, obstetrics, and the other specialties; the clinical records of patients, free and pay, to be the basis for such review and analyses.

4. That accurate and complete records be written for all patients and filed in an accessible manner in the hospital—a complete case record being one which includes identification data; complaint; personal and family history; history of present illness; physical examination; special examinations, such as consultations, clinical laboratory, X-ray and other examinations; provisional or working diagnosis; medical or surgical treatment; gross and microscopical pathological findings; progress notes; final diagnosis; condition on discharge; follow-up and, in case of death, autopsy findings.

5. That diagnostic and therapeutic facilities under competent supervision be available for the study, diagnosis, and treatment of patients, these to include at least (a) a clinical laboratory providing chemical, bacteriological, serological, and pathological services; (b) an X-ray department providing radiographic and fluoroscopic services.

---

*Source: Reprinted with permission from the *Bulletin of the American College of Surgeons*, Vol 8, p. 4 © 1924.

this process: the development of reasonable standards that every organization should be expected to meet and that the health professions agree will have a positive effect on improving the quality of patient care; the voluntary request for survey and approval by a health care organization; the survey of the organization by professionals who assess compliance with the standards and provide consultation to support achievement of greater levels of compliance; and that subsequent efforts of organizations to use the standards and survey results to improve patient care.

The Minimum Standard was considered to be a beginning. The College knew that hospitals would advance and change, and it expected the Hospital Standardization Program to evolve with them. Ensuring that the standards and the accreditation process remain responsive to conditions in health care organizations and focused on issues that will protect and promote quality of care has proved to be one of the greatest challenges to the health professions.

The Hospital Standardization Program had a strong beginning, and the value of the program became broadly apparent. The case records submitted to the College by surgeons in approved hospitals provided an acceptable basis for evaluation, and the quality of care in these hospitals improved noticeably. As news of the program's success spread, more and more hospitals sought approval. The number of approved hospitals rose from 89 in 1919 to 3290 in 1950, over half of the hospitals in the United States.

By 1950, the size and scope of the program had increased significantly, and the College, which had already invested $2 million in the Hospital Standardization Program, was having difficulty in supporting the effort alone. In addition, the increasing sophistication of medical care, the growing number and complexity of modern hospitals, and the rapid emergence of nonsurgical specialties after World War II required that the standards be revised, expanded, and updated, and that the scope of the survey be extended. These considerations clearly suggested that the Hospital Standardization Program needed the support of the entire medical and hospital field. Consequently, the College solicited the support and participation of other national professional organizations in the creation of an independent organization that could devote all of its efforts to improving and promoting voluntary accreditation.

After considerable deliberation, the American College of Physicians, the American Hospital Association, the American Medical Association, and the Canadian Medical Association joined the American College of Surgeons on December 15, 1951, to form the Joint Commission on Accreditation of Hospitals as an independent, nonprofit organization. The Canadian Medical Association withdrew in 1959, to participate in the development of its own program, the Canadian Council on Hospital Accreditation. The College officially conveyed its program to the Joint Commission on December 6, 1952, and the Joint Commission began to offer accreditation to hospitals in January 1953.

In addition to carrying on the College's program, the Joint Commission preserved the traditions established by the College. The accreditation process remains voluntary, the standards continue to represent what health professionals agree is most conducive to the provision of quality care to patients, and the accreditation survey still provides an evaluation that achieves its most beneficial effects through a combination of evaluation, education, and consultation. Also, as in the past, the information obtained in the survey process is still held in confidence between the Joint Commission and the organization surveyed. [Under public pressure, the JCAHO has since changed its policy and now releases information related to the most recent survey, such as an organization's accreditation status including any designation attached to that status; scores for each performance area evaluated and national comparisons to scores; and performance areas with recommendations for improvement, as well as efforts made to correct deficiencies from the most recent survey.]

The Joint Commission today is directed by a 22-member Board of Commissioners. Seven commissioners are appointed by the American Medical Association; seven by the American Hospital Association; three by the American College of Physicians; three by the American College of Surgeons; one by the American Dental Association, which accepted an invitation to become a corporate member in 1979; and one is a private citizen appointed annually by the rest of the board.

Under the direction of the Board of Commissioners, the Joint Commission continued to expand the College's program, which was now called the Hospital Accreditation Program. It hired and trained a cadre of experienced surveyors and focused the survey on medical staff and patient care issues; and just as the College of Surgeons had done, it periodically revised the standards to reflect the evolution of hospital care.

In August 1966, the Joint Commission board made a major decision to undertake a complete revision of the standards to reflect an optimal achievable rather than a minimal essential level of care. This decision, which redefined the Joint Commission's role in health care, was made for two reasons. First the majority of hospitals in the country had achieved and were maintaining the minimum standards, and because of this, the standards no longer challenged hospitals to reach for the levels of quality care the Board of Commissioners thought could now be achieved. The second reason was even more compelling. Dr. John Porterfield, who was then the director of the Joint Commission, described it as follows:

> In the mid 1960s the Joint Commission found itself no longer the advanced and lonely leader. The Federal government wrote its conditions for participation in Medicare. State after state with new and refurbished licensing authority wrote regulatory codes, where

there had been few or none before. They did have some premise
on which to build and it is more than coincidence that the federal
conditions and, more particularly, the state codes bore a strong
family resemblance to the Joint Commission's accreditation standards. From advanced leader, the Joint Commission seemed almost overnight to be struggling to stay even in the vanguard of
progress. And it was challenged, most seriously, as being no longer
necessary because now everybody was beginning to do what it
had once done alone.[11]

When the government moved toward usurping the Joint Commission's
role as the definer of the minimal acceptable level of hospital care, it became
necessary and appropriate for the Joint Commission to become the definer of
the optimal achievable level of care. In doing so, the Joint Commission was
not only realizing the intentions of the founders of hospital standardization,
but also assuming a role that was more compatible with the ideals of the health
professions that supported voluntary accreditation.

The publication of the optimal achievable standards in the 1970 *Accreditation Manual for Hospitals* was a landmark.[12] In little more than 50 years, the
one-page set of standards that specified a minimal essential level of performance had developed into a 152-page manual of state-of-the-art standards.
The Joint Commission did not intend the term *optimal achievable* to mean the
ideal. It meant the best that could be achieved at the time, given the legal and
other concerns that must be accommodated in national standards to make them
as effective as possible.[13] The publication of these standards was a clear indication of the tremendous progress hospitals had made since the beginning of
this century and of the impact of voluntary accreditation on the quality of
hospital care.

In the early 1960s, concern for the quality of care provided in other types
of health care organizations that were proliferating throughout the country led
the Joint Commission and other national professional organizations to discuss
the possibility of developing new accreditation programs. The expansion of
the Joint Commission to include programs for other types of health and health-
related organizations seemed only natural after the successful leadership it
had demonstrated in improving hospitals. The Joint Commission had experience and expertise, and it had national scope and acceptance. A principal organization for voluntary accreditation would also give unity and strength to
new accreditation efforts and would afford the greatest opportunities for the
coordination of efforts and consistency among approaches to accreditation.

Working with an ever-expanding number of national professional organizations, the Joint Commission developed standards and accreditation programs
for a broader variety of health care settings. An accreditation program for long-
term care facilities was established in 1965, for organizations serving devel-
opmentally disabled persons in 1969, and for psychiatric facilities, substance

abuse programs, and community mental health programs in 1970. An accreditation program for ambulatory health care programs was established in 1975 and for hospices in 1983.

During the expansion, the Joint Commission established what are now called Professional and Technical Advisory Committees. One of these committees advises each Joint Commission accreditation program on standards development and survey procedures. Each committee is composed of approximately 15 individuals who are usually appointed as representatives of national organizations having expertise relevant to the particular accreditation program. In addition, approximately 15 experts on education and publications and 15 on health care safety serve on committees that advise the Joint Commission in these areas. All Joint Commission accreditation services are supported by education, publications, and research activities.

Through its Board of Commissioners, the various committees that advise the Joint Commission on a regular and ad hoc basis, the thousands of facilities that participate in the accreditation process and a standards development process that includes extensive review by the field, the Joint Commission maintains close working relationships and continuous communications with health professionals. Through these mechanisms, the Joint Commission monitors the health care environment and has access to the best advice available in health care. This is of incalculable value in the Joint Commission's efforts to maintain state-of-the-art standards and survey processes, as well as education programs and publications. These mechanisms also give the Joint Commission a large measure of assurance that current issues and trends will be fully discussed before important decisions are made.

In addition to its close working relationships with the health professions, the national professional organizations that represent them, and the wide array of accredited organizations, the Joint Commission has important relationships with government. These relationships began in 1965, when Congress passed Public Law 89-97, the Medicare Act. Written into this law was a provision that hospitals accredited by the Joint Commission were "deemed" to be in compliance with most of the Medicare *Conditions of Participation for Hospitals*[14] and, thus, deemed to meet eligibility requirements for participation in the Medicare program. Because a hospital that was certified for Medicare was also considered certified for Medicaid, hospitals accredited by the Joint Commission were similarly eligible for Medicaid participation. Consequently, hospitals that desired to participate in the Medicare and/or Medicaid programs could undergo either a certification inspection by a state agency or an accreditation survey by the Joint Commission.

Government oversight and responsibility were added to this system in 1972 through amendments to the Social Security Act, Public Law 92-603. These amendments required the Secretary of the Department of Health and Human Services to validate Joint Commission findings on a selective sample basis or on the basis of substantial complaint. The law also required the Secretary to include an evaluation of the Joint Commission accreditation process, as gleaned from validation surveys, in his annual report to Congress on Medicare.

Accredited psychiatric and tuberculosis hospitals were not accorded deemed status by the Social Security Act. Instead, the Act required that such hospitals be accredited by the Joint Commission to participate in Medicare and Medicaid. Because this requirement impinged on the voluntary nature of the accreditation process, the Joint Commission sought and finally succeeded in obtaining elimination of this mandate in the Deficit Reduction Act of 1984, Public Law 98-369.

The Joint Commission also has developed relationships with state governments. Today, 39 [now 44] states and the District of Columbia have incorporated the Joint Commission's hospital accreditation requirements, in whole or in part, into their hospital licensure systems. In most of these states, however, licensure is not granted merely on the basis of accreditation, but rather on the basis of an acceptable review of Joint Commission findings by the state licensing agency. All of the affected states have retained the enforcement powers that accompany responsibility for licensing hospitals. Even though a hospital is considered licensable if it is accredited, the hospital must still comply with licensing laws and regulations.

Accredited hospitals have been considered to meet Medicare health and safety standards for over 20 years now, and the Joint Commission has considerable experience with state licensure programs. Through this time, there is no evidence that these arrangements have had any negative effects on Joint Commission standards and survey processes. On the other hand, there is considerable evidence that these cooperative relationships with government have had synergistic effects that benefit all concerned.

The combination of private sector and public sector responsibilities has served as a stimulus for the Joint Commission to improve its accreditation process. A two-year study of the Joint Commission, state agencies, and what was then the Department of Health, Education, and Welfare, was conducted by the General Accounting Office and reported to Congress on May 14, 1979, in publication HRD-79-37, *The Medicare Hospital Certification System Needs Reform.*[15] Although the report identified deficiencies in the procedures of all three organizations, it praised the Joint Commission for the consistency, effectiveness, and economy of its standards-setting, surveyor-training, accreditation-survey, and decision-making processes.

At the state level, cooperative arrangements with the Joint Commission have provided states with an alternative perspective on the strengths and weaknesses of the hospitals under their jurisdiction and have enabled them to concentrate their resources and enforcement efforts on problem facilities. These arrangements have reduced the number of surveys that hospitals have had to undergo and, consequently, there have been considerable savings of time, effort, and money for these hospitals.

No history of the Joint Commission's voluntary accreditation program effort would be complete without a discussion of quality assurance. The first national requirements calling for regular review and evaluation of the quality of care provided to patients in hospitals were part of the minimum standards of the American College of Surgeons. After the Joint Commission assumed responsibility for the College's program, efforts were undertaken to develop standards for the various services in modern hospitals. These standards paralleled the minimum standards with regard to their emphasis on review and evaluation of the quality of care provided. However, most in-hospital evaluations that were conducted were informal and subjective and were based on an individual practitioner's knowledge and experience in evaluating records and in observing the performance of others.

At the same time, those involved in quality assurance research were developing methods to make the review and evaluation process more structured and objective. While various approaches were proposed, all involved two common elements. These focused on the use of systematic review procedures and the development of objective and valid criteria for measuring the actual quality of care being provided. Both of these elements constituted the essence of a medical audit methodology that the Joint Commission began promoting in the early 1970s. As a result, retrospective outcome-oriented audits were conducted throughout the country. Medical audits even became requirements of the Professional Standards Review Organizations legislated in 1972, in Public Law 92-603.

While encouraging the medical audit as a method of reviewing quality of care, the Joint Commission also directed attention to enhancing and clarifying other quality assurance standards. Requirements concerning medical staff monitoring functions were consolidated and clearly defined as surgical case, pharmacy and therapeutics, blood and antibiotic usage, and medical records review. Standards were also adopted that called for review and evaluation of both the quality and appropriateness of care provided by medical and support service departments. Safety management, infection control, and utilization review standards were also strengthened. Finally, the Joint Commission adopted standards that asked hospitals to consider relevant results of quality assurance activities in reviewing the credentials and delineating the clinical privileges of medical staff members. This was the first explicit reference in Joint Commission standards to the important relationship between quality assurance activities and the delineation of clinical privileges.

Despite this quality assurance focus, most relevant hospital activities consisted of formal audit studies. In too many cases, these studies became paper exercises conducted to meet Joint Commission or Professional Standards Review Organization requirements. Because of this, the quality assurance effort was compromised and failed to effect the desired intent. Preoccupation with the audit requirement rather than quality of care had left hospitals at the periphery of meaningful quality assurance activities.

To address this problem, the Joint Commission developed a new quality assurance standard in 1979, which eliminated the numerical audit requirements and directed hospitals to develop a hospital-wide program that integrates all quality assessment activities. The purpose of the standard was to shift the attention of hospitals toward a systematic quality assessment process, the central element of which was the monitoring and evaluation of all important aspects of patient care to identify and correct patient care problems.

Since adoption of the new quality assurance standard for hospitals in 1979, the Joint Commission has established similar standards for all of the other types of health care organizations that it accredits. Through this standard, the Joint Commission intends to foster the integration of quality assurance mechanisms into the core management systems of accredited facilities. Clearly, quality assurance activities are increasingly linked to the processes of planning, budgeting, and tracking the utilization and cost of limited resources in many health care organizations today.

The evolution of voluntary accreditation has spanned most of the 20th century and is an integral feature of the era of modern medicine. Beginning with the commitment of the American College of Surgeons, the process has steadily gained the support of the hospital and medical fields. Today, the Joint Commission accredits approximately 5000 of the 6500 hospitals in the United States and 2800 other health care organizations. Approximately 1% to 2% of those who seek accreditation do not achieve this status—a reflection of the strong professional motivation of those seeking accreditation to meet the established standards.

Since the Joint Commission began, the voluntary accreditation movement has spread to Canada and Australia and in 1981, the Catalonia province of Spain implemented the first hospital accreditation program in Europe. Interest in voluntary accreditation and quality assurance systems in health care is now spreading rapidly to other countries.

Since 1917, the voluntary accreditation movement has been a consistent and persistent voice for quality in health care. The future holds its own challenges, but as in the past, meeting those challenges provides substance to the merits of voluntarism—of the willingness of the health professions to regulate themselves on the basis of their ideals, integrity, and commitment to patient care.

THE JCAHO'S AGENDA FOR CHANGE

In 1987, the JCAHO launched the "Agenda for Change," a set of initiatives the objective of which is to modernize the accreditation process to one that places primary emphasis on the actual performance of the health care facility. Included in the initiatives of the Agenda for Change were revision and reorganization of the JCAHO standards to focus on organizational performance of important functions; redesign of the survey process to provide more interactive onsite evaluation and education; and development of an indicator-based monitoring system.

The JCAHO's indicator monitoring system (IMSystem®) is a national database resource to support performance improvement in hospitals and other patient care settings. As initially proposed, hospitals were expected to use clinical indicators developed by expert task forces assembled by the JCAHO, and feed their information into the JCAHO's indicator databases. Hospitals would then receive back their indicator results and aggregate, comparative data from other hospitals. But hospitals balked at using the JCAHO's costly and inefficient programs to measure clinical outcomes. Many alpha and beta test site hospitals dropped out the of project because it was "too complicated, labor intensive and costly to justify what little benefit they received."[16] Many facilities had developed their own data collection and measurement systems and found the IMSystem® inferior.

The JCAHO continued to pursue the objective of including performance measurement as a requirement in the accreditation process, but backed away from the original mandate that all facilities use the IMSystem®. In 1997, JCAHO announced that health care organizations are required to participate in the ORYX initiative. The ORYX requirement calls for accredited organizations, beginning with hospitals and long-term care providers, to collect and send performance data to the JCAHO. By the first quarter of 1999, these organizations must track at least two clinical areas—such as Caesarean section rates— that reflect the needs of 20 percent of their population. Health care organizations must submit this data to a performance measurement system, which will then report the results to the JCAHO. In 1997, the JCAHO published a list of software vendors whose measurement systems will satisfy the ORYX requirement. Within the next five years, the JCAHO could require hospitals and long-term care providers to track eight indicators that cover 80 percent of their patient population. Performance measurement information will supplement standards compliance information from JCAHO surveys.[17]

In July 1994, the JCAHO published the *Comprehensive Accreditation Manual for Hospitals*, a revised manual with 11 functional and four structural chapters of standards. The 11 functions that make up the key standards for hospitals are grouped into two sections: patient-focused functions and organization-focused functions. Patient-focused functions include: patient rights and organization ethics; assessment of patients; care of patients; patient and family education; and continuum of care. Organization-focused functions include: improving organization performance; leadership; management of the environment of care; management of human resources; management of information; and surveillance, prevention and control of infections. The four structural chapters of the manual include: governance, medical staff, nursing, and management.

The JCAHO performance improvement standards require officials at all accredited health facilities to institute a "planned, systematic organizational-wide approach to designing, measuring, assessing and improving...performance." The shift to a performance focus is a cornerstone of the JCAHO's Agenda for Change.

The Survey

The JCAHO survey has changed to one that focuses on talking to people about what they do rather than on reviewing documents. Surveyors now spend the majority of their time questioning survey participants instead of reading bylaws, minutes, policies and procedures, and other documents. Hospital leaders and all employees, volunteers, and physicians must be prepared to be questioned by the surveyors about compliance with the standards and the facility's performance improvement activities.

The hospital survey lasts from two to five days, depending on the number of beds and extent of hospital patient care activities. Smaller hospitals may have two surveyors (physician and nurse) and larger hospitals have three surveyors (physician, nurse and administrator). Most surveys include an opening conference with key leaders, a presentation on the facility's performance improvement activities, documentation review of specifically requested documents, interviews with organization leaders, visits to patient care settings, interviews with staff members relating to specific functions, medical record review, and a leadership exit conference. The surveyors now use laptop computers to enter results of their surveys in order to expedite the final report.

The hospital's accreditation decision is based on how well it complies with the standards. Each standard surveyed is given a score of one to five, with one being the highest score. Using a complex decision grid and formulas to consolidate scores, the hospital is given a summary grid score. The accreditation decision depends on how well a hospital scores. A hospital may receive accreditation with commendation when exemplary performance in complying with the standards has been demonstrated. Accreditation without any follow-up monitoring is awarded to hospitals that have substantially complied with the standards. Accreditation with type I recommendations, which will require some follow-up (either a written progress report or a focused survey), results when an organization receives at least one recommendation addressing insufficient or unsatisfactory standards compliance in a specific performance area. Conditional accreditation with follow-up monitoring is assigned when an organization is not in substantial compliance with the standards but is believed to be capable of achieving acceptable compliance within a stipulated time period. Provisional accreditation is awarded to new hospitals. Preliminary non-accreditation results when an immediate threat to patient or public health and safety exists within an organization. Organizations that do not comply with the standards receive a non-accreditation status. Accreditation watch is assigned when a sentinel event (a serious accident or patient care event) has occurred and it has been determined there is a reasonable potential for improvement in the organization.

The full accreditation survey occurs every three years; however, five percent of hospitals are subject to a random unannounced survey at the midpoint of the accreditation cycle. There is an appeals process for hospitals that wish to challenge any portion of the survey report or the decision to deny accreditation. A facility that receives a preliminary non-accreditation decision has the right to make a detailed presentation before a review hearing panel. The report of the review hearing panel may be appealed to the board appeal review committee. The final decision is made by the accreditation committee.

Sentinel Event Reporting

The JCAHO is concerned about accidents or patient care errors (sentinel events) that lead to death or major injury to hospitalized patients, and instituted a policy in early 1998 requiring hospitals to voluntarily report these events. Sentinel events are defined by JCAHO as: any event that leads to a patient's unanticipated death, major permanent loss of bodily function, an infant abduction or discharge to the wrong family, rape by a patient or staff member, hemolytic transfusion reaction, or surgery on the wrong patient or body part. The facility is then expected to undertake a root-cause analysis to determine the reasons for the event and take corrective measures accordingly. In accordance with this policy, hospitals that report sentinel events would not be placed on accreditation watch.

Announcement of this requirement resulted in warnings from hospital associations, attorneys, insurance companies, and risk managers, that hospitals may lose confidentiality protection provided by state statutes if they voluntarily report sentinel events to the JCAHO. Federal legislation protecting this type of reporting to the JCAHO has been proposed. Additionally, in response to concerns over legal protection of sentinel event reports, JCAHO changed the policy in April 1998, to allow for an on-site review of the root-cause analysis by a specially trained surveyor rather than requiring the hospital to send in the analysis. At this writing, the outcome of this controversial requirement is unknown.

The American Osteopathic Association (AOA)

The AOA Committee on Accreditation is the accrediting agency for designated osteopathic hospitals. A hospital with a medical staff composed of both allopathic and osteopathic physicians may become accredited by the AOA but need not be designated as osteopathic.

To achieve AOA accreditation, hospitals must comply with standards addressing the following: governing body; patient rights and advance medical directives; physical plant; quality assurance program; professional staff; required facilities and services; optional facilities and services; and allied health professionals.

The survey team includes an osteopathic physician, a hospital administrator, and pathologist. Hospitals are awarded three-year accreditation, two-year accreditation or one-year accreditation. Hospitals with one-year accreditation must have an AOA-approved consultant advise them on correcting areas of non-compliance with the standards, unless this requirement is waived by AOA. Additional on-site surveys may also be conducted for hospitals non-compliant with the standards. There is an appeals process for hospitals that have been denied accreditation.

MANAGED CARE ORGANIZATION ACCREDITATION

National Committee on Quality Assurance (NCQA)[18]

In 1979, two major managed care trade associations, the American Managed Care and Review Association and the Group Health Association of America, formed a joint venture to create the the National Committee on Quality Assurance. NCQA accredits managed care organizations (MCOs), managed behavioral health care organizations, credentials verification organizations (CVOs) and physician organizations. The NCQA Board includes employers, consumer and labor representatives, health plans, quality experts, regulators, and representatives from organized medicine. NCQA's mission is to provide information on the quality of health care plans so that purchasers and consumers of managed health care can distinguish among the plans. The NCQA's activities center around two activities: accreditation and performance measurement.

MCO Accreditation

NCQA began to accredit managed care organizations in 1991 in response to the need for standardized, objective information about the quality of those organizations. NCQA surveys Health Maintenance Organizations, Networks, Preferred Provider Organizations, and Physician-Hospital Organizations. During an accreditation survey, plans are reviewed against more than 50 different standards, each of which focuses on an important aspect of the health plan. Standards address the following areas: quality improvement; physician credentials; members' rights and responsibilities; preventive health services; utilization management; and medical records.

Performance Measurement—HEDIS

NCQA's performance measurement tool for managed care is the Health Plan Employer Data and Information Set (HEDIS). These are a set of standardized measures used to compare health plans. NCQA collects HEDIS data and accreditation information in a national database called Quality Compass. Quality Compass allows NCQA to generate national and regional averages and to identify benchmarks which are useful for comparative purposes. HEDIS assesses how effectively health plans care for acute and chronic illnesses, and includes measures that address many of the nation's most serious health problems, such as cancer and heart disease.

Beginning in 1999, MCOs will be required to implement HEDIS and submit audited HEDIS performance results to NCQA. Like the JCAHO, NCQA will consider performance results as a part of the accreditation process. To ensure that quality and performance are maintained between on-site surveys, health plans will be required to submit independently audited HEDIS results to NCQA annually. Should these results suggest a lapse in quality, NCQA may elect to resurvey the health plan.[19]

The Survey

The MCO survey lasts from three to five days and is conducted by a physician and administrator. The survey generally includes a review of documents and records, on-site observation, interviews with members of the organization, medical records review, and an assessment of the member service systems, such as the provisions for complaints and grievances.

Managed care plans receive full accreditation for three years, one-year accreditation, provisional accreditation, or denial, depending on their continuous quality improvement programs and how well they meet the standards. Beginning in July 1999, NCQA will implement the following levels of accreditation: Excellent, Commendable, Acceptable and Denied.[20] There is an appeals process for MCOs that have been denied accreditation.

CVO Certification

In 1996, NCQA began reviewing and certifying credentials verification organizations (CVOs), organizations that gather verification of physician credentials for managed care plans and hospitals. The standards for certification were developed with the assistance of representatives of the verification industry and managed care organizations. Certified CVOs must meet these standards as well as applicable credentialing standards from NCQA's *Standards for Accreditation of Managed Care Organizations*.

The CVO Certification survey has two components: determination of compliance with the CVO standards and an audit of completed credentials files. During the survey the following are reviewed: policies and procedures for credentials verification; mechanisms for maintaining credentials data integrity and confidentiality; capabilities for ongoing data collection; physician application components; and reporting of physician disciplinary actions.

Certification is awarded to participating organizations on an individual credentials element basis. Organizations may be certified for all, some, or none of the following 10 credentials elements addressed in the NCQA standards:

> Licensure
> Hospital Privileges
> Drug Enforcement Agency Registration
> Medical Education and/or Board Certification
> Malpractice Insurance
> Liability Claims History
> National Practitioner Data Bank Queries
> Medical Board Sanctions
> Medicare/Medicaid Sanctions
> Provider Application.

In order to be certified for any of the 10 credentials elements reviewed by NCQA, a CVO must achieve a minimal level of compliance with each of the six areas of CVO Standards noted above. If a CVO meets these criteria it may be certified for any of the credentials elements for which it achieves 90 percent compliance in the audit of completed credentials files.

CVO surveys last one to two days and are conducted by two surveyors—a representative of NCQA and the National Association Medical Staff Services. Initial certification is for one year. Following a second successful survey, certification may be extended to three years.

Physician Organization Certification

In 1997, NCQA released standards for a Physician Organization Certification (POC) program. The program helps streamline NCQA's accreditation process for managed care organizations by substituting a single NCQA survey of each participating organization for the overlapping annual reviews from MCOs seeking NCQA accreditation.

The POC standards are comprised largely of a subset of NCQA's 1997 MCO Accreditation Standards. Although a few new program-specific standards were added, no significant changes were made to the existing MCO standards in order to apply them to physician organizations. The standards fall into the following categories: quality management and improvement; utilization management; credentialing and recredentialing; preventive health; members' rights and responsibilities; and medical records.

Physician organizations may seek certification for any subset of the categories, from one to all six. MCOs must continue to exercise some oversight of NCQA-certified physician organizations, but they will not be required to conduct an annual on-site audit of the activities for which the groups have been certified. Eligible physician organizations include: primary care, multispeciality groups and networks; physician hospital organizations; independent practice associations; integrated delivery systems; and those that provide management services only.

The surveys will generally consist of an on- and off-site review of the organization by a two- or three-person team of physicians and managed care experts. Surveys will last one to three days depending on the size of the organization. Initial certification will last for one year. Following a second successful survey, certification may be extended to three years.

The American Accreditation Healthcare Commission, Inc.[21]

In addition to NCQA, the American Accreditation HealthCare Commission, Inc. (AAHCC), formerly the Utilization Review Accreditation Commission, or URAC, accredits networks, CVOs, and utilization review programs. Founded in 1990, its initial focus was on standardizing utilization review procedures. In 1994, AAHCC acquired the American Accreditation Program, Inc., which accredited preferred provider organizations (PPOs). AAHCC then expanded its managed care accreditation program to include HMOs, PHOs, IPAs, independent delivery networks, management service organizations, and single specialty networks. The AAHCC board of directors is represented by managed care associations, health care providers, and the public.

The AAHCC network standards essentially address the same areas as those of NCQA. Network surveys are conducted by nurse and network surveyors, often physicians. Organizations are either accredited for two years or are denied accreditation.

AAHCC also accredits utilization review (UR) and workers' compensation programs. The standards address the areas of confidentiality, UR program staff qualifications and credentials, program qualifications, quality improvement programs, accessibility and on-site review procedures, information requirements for UR organizations, UR procedures, and appeals. Surveys are conducted by a nurse and a physician. Two-year accreditation is awarded upon successful survey or is denied.

In 1998, AAHCC introduced an accreditation program for CVOs (see Chapter 9).

JCAHO Network Accreditation

In addition to its hospital accreditation program, the JCAHO accredits health care networks including HMOs, IPAs, integrated health care delivery systems, PHOs, and specialty services systems.

The JCAHO surveys networks on standards addressing the following areas: rights, responsibilities and ethics; continuum of care; education and communication; leadership; management of human resources; management of information; and improving network performance. In addition to surveying the central network office, up to eight practitioner sites are surveyed. The survey lasts from one to two days, depending on the organization, and there are from one to three surveyors. Accreditation decisions are the same as those noted in the hospital accreditation section.

PHYSICIAN ACCREDITATION PROGRAMS

Both the American Medical Association (AMA) and the American Osteopathic Association (AOA) have announced plans for programs to accredit individual physicians. The concept is that these organizations will act as national credentials verification organizations, verifying all of a physician's credentials, maintaining the information and making it available to hospitals and managed care organizations that request it. The concept is good and would eliminate an enormous amount of duplication of effort by hospitals and managed care organizations in the credentialing process. The AMA's program has been dubbed the American Medical Accreditation Program (AMAP) and the AOA's, the American Osteopathic Accreditation Program (AOAP).

In order to be accredited by AMAP, a physician must meet all required standards and score at least 11 out of 22 points on the supplemental standards. A physician can meet 10 of the 11 points through the board certification process. The AMAP standards will address medical education and training; licensure; ethical violations; felony or fraud convictions; state or federal disciplinary action within the past five years; and review of the medical office site. Supplementary standards include specialty board certification and recertification; professional liability claims experience; continuing education; and participation in data systems for evaluation of clinical performance and patient care results. The standards for clinical performance and patient care results have not yet been announced by the AMA and are expected after the year 2000.

Announcement of these plans has been met with a great deal of skepticism and resistance. The AMAP will obtain the basic credentials information from the AMA Physician Masterfile, which for years has been inaccurate and suspect as a tool for credentials verification. Additionally, Hugh Greeley, Chairman of The Greeley Company of Marblehead, Massachusetts states:

for any single organization in America to assume that it has the capability to evaluate the quality and appropriateness of all physicians' work is ridiculous.

The program has raised concern among the medical specialty boards about AMAP's impact on board certification. Greeley notes that the 24 American Board of Medical Specialties-approved specialty boards grant certification to physicians based on a careful assessment of their education, training, cognitive knowledge, and ability to respond to clinical questions.[22]

Further, the program has run into difficulties with state medical association credentials verification organizations, although 10 or 12 state medical societies signed letters of intent to participate. As of this writing, the AMA has not worked out the way it will compensate the participating medical societies.[23] Whether this program will be successful remains to be seen.

The AOAP program, which is planned for implementation sometime in 1998, is similar to the AMAP but also has major differences. It will be offered as a membership benefit rather than as moneymaking entity like the AMAP. The AOA hopes to save its members from having to duplicate the credentialing process with the many managed care plans in which they participate. The AOAP will address education and training, board certification, continuing medical education, and will eventually include office site inspections, clinical performance measures, self-assessments, and patient satisfaction measures.[24]

AMBULATORY CARE ACCREDITATION[25]

Accreditors for these facilities include the American Association for Accreditation of Ambulatory Surgery Facilities, the Accreditation Association for Ambulatory Health Care and the JCAHO.

American Association for Accreditation of Ambulatory Surgery Facilities (AAAASF)

The American Association for Accreditation of Ambulatory Surgery Facilities (AAAASF) accredits single and multispecialty ambulatory surgery facilities, including centers that perform minor surgical procedures using local, regional or topical anesthesia; and centers that perform major surgical procedures using sedation or general anesthesia by intubation. The Board of Directors is comprised of 12 physician members.

The standards address the following areas: physical layout, patient and personal records; peer review and quality assurance; operating room personnel, management, operations, and equipment; and sanitation/infection control in the operating suite or office complex.

Surveyors are board certified surgeons who own and/or direct AAAASF-accredited surgical facilities. The surveyors assess how well the facility complies with the standards as well as the scope of procedures being performed at the facility to ensure the surgeon(s) has comparable hospital privileges.

Facilities are awarded accreditation, provisional accreditation, or denial of accreditation. The length of accreditation is three years and facilities must complete a self-evaluation during the second and third years of each accreditation cycle.

Accreditation Association for Ambulatory Health Care, Inc. (AAAHC)

The AAAHC accredits ambulatory clinics, surgery centers, single and multispecialty group practices, health maintenance organizations, birthing centers, college and university health services, urgent and immediate care centers, office based surgery centers and practices, and networks and groups of ambulatory care organizations. Members of the governing board of the AAAHC are appointed from a number of professional medical academies and societies as well as college and community health centers. The AAAHC has deemed status for Medicare.

The standards cover governance, administration, quality of care provided, quality management and improvement, clinical records, professional improvements and facilities and environment. The on-site survey lasts up to two days, depending on the size and type of organization. Facilities are granted three-year accreditation, one-year accreditation or deferred accreditation.

JCAHO

The JCAHO accredits outpatient surgery centers, rehabilitation centers, infusion centers and group practices. The standards for ambulatory care facilities are the same 11 functions listed in the information addressing hospital accreditation. The survey lasts from a day and a half to over a week, depending on the size of the facility and scope of service. The survey is conducted by a physician and an administrator. The types of accreditation decisions are the same as those described for hospital surveys.

REHABILITATION FACILITY ACCREDITATION[26]

The JCAHO accredits rehabilitation hospitals under its hospital accreditation program and CARF...The Rehabilitation Commission (CARF) accredits the rehabilitation program of the hospital. CARF also accredits outpatient rehabilitation programs. Since 1997, CARF and JCAHO conduct their surveys concurrently in a combined process.

CARF...The Rehabilitation Accreditation Commission (CARF)

CARF was established in 1966 and accredits medical rehabilitation programs in rehabilitation hospitals, hospitals providing rehabilitation as part of acute care services, spinal cord injury rehabilitation facilities, pain management programs, brain injury programs, outpatient medical rehabilitation programs, occupational rehabilitation programs, health enhancement programs and pediatric family-centered rehabilitation programs. The board of directors is composed of representatives of 26 medical academies and associations, and at large trustees.

Medical rehabilitation programs must meet CARF standards on promoting organizational quality; promoting program quality; promoting outcome measurement and management; and program standards. Program standards address areas for each of the different programs and facilities noted in the paragraph above. There are two surveyors, an administrator and an MD.

Rehabilitation programs receive three-year accreditation, one-year accreditation, provisional accreditation, or non-accreditation from CARF. There is an appeals mechanism for organizations denied CARF accreditation.

THE SOCIAL SECURITY ACT—MEDICARE

Title XVIII of the Social Security Act, Health Insurance for the Aged, is commonly known as Medicare. The legislation was passed in 1965 and went into effect in 1966. The Medicare program is operated by the Department of Health and Human Services—Health Care Financing Administration (HCFA).

Hospitals receiving Medicare reimbursement must satisfactorily comply with the Conditions of Participation, which are federal regulations delineating standards for health care delivery, similar to standards of the JCAHO. As stated earlier, hospitals accredited by the JCAHO or the AOA are "deemed" to meet the conditions.

The Conditions of Participation recently have been revised to closely resemble the JCAHO's patient-centered care standards. The medical staff condition has been eliminated and is now included as part of the human resources condition. The controversial and misunderstood language prohibiting hospitals from making board certification the only criterion for privileging decisions also has been eliminated. The conditions now allow the hospital to decide how to structure the medical staff as well as which types of allied health professional to appoint to the medical staff. [27]

State departments of health conduct Medicare validation surveys or may perform unannounced surveys of hospitals in response to a patient or family complaint. These surveys can be very stringent and thorough, so attention to the requirements of both the voluntary accrediting body and Medicare is a must.

PREPARING MEDICAL STAFF SERVICES FOR AN ACCREDITATION SURVEY

As discussed in this chapter, there are several agencies that accredit health care institutions. As the majority of hospitals in the country are JCAHO accredited, this section will address preparing for a survey by that agency. As all accreditation surveys are similar, these suggestions will serve as a guide for surveys by other accrediting bodies as well.

The health care facility initiates the accreditation survey by applying to the JCAHO for an on-site survey. A detailed questionnaire related to the standards is mailed to the hospital for completion prior to the survey and is returned to the JCAHO for analysis.

It is helpful for the health care facility to conduct a self-survey, using the accreditation scoring guidelines published by the JCAHO. Areas that are deficient or weak can be identified and improved prior to the survey using this tool. This must be done at least a year in advance of the survey, however, in order to establish a minimum 12-month track record of compliance with the standards. It is also helpful to spend some time with physician leaders several weeks prior to the survey making sure they are prepared to answer questions the surveyors may pose to them.

The on-site survey is scheduled in advance and the hospital is notified of the dates and names of the survey team members. The team usually consists of a physician, a registered nurse and an administrator, although other health care professionals may be used to supplement the survey team, based on the facility's scope of services. In some states, a cooperative survey is conducted simultaneously by representatives of the state hospital licensing agency and the JCAHO. In at least one state (California) representatives of the state medical association also conduct various parts of the survey and each accepts the other's findings. In 44 states, however, the state hospital licensing agency accepts the findings of the JCAHO, with a sample validated by independent survey.

During an accreditation survey the medical staff organization receives primary attention. The physician member (or members) of the survey team devotes his or her time exclusively to (1) observing and reviewing matters relating to the function of the medical staff organization and (2) interviewing the medical staff leadership. The medical staff services professional also must be available to the physician member of the survey team in order to provide requested documentation and answer questions or clarify practice relating to the particular medical staff being surveyed. It is not unusual for the medical staff services professional to spend the entire three days (in larger hospitals) with the physician surveyor, even accompanying him or her on the inspection tour of hospital departments that have medical direction.

Documents Needed for the Survey

When the hospital receives written notice of an impending accreditation survey, a list is included of documents the surveyors will want to review. Those related to survey of the medical staff include the medical staff bylaws, rules and regulations and related policies; credentials files (records of appointments and reappointments, including results of quality improvement activities); and minutes of medical staff committee and department meetings.

The surveyor will provide at the time of the survey a list of the credentials files he or she wishes to review. The list usually includes a practitioner from each specialty represented on the medical staff membership and several allied health professionals. Sometimes the surveyor requests the credentials files of each of the department chairs and each medical director of clinical support services. Prior to the survey, the medical staff services professional should plan for the credentials files to be presented, assuring that they are in good order and contain evidence of current licensure and narcotics registrations, and any other documentation required by the medical staff bylaws or JCAHO standards. If results of quality improvement activities relating to specific practitioners are maintained in files separate from the credentials file, these files should also be prepared.

In addition to looking for documentation of current licensure, the surveyor checks the files for adequacy of privilege delineation and appropriate source verification of education, training, and experience. Reappointment documentation is checked to determine whether there is a profile of physician performance information that supports the clinical privileges exercised by the staff member. Reappointment dates are also carefully checked to determine whether the staff member has been reappointed within two years of the last appointment.

Minutes of medical executive committee, credentials committee and department meetings (unless they are with the executive committee minutes) from the past three years must be made ready for review and should be presented in an organized, professional manner. Most hospitals store meeting minutes in three-ring binders. In the front of the binder a record of attendance of the group is maintained and minute sets are divided by month. Although a full accreditation survey occurs once every three years, the surveyor usually focuses review on documentation from the past year. Minutes for the three-year period being surveyed must be available readily if requested, but the surveyor will probably review records from the past year or two only due to time constraints.

Other Arrangements Prior to the Survey

Because of the large volume of documentation that will be reviewed by the surveyors, a meeting room should be scheduled for the survey of records that will accommodate all of the minute books and other documents. A comfortable setting should be arranged for the surveyors as they will use this room to confer with each other throughout the survey in addition to looking through documents.

It is critical that medical staff leadership be available for the survey. The physician surveyor will schedule two sessions with medical staff leaders. In one session, the surveyor will interview physician leaders about the vision and mission of the hospital, performance improvement activities, and the medical staff's involvement in various hospital operations. A luncheon meeting is also held with members of the medical executive committee to discuss survey findings.

Avoiding Last-Minute Panic

Panic and pandemonium in the hospital always seem to precede an accreditation survey. In the experience of the author, some hospital employees stay up the entire night before a survey doing things at the last minute that should have been done weeks or months before. While some tidying up of records and files is important prior to a survey, this should not be left undone until the night before. If the documentation necessary for an accreditation survey has not been appropriately maintained all along, it is doubtful that it can be produced at the last minute.

The Survey

The hospital is surveyed for substantial compliance with the accreditation standards. As stated earlier, surveyors now spend a great deal of their time talking to hospital employees and physicians about standards requirements in addition to a documentation review session. The physical environment of the hospital is also inspected for safety issues. If a surveyor finds that a particular area is not in substantial compliance or needs improvement, he or she may well offer sample documents from other surveyed hospitals or advice and recommendations for improvement. It behooves the medical staff services professional to graciously accept any proffered advice or sample documentation from other sources.

At the end of the survey an exit conference will be held with the surveyors and senior hospital management and medical staff leaders. Since the surveyors now have laptop computers to assist them with scoring, the hospital will receive information at this time about problems identified in the course of the survey. A written report of survey findings and the accreditation decision will be mailed to the hospital at a later date.

Common Accreditation Problems

According to *Briefings on JCAHO*,[28] the following areas relating to function of the medical staff organization were most frequently cited as deficient by JCAHO in 1997 (see Table 2-2).

Table 2-2. Deficient Areas Relating to Medical Staff Organizations in 1997.

Grid Element	Standard	% Hospitals receiving score of 3, 4 or 5
Bylaws, Rules & Regulations	Bylaws define conditions & mechanisms for removal of officers	5.6%
Credentialing	Department recommendations form the basis for membership and privileges	4.5%
Credentialing	Information about challenges/voluntary loss of licensure/registration is requested	3.9%
Credentialing	The medical staff develops and uses autopsy criteria	3.5%
Credentialing	Information about voluntary/ involuntary changes in member- ship & privileges is requested	3.4%

Source: Data from *Briefings on JCAHO*, October, 1997.

Since the requirement to define criteria in Bylaws for removal of medical staff officers has existed since the mid-1980s, it is hard to believe there are facilities that still have not done this. The requirements to query practitioners about the voluntary (as well as involuntary) loss of licensure, privileges, or membership also have existed since the mid-1980s, as has the requirement for autopsy criteria. It is even more surprising that 4.5 percent of hospitals failed to have the clinical departments make recommendations for membership and privileges. This requirement has existed for 30 years or more.

These findings should make it clear that the medical staff services professional should read the JCAHO standards and be prepared to show documentation of compliance.

NOTES

1. *The Health Care Accreditation Industry Report* (Marblehead, MA: Opus Communications, 1997): 5.

2. E.A. Codman, "An Autobiographic Preface," in *The Shoulder: Rupture of the Subraspinatus Tendon and Other Lesions in or About the Supracromial Bursa* (Boston: Thomas Todd, 1934), v- vi.

3. J.A. Hornsby, "Hospitals as They Are: The Hospital Problem of Today - What Is It?" *Bulletin of the American College of Surgeons* 1 (1917): 4-11.

4. L. Davis, *Fellowship of Surgeons: A History of the American College of Surgeons* (Chicago: American College of Surgeons, 1973).

5. C.P. Schlicke, "American Surgery's Noblest Experiment," *Archives of Surgery* 108 (1973): 379-85.

6. Hornsby, "Hospitals as They Are."

7. Davis, *Fellowship of Surgeons*, 226.

8. Ibid., 489-90.

9. F.H. Martin, *Fifty Years of Medicine and Surgery: An Autobiographical Sketch* (Chicago: Lakeside Press, 1934), 338.

10. G.W. Stephenson, "The College's Role in Hospital Standardization," *Bulletin of the American College of Surgeons* 66 (1981): 17-29.

11. J.P. Porterfield, "From the Director's Office," *Bulletin of the Joint Commission on Accreditation of Hospitals* 4 (1972): 1-2.

12. Joint Commission on Accreditation of Hospitals, 1970 *Accreditation Manual for Hospitals* (Chicago: Joint Commission on Accreditation of Hospitals, 1969).

13. J.P. Porterfield, "Mechanisms for Hospital Standards," *Bulletin of the Joint Commission on Accreditation of Hospitals* 48 (1968): 1-4.

14. U.S. Department of Health, Education, and Welfare: *Conditions of Participation for Hospitals*, (Washington, D.C.: Social Security Administration, 1966).

15. U.S. General Accounting Office: *The Medicare Hospital Certification System Needs Reform: Report to Congress* (Washington, D.C.: U.S. General Accounting Office, 1979).

16. David Burda, "JCAHO Hits a Wall With Plan on Indicators," *Modern Healthcare* 24 (March 14 1994): 30-35.

17. *ORYX: The Evaluation Process*, (Marblehead, MA: Opus Communications, July 1997): 2.

18. *National Committee for Quality Assurance - An Overview*, (Washington, DC: National Committee for Quality Assurance Web site). Available at: http://www.ncqa.org. Accessed March 3, 1998.

19. Ibid., Accessed June 15, 1998.

20. Ibid., Accessed June 15, 1998.

21. American Accreditation HealthCare Commission, Inc. "About URAC," (Washington, DC: American Accreditation HealthCare Commission, Inc. Web site). Available at http:\\www.urac.org. Accessed May 28, 1998.

22. Hugh Greeley in "Observers Applaud AMAP Concept, But Question Ability to Carry it Out," *Briefings on Credentialing* 6 (July 1997): 4.

23. "AMAP Soldiers on Despite Struggles," *Medical Staff Briefing* 8 (March 1998): 9.

24. Ibid., 7.

25. *The Health Care Accreditation Industry Report* (Marblehead, MA: Opus Communications, 1997): 17-27.

26. Ibid., 191-202

27. "Proposed COP Echoes JCAHO's Emphasis on 'Patient-Centered Care,'" *Medical Staff Briefing* 8 (March 1998): 1, 4.

28. "The Top 40 Findings in 1997," *Briefings on JCAHO* 8 (October 1997): 6-7.

Chapter 3

Medical Staff and Provider Organizations

Richard E. Thompson, MD

Caring for patients continues to be the nucleus of activity
around which all health care organization functions revolve.

(Physician leaders) are intricately involved in carrying out, and in
providing leadership in, all patient care functions conducted by
individuals with clinical privileges.[1]

—Joint Commission on Accreditation of Healthcare Organizations

INTRODUCTION

To individuals who are new to the Medical Staff Services Profession:
Welcome to a unique and valuable profession.

To the experienced Medical Staff Services Professional (MSSP): Boot up
your brain and put in a fresh, blank, disk. The entering student has an advantage over you, because he or she has less to *un*learn. Things are different now
than when you first entered this field, and the differences go far beyond results of the recent "re-structuring" era.

Organizational Role of The Medical Staff Services Professional

The usual role of the MSSP is to support and coach responsible physician
leaders who work on the dependable performance ("quality") side of the "value"
equation.

The MSSP's title might be director or coordinator of the medical staff
office, network credentialing coordinator, or some similar title reflecting both
the MSSP's job description and specific organizational structure. If the bad
news is that the MSSP ordinarily occupies a staff position instead of a line
position, the good news is that the MSSP borrows and reflects the power of
influential physician leaders.[2]

Physician leaders include a hospital's medical staff president, credentials chair, performance improvement chair, and chairs of clinical departments, a network's medical director and directors of clinical departments and their designees, and members of a health care system's medical advisory board.

The MSSP's role is critical because some physician leaders do not yet fully understand the difference between organizational leadership and political leadership. Indeed, effective on-the-job orientation of physician leaders by MSSPs over the last few years is one major reason that "physician leader" is no longer an oxymoron.

Critical Importance of the MSSP/Physician Leader Team

Value means that dependable services (from the viewpoint of the patient and family member) are provided at reasonable cost. In choosing to focus on *dependable performance*, the editors and publishers of this book provide a unique resource which counter-balances the plethora of resources focusing on the *cost and profit* side of the value equation.

Value is today a common management buzzword. That is because those holding health care dollars seem eager to award contracts on the basis of cost *plus* quality (value). This trend was predictable because "End the practice of awarding business on the basis of price" is W. Edwards Deming's Continuous Quality Improvement (CQI) Principle Number Four![3]

Indeed, the most successful health care executives appreciate that profits cannot be generated in the health care business unless high priority is given to credentialing independent practitioners including physicians, obtaining and heeding the input of frontline clinical practitioners, and generating data confirming dependable practitioner performance. And such activities cannot go forward without an adequate number of well-qualified MSSPs.

A Caveat

Incidentally, if the dependable performance focus of an MSSP's activities does not match the true interests of the reader, then he or she would be well-advised to consider entering another field or seeking another position within the organization. For example, if the reader is primarily interested in being in a position in which the results of his or her efforts can be quantified in terms of profit (or loss) to the organization, then he or she should start out on a track that might lead to becoming vice president of marketing or finance. Working in medical staff services certainly brings value to the organization but not in dollars made or lost.

"Physician Leader" Defined

In the context of this chapter, *physician leader* means an MD or DO who chooses to remain primarily a clinician, yet accepts a position of organizational leadership. A good physician leader has come to understand that "patient care" now means much more than "me and my patient." This physician leader, often as a result of coaching by a skilled and experienced MSSP, also knows how organizations work, so he or she effectively adds the dimension of clinical reality to organizational activities such as credentialing and performance improvement.

For information about working with a full-time Vice President for Medical Affairs (VPMA), the reader is referred to resources already available.[4] (See also Chapter 4.)

The MSSP as True Partner

The medical staff services profession has evolved over the years from a position in hospitals that was first known as "medical staff secretary." A major difference in today's organizational scenario and that of previous generations is that the MSSP is no longer the handmaiden of the physician. Rather, the knowledgeable, skilled, and committed MSSP is the physician leader's true partner, coach, and internal consultant.

Two General Structures

First we'll take a look at the MSSP/physician leader partnership in the hospital. Then, since the hospital is now usually one component of an integrated delivery network (IDN), we'll look at the MSSP/physician leader partnership in networks. A third type of organizational structure, which is groups of physicians organized for the purpose of obtaining contracts with IDNs, is an area in which there are growing opportunities for MSSPs.

Remember that we are focusing on "quality" functions. This emphasis does not require a discussion of technical, legalistic structural differences between a health maintenance organization, independent practice association, health delivery network, integrated delivery system, and so on. That is because today's "pretend you are the patient" approach to physician leader functions is the same in all varieties of health care organizations. Readers interested in technical structural variations between this health care delivery network and that one should consult resources already available.[5]

Neither is it necessary to detail the difference between a profit-oriented managed care organization (MCO) and a service-oriented IDN.[6] It is important to note, however, that if profit-oriented MCOs do not begin placing greater emphasis on dependable performance ("quality"), there is a risk that existing U.S. health care policy, which encourages profit-taking, might be replaced by some other policy.[7]

THE MSSP/PHYSICIAN LEADER TEAM IN THE HOSPITAL/ MEDICAL CENTER

Brief History of the Organized Medical Staff

Knowing a little history of the medical staff organization can help the MSSP understand and resolve many problems encountered by anyone responsible for working with physician leaders.[8]

Until about the time of World War I, each doctor practicing in the United States had a unique individual relationship with the superintendent of the local hospital, and had the authority to give orders to nurses working in that hospital. Completely independent and autonomous, each physician enjoyed unbridled freedom to order whatever came to mind for the diagnosis and treatment of hospitalized patients. The doctor could also perform whatever operation a patient needed, whether or not he had seen or done that operation before.

Then, in 1919, the American College of Surgeons (ACS) responded to two separate but related studies.[9,10]   Taken together, these studies suggested that results of marked variations in the practice habits of generally-trained physicians were not really known but might need to be improved. So the ACS created a one-page list of Hospital Standards.[11] Designees of the ACS (practicing surgeons) then visited, inspected, and accredited worthy hospitals, using the list of standards.

ACS's standards required, among other things, that "doctors practicing in the hospital be organized as a definite group or staff...restricted to physicians and surgeons...and that the staff initiate and, with the approval of the governing board of the hospital adopt rules, regulations, and policies governing the professional work of the hospital."[11] Thus was born the modern "organized medical staff" in U.S. hospitals.

Note, by the way, that the term *bylaws* is not used in this initial list of hospital standards. In fact, since the ACS's initial accreditation effort arose from concern for patients expressed by one of its members (Dr. Codman[10]), it is likely that the surgeons intended to use such terms as *standards*, *rules*, and *policies* in the sense of professional guidelines rather than in the sense of *absolute, legal standards* to be relied upon in a court of law and other legal proceedings.

Activities that grew out of the ACS accreditation effort included peer review and credentialing. Initial methods are ancestors of today's systems for credentialing and privileging independent clinical practitioners, and for developing data confirming current dependable performance.

Physician leaders enlisted the medical records librarian to be their chief peer review assistant. And they created the position of medical staff secretary. This person, the forerunner of today's MSSP, kept medical staff members' credentials files, typed minutes of meetings, collected staff dues, and planned the annual medical staff Christmas party.

In 1951, the ACS enlisted the help of other organizations in the hospital accreditation effort. The ACS got together with the American Medical Association (AMA), the American Hospital Association (AHA), the American College of Physicians (ACP), and the Canadian counterparts of all four organizations to form the *Joint* Commission on Accreditation of Hospitals (JCAH). Over the years, Canadian associations dropped out and formed their own accrediting agency, and other professional associations joined the JCAH effort. JCAH expanded its hospital accreditation effort to other entities, and became JCAHO, the Joint Commission on Accreditation of Healthcare Organizations.

Today, JCAHO's senior leaders are at the leading edge of innovation in the structure and activities of the MSSP/physician leader team.[12,13]

TRADITIONAL MODEL OF THE HOSPITAL'S ORGANIZED MEDICAL STAFF

Believe it or not, the entering MSSP will still encounter remnants of the original 1919 medical staff organizational model in today's modern hospitals.

The central elements of this old model were medical staff officers (president, vice president, and secretary-treasurer of the medical staff) and the general medical staff, meaning all the doctors who admitted patients to the hospital. Organizational elements included categories, departments, and committees.

The general medical staff met monthly. Officers, committee chairs, and department chairs were not allowed to do much without first saying, "May I?" in a general medical staff meeting. The whole staff would then vote on how much of what kind of leadership their elected "leaders" were allowed to exercise.

The medical staff/governing board/administration relationship was characterized as a "three-legged stool." *Governing board members* sought to avoid financial failure, including making up budget deficits from their own personal funds. *Hospital "administrators"* were responsible for day-to-day management of such matters as personnel, integrity of the physical hospital plant (the building), and staying within budget. Meanwhile, *the medical staff* was pretty much left alone to do its own thing. The theoretical authority of the governing board over the medical staff was acknowledged, but reports and requests to the board were ordinarily rubber-stamped.

The products of this organizational model were meetings and minutes. Additional products included apathy, conflict, attorney control of medical staff functions, and unfair expectations of the medical staff coordinator.

Most physicians cared little about the organized medical staff's activities. Attendance at meetings was so minimal that it was hard to enforce the usual requirement that medical staff members attend a certain number or percent of meetings each year.

The more administrators and boards tried to force participation of every medical staff member in hospital matters, the more physicians resisted. Seminars on "how to resolve hospital/medical staff conflict" were in vogue.

Administrators sought help from attorneys on how to prevail in conflicts with the medical staff. So attorneys became key players in controlling the activities of the organized medical staff and its members. Relevant state statutes and judicial precedents over-shadowed professional guidelines as determinants of the activities of the MSSP/physician leader team.

Meanwhile, as this power struggle raged, the medical staff coordinator was expected to accept responsibility for such activities as proving to JCAHO surveyors that physician leaders, board members, and the CEO, in spite of appearances, were actually focused on "assuring quality."

Readers interested in additional historical detail can consult other available resources.[14, 15, 16]

This organizational model could not have survived much longer, even without the managed care revolution and the coming of a new millennium.

RESULTS OF THE RE-STRUCTURING ERA (1996–THE PRESENT TIME)

For the past few years, the MSSP/physician leader team has been busy re-engineering, re-structuring, and down-sizing the organized medical staff. Results of this era, still in progress at this writing, include

1. The focus now being on individual physician leaders, such as department chairs and their designees, functioning day-by-day, as opposed to waiting for a committee meeting to analyze a problem and design a solution;

2. The focus now being on function, rather than primarily on structure as in previous years. For example, the name of the medical staff game once was: "Do we have enough committees to be sure that every active medical staff member is on two or three and can thus pull their share of the load?" But the questions today are: "What is the task to be accomplished, or the ongoing function to be maintained? What is the most effective and efficient way to do that?" The answer, by the way, is very rarely, "Appoint a committee, add staffing it to someone's job responsibilities, try to get the doctors to come to

the meetings, and focus on two goals which are referring problems to some other committee and developing minutes to confirm that you have dealt with the problem."

3. The focus on the professional aspect of MSSP/physician leader activities and these activities as a winning organizational strategy. That is in contrast to the former primary emphasis on legalities and compliance with JCAHO standards, which effectively prevented adequate attention to demonstrating patient-oriented professionalism (which today is the major key to both avoiding legal hassles and complying with JCAHO!)

4. In the traditional model, Medical *Executive* Committees acted more like Medical *Legislative* Committees. Today, many physician leaders understand the medical executive function as similar to the executive function in any organization.

5. The activities of the MSSP/physician team being increasingly appreciated as valuable (therefore rewardable) far beyond the goal of satisfying JCAHO.[17]

TODAY'S ORGANIZATIONAL MODEL

Figure 3-1 summarizes today's hospital medical staff organizational model, including the medical staff's relationships to other organizational components of the hospital.

Some MSSP/physician leader team activities, such as interpreting and using clinical information supplied by the performance improvement office, are now accomplished effectively and efficiently on a day-to-day basis instead of inefficiently and ineffectively, or not at all, by a committee that met only once a month.

However, no matter how many organizational charts you look at you will never see another one like that shown in Figure 3-1, because elements of the newer, streamlined organizational model exist side-by-side with remnants of the old 1919 model.

For example, one might expect a vice president of medical affairs (VPMA) to be a member of the hospital's executive staff, similar to the vice president of finance. That is the reporting relationship to the chief executive officer (CEO). Yet with respect to the organized medical staff, the VPMA often has no direct authority. Medical executive authority still resides in a medical executive committee (MEC) or, at best, some combination of the MEC, medical staff president, and VPMA.

Also, one might expect a department chair or director (see Figure 3-1) to be selected because of good organizational skills and to hold a relatively permanent position. But it is still common to find department chairs who are elected or serve in rotation, and serve only two-year "terms."

Figure 3-1. Hospital Medical Staff Organizational Components and Their Relationships.

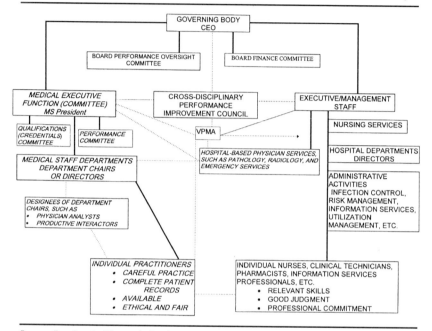

Source: Reprinted with permission from Thompson, Mohr and Associates, Inc., © 1998.

PHYSICIAN LEADERS IN TODAY'S HOSPITAL MEDICAL STAFF ORGANIZATIONAL STRUCTURE

The success of the MSSP/physician leader team must begin with careful selection, adequate orientation, and periodic evaluation of physician leaders. (Evaluation in this context means *as leaders.* Evaluation as a clinician is a separate matter.)

Physician leaders in today's hospital medical staff organization include clinical department chairs, designees of department chairs, and the medical staff president.

Chair of Each Clinical Department

Responsibilities of the department chair ordinarily are to[18]

1.   Develop, review, revise as necessary, follow, and summarize at a regular or special department meeting, a department guidelines, policies, and methods manual;

2.   Participate in, or provide designees to participate in, relevant activities of the hospital's performance assessment and improvement program;

3.   Act as spokesperson for the department to such groups as the MEC and other medical staff committees, departments, and sections, hospital executive/management staff, nursing and other hospital departments, and to the medical center board;

4.   Serve as a coordinating point by providing information about medical center and medical staff affairs to members of the department;

5.   Analyze information, including but not limited to, applications for membership and clinical privileges of individuals who are members of or who are likely to be assigned to the department, patient care information resulting from performance assessment and improvement activities, capital improvement needs of the department, staffing needs, and the relevancy of departmental policies and guidelines;

6.   Interact with members of the department when there are questions about clinical performance, disregard for reasonable departmental or hospital rules, lack of respect for co-workers, inefficient practice, suspected impairment, or practicing outside the limits of clinical privileges that have been awarded;

7.   Act as primary spokesman for the department with outside agencies, where applicable, such as during the hospital's survey by the JCAHO;

8.   Evaluate causes for, and participate in response to, untoward incidents involving members of the department;

9.   Occasionally, with the help of relevant support personnel, plan and conduct meetings of the department.

Designees of Department Chairs

Note: The MSSP will find that the useful organizational principle of lending one's authority to another (delegating) is not part of the experience of frontline clinicians. It is not wise for a skilled surgeon to send someone else to perform operations in his stead on a patient for whom the surgeon is responsible. So, the MSSP may have to coach some physician leaders in the fine art of delegation, including how to determine that an assignment has been adequately completed in a timely fashion.

One example of a physician leader designee is the *physician analyst*.[19] A physician analyst is a person who agrees to analyze and suggest conclusions from data and daily observations developed in the course of performance assessment and improvement activities. The physician analyst and department chair work together to compile positive data, and to react to needs for improved performance in a timely manner.

The physician analyst concept is also valuable in credentialing. Prior to action on applications, a physician credentials analyst should read the application with the MSSP, and they should suggest (to the credentials chair or medical staff president, depending on exact organizational structure) additional information that may be needed.

Medical Staff President

The duties of the medical staff president ordinarily are to[20]

1. Act in coordination and cooperation with the VPMA and CEO in all matters of mutual concern within the hospital;
2. Call, preside at, and be responsible for the agenda of all general medical staff meetings (Note: Annually, plus any special meetings);
3. Serve on the medical executive committee and serve as its chair;
4. Serve as ex-officio member of all other medical staff committees;
5. Be responsible for seeking compliance of practitioners with medical staff and medical center rules;
6. Appoint committee members to all standing, special, and multidisciplinary committees except as otherwise provided;
7. Present the views, policies, and needs of the medical staff to the board and CEO;
8. Interpret the policies of the board to the medical staff, and report to the board on performance and maintenance of dependable and efficient care;
9. Be responsible for seeing that continuing education activities are provided;
10. With the VPMA and MEC, oversee the work of department chairs.

Members of the Medical Executive Committee

Members of the medical executive committee, together with the medical staff president and VPMA, are responsible for the medical executive function which should be similar to the executive function in any organization. The following language is from a sample set of medical staff bylaws:[21]

The Executive Function Defined
The executive function in organizations means that an individual or group is authorized to execute, carry out, on a day-to-day basis,

the policies of the organization, and is entrusted with the responsibility to act on a daily basis to direct the organization's activities.

The Medical Executive Function
The medical executive function of this medical staff is entrusted to a medical executive committee, members of which work in concert with the medical staff president and vice president of medical affairs.

Medical Staff Categories

The purpose of medical staff categories is to relate the individual's *membership* prerogatives and obligations to the frequency with which the individual engages in *clinical* activities at this hospital.

Once upon a time, a medical staff member was appointed to a category such as either active or courtesy, and the clinical privileges that could be exercised were related to the category assignment. For example, an active category staff member would have more clinical privileges than a courtesy category member.

Today, in addition to confirming the individual's identity, current state licensure, acceptable liability (malpractice) history, and so on, a first key step is awarding individual-specific clinical privileges. Over time, the individual's category assignment comes to reflect the frequency with which those clinical privileges are exercised at this hospital.

This distinction between *membership on or appointment to* the medical staff organization on one hand, and *clinical privileges* on the other, is today a major key to resolving several common credentialing and privileging issues.[22]

For example, a category such as "managed care affiliate" is useful for accurately describing the relationship to the hospital of an IDN physician engaged only in outpatient care.

THE MSSP/PHYSICIAN LEADER TEAM'S PORTFOLIO: NEEDED DOCUMENTS

Once upon a time, medical staff bylaws, rules and regulations were the documents governing activities of physician leaders. But today, while medical staff bylaws remain important, the central focus is on professional guidelines rather than on absolute legal standards.

Any statements, rules, or provisions intended to be relied upon in a court of law or other legal proceeding should be placed in documents called bylaws, rules, and policies. But other important documents, not requiring legal review, can contain flexible professional guidelines and plain-language methods descriptions.

Examples of such documents are[23]

1. a guidelines and methods manual for each clinical department (which may be a supplement to a policy manual for each clinical department);
2. a guidelines and methods manual for the MEC;
3. step-by-step descriptions of methods used in activities such as performance awareness and improvement, credentialing and privileging, and planning continuing medical education sessions;
4. descriptions of needed clinical committees (which need not be described in medical staff bylaws).

THE PHYSICIAN LEADER AND MSSP IN THE INTEGRATED DELIVERY NETWORK (IDN)

Contrast Figure 3-2, the organizational model in a health care network, with Figure 3-1, the existing organizational model in hospitals. In the model seen in Figure 3-2, the medical director (or the title may be vice president of medical affairs) is a physician vice president, with direct authority over MD or DO department chairs, who in turn have direct authority over frontline physicians.

The key to success in implementing this organizational structure is to recognize that a salaried family physician, for example, may be subordinate to management, but the same family physician is the CEO in the context of caring for an individual patient.[24]

Credentialing as an Example of the MSSP/Physician Leader Partnership in Networks

In the hospital, credentialing and privileging applications still take a traditional route from the applicant to the board, passing through several stops including the department chair's report, the credentials committee's recommendation to the MEC, and the MEC's recommendation to the board or relevant board sub-committee. That process is often delayed by waiting for meetings of committees, then by having committee members ask for additional information, which cannot be considered until the next meeting a month later. (Some hospitals are now doing "fast-track" credentialing, in which the steps once accomplished by committees are now accomplished by responsible physician leaders in a much shorter time.)

One might expect to learn that the contrasting model in an IDN is that physician hiring and firing can be handled by a human resources department, just like other personnel. That probably is not going to happen anytime soon. Note, for example, that at this writing, employees who do not perform up to

Figure 3-2. Organizational Relationships of Physicians and Physician Leaders in an Integrated Deliver Network (IDN).

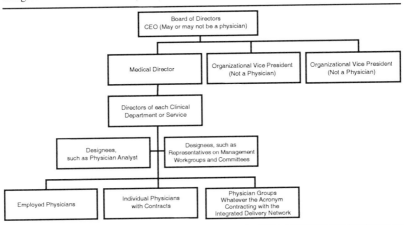

expectations are *fired* but physicians whose performance is not adequate must be *de-selected.*

So it is necessary to seek a structural model of credentialing for IDN's. In doing so, three mistakes may be made. One is simply to forward the old, traditional, committee-based, legalistic credentialing process from hospitals to the IDN. The second mistake is to make the first mistake more than once, trying to set up a separate credentialing process in each of the IDN's components. And the third mistake is for those responsible for the duplicate credentialing processes to set up conflicts with each other over needed information and credentialing requirements!

Figure 3-3 provides an example of a reasonable IDN credentialing process. This process is designed to simultaneously protect patients, practitioners, and the relevant organizations and components of the "integrated" delivery network. The process is reminiscent enough of the old hospital process to be acceptable to most, yet avoids duplicate effort, and offers points at which inter-component conflicts can be resolved.

In passing, note that Figure 3-3 is one example of using the principle of *separating* membership issues from clinical credentialing issues to find a solution to a credentialing problem.

The System or IDN Medical Advisory Board

Successful health care systems and integrated delivery networks usually have a medical advisory board which includes, along with other members, physician leaders from all components of the system or network.

As the name suggests, a medical advisory board has no direct authority. However, this group can be very successful in influencing decisions of the board of directors and executive staff.

In fact, in some instances, the input of these knowledgeable clinicians can result in avoiding expensive management mistakes. For example, if early managed care organizations had listened to their physician leaders, there never

Figure 3-3. Physician Credentialing Account for All Organizational Components.

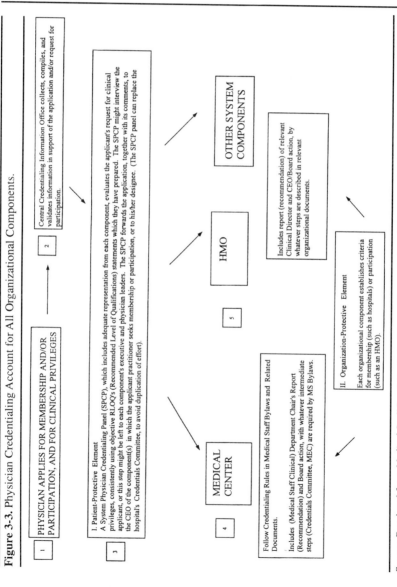

1 — PHYSICIAN APPLIES FOR MEMBERSHIP AND/OR PARTICIPATION, AND FOR CLINICAL PRIVILEGES

2 — Central Credentialing Information Office collects, compiles, and validates information in support of the application and/or request for participation.

I. Patient-Protective Element
A System Physician Credentialing Panel (SPCP), which includes adequate representation from each component, evaluates the applicant's request for clinical privileges, consistently using objective RLOQ's (Recommended Level of Qualifications) statements which they have prepared. The SPCP might interview the applicant, or this step might be left to each component's executive and physician leaders. The SPCP forwards the application, together with its comments, to the CEO of the component(s) in which the applicant practitioner seeks membership or participation, or to his/her designee. (The SPCP panel can replace the hospital's Credentials Committee, to avoid duplication of effort).

3 — Follow Credentialing Rules in Medical Staff Bylaws and Related Documents.
Includes (Medical Staff Clinical) Department Chair's Report (Recommendation) and Board action, with whatever intermediate steps (Credentials Committee, MEC) are required by MS Bylaws.

4 — MEDICAL CENTER

5 — HMO

OTHER SYSTEM COMPONENTS

Includes report (recommendation) of relevant Clinical Director and CEO/Board action, by whatever steps are described in relevant organizational documents.

II. Organization-Protective Element
Each organizational component establishes criteria for membership (such as hospitals) or participation (such as an HMO).

Source: Reprinted from *Medical Staff Portfolio*, 2nd edition, with permission of Thompson, Mohr and Associates, Inc., Dunedin, FL, © 1996.

would have been any such thing as a "gag order."[25] The entire health care industry is still recovering from the poor public image that this management mistake created.

An MSSP may have the task of providing staff support to the medical advisory board.

WHAT IS NEXT FOR THE STRUCTURE WITHIN WHICH MSSP/ PHYSICIAN LEADER TEAMS FUNCTION?

As more and more physicians develop leadership skills and occupy positions of senior management in IDN's and their hospital components, and as market forces and public opinion force hospitals and networks to remember the social contract which they must fulfill,[26] streamlining of organizational structures will continue.

No one knows exactly what form these new structures will take. But one thing is certain: The work of skilled and committed MSSPs has been a critical factor in recent improvements in structural models. And MSSPs are primary players in molding the organizational structures of the new millennium.

NOTES

1. Joint Commission on Accreditation of Healthcare Organizations, "Introduction to MS.6, Care of the Patient," *1998 Hospital Accreditation Standards* pocket-size edition (Oakbrook Terrace, IL: Joint Commission on Accreditation of Healthcare Organizations, 1997): 263.

2. Richard E. Thompson, MD, "How to Exercise Power When you Have Limited Authority," *Family Practice Management* 5 (1998): 82.

3. Mary Walton, *The Deming Management Method* (New York: Perigee Books, 1986): 34.

4. Publications and services of the American College of Physician Executives (ACPE), Tampa, FL.

5. David Nash, MD, MBA, *The Managed Care Manual* (Boston: TLC Medical Publishing, a division of Total Learning Concepts, Inc., 1997).

6. Richard E. Thompson, MD, *So You've Been Integrated: Now What? Opportunities for Physicians Practicing in Managed Care Settings* (Tampa: American College of Physician Executives, 1996).

7. Richard E. Thompson, MD, *Health Care Reform as Social Change* (Tampa: American College of Physician Executives, 1993).

8. Richard E. Thompson, *Keys to Winning Physician Support* (Tampa: American College of Physician Executives, 1991).

9. Abraham Flexner, *Medical Education in the United States and Canada* (New York: Carnegie Foundation for the Advancement of Teaching, 1910).

10. E.A. Codman, MD, "The Product of a Hospital," *Surgery, Gynecology, and Obstetrics* 118 (1914): 491-496.

11. American College of Surgeons, "The Minimum Standard," 1919.

12. Joint Commission on Accreditation of Healthcare Organizations, *1998 Comprehensive Accreditation Manual for Hospitals* (Oakbrook Terrace, IL: Joint Commission on Accreditation of Healthcare Organizations, 1997).

13. Richard E. Thompson, MD, *Compliance Guide to the Joint Commission's Medical Staff Standards*, 2nd ed. (Marblehead, MA: Opus Communications, 1998).

14. Malcolm T. McEachern, *The Medical Staff in the Hospital*, 2nd ed. (Chicago: Physicians' Record Company, 1953).

15. C. Wesley Eisele, ed., *The Medical Staff in the Modern Hospital* (New York: McGraw-Hill, 1967).

16. C.W. Eisele, MD, W.R. Fifer, MD, T.C. Wilson, MPA, *The Medical Staff and the Modern Hospital* (Englewood, CO: McGraw-Hill, 1967).

17. Martin Merry, MD, *The Shifting Quality Focus* (LaJolla, CA: The Governance Institute, 1996).

18. The TMA Press, "Medical Staff Bylaws Document," *Medical Staff Portfolio* (Dunedin, FL: The TMA Press, 1997).

19. Richard E. Thompson, MD, "Developing and Using Information Confirming Dependable Performance, *The Medical Staff Leader's Practical Guidebook*, 3rd ed. (Marblehead, MA: Opus Communications, 1998): 52.

20. The TMA Press, *Medical Staff Portfolio*.

21. Ibid.

22. Richard E. Thompson, MD, "Credentialing (Confirmation of Entry-Level Qualifications)," *Compliance Guide to the Joint Commission's Medical Staff Standards*, 2nd ed. (Marblehead, MA: Opus Communications, 1998): 55.

23. The TMA Press, *Medical Staff Portfolio*.

24. Thompson, "How to Exercise Power When You Have Limited Authority."

25. Gag orders = Agreements that some managed care companies aksed physicians to sign, preventing physicians from telling patients that they should have certain costly diagnostic tests, treatments or operations.

26. Thompson, *HealthCare Reform As Social Change*.

Chapter 4

Physician Executives

Vicki L. Searcy

Special thanks to the following physicians who provided information used in this chapter:

- *Charles R. Mathews, MD, Former Medical Director; Sarasota Memorial Hospital, Sarasota, Florida*

- *Merrill N. Werblun, MD, Vice President, Medical Affairs; The Queen's Medical Center, Honolulu, Hawaii*

- *Gary Mihalik, MD, President, The Mihalik Group; Chicago, Illinois*

HISTORICAL PERSPECTIVE

Many physicians practicing today have fond memories of less complicated times, before diagnostic-related groups (DRGs) and professional review organizations (PROs), before managed care and the resulting new types of organizations and relationships (preferred provider organizations [PPOs], independent practice associations [IPAs], physician-hospital organizations [PHOs], to name a few); of times when *marketing* was not a health care verb and malpractice liability and competition were on the periphery of professional awareness.

The relationship of physicians to their hospitals seemed similarly uncomplicated: A lone secretarial type usually manned the minuscule medical staff office, processing the one- or two-page applications for medical staff membership and keeping a calendar of the meetings.

In those untroubled years, physicians and "administration" coexisted in a stance of polite non-intimacy, while they reaped their portions of the green harvest of Medicare charge-based reimbursement. Practitioners performed their healing arts in their hospital "workshops," filling the beds (often straining the bed capacity), while the administrators kept the shop running. The infrequent contacts between the two groups usually arose from requests by the physicians for more equipment or services, which were usually forthcoming since third-party payers picked up the tab.

Into the seventies, the organizational structure of the typical medical staff was relatively straightforward, governed by a pyramidal hierarchy consisting of committee chairs, heads of clinical departments, and a chief of staff at the apex. In the community hospitals, top medical staff leaders typically were elected and held office for one or two years.

In most hospitals, the time-tested laissez-faire model persisted into the early eighties, at which time a number of forces converged to irreversibly alter the delivery of health care services in hospital and non-hospital settings, including the physicians' office practices.

HOSPITAL TRUSTEE ACCOUNTABILITY

Beginning with the landmark *Darling* case in 1965, the courts and the various regulatory and accrediting bodies have increasingly held hospital governing boards accountable for the quality of care delivered in their institutions. Trustees are no longer simply public-spirited citizens, contributing time and fund-raising abilities to their hospitals of choice. They now typically assume fiduciary roles that encompass the responsibility for the practitioners' performance in patient care. Rarely, however, are trustees medically sophisticated, and they heavily rely upon the medical staff not only to deliver an acceptable level of care but to document and report to the governing body information about the quality and appropriateness of such care. Although the governing board has historically, of necessity, delegated the monitoring of quality (quality assurance) to the medical staff, the pattern of "arms length" delegation became unacceptable in the eighties—the age of accountability.

HOSPITAL REIMBURSEMENT

The institution of the prospective payment system, with its DRGs, in 1983 signaled the end of the financial cornucopia for hospitals. The Medicare and other third-party spigots were tightened, resulting in an abrupt change in hospital admission patterns. As the medical staff learned that "groupers" were not a variety of fish, length of patient stay dropped dramatically. Many procedures previously performed comfortably within the walls of the hospital suddenly became outpatient procedures. Case mix changed: The patients admitted were sicker and required greater intensity of care. To monitor Medicare admissions, a professional review organization (PRO) appeared in every state by congressional mandate. Initially, the PROs monitored only the financial aspects of the admissions, but subsequently the monitors included quality of care. At the same time, there has been progressive "ratcheting down" of the reimbursements, with the result that hospitals must be managed efficiently or risk losing money on their Medicare admissions.

In addition, the advent of managed care and the contractual arrangements of health plans with hospitals have resulted in the necessity to manage all hospitalized patients efficiently, not just Medicare patients.

PROBLEMS OF TRADITIONAL HOSPITAL MEDICAL STAFF LEADERSHIP

Time Commitments

Physicians have typically assumed medical staff leadership positions during their most active practice years. Always demanding, the increasing responsibilities and time commitments have made it very difficult in all but the smallest hospitals for a practitioner to perform the functions of a chief of staff or departmental or committee chair, without the skilled assistance of a full-time or part-time physician executive: the medical director.

Dual Roles

The dual roles of elected medical staff leaders are often not fully appreciated by the governing board, nor by the elected leaders themselves or the medical staff organization members. In one capacity, the chief of staff is the "president" or chief executive of the medical staff. As such, the chief of staff exercises the authority and assumes responsibility for the functions of the medical staff. The chief of staff also represents the interests of the staff vis-a-vis the hospital administration and to the governing board.

At the same time, whenever the chief of staff, departmental or committee chairs, or any other officers of the medical staff are performing their official functions, they are acting on behalf of the governing board and as such are in effect "officers" of that board, with derivative authority, accountability and fiduciary responsibility.

Lack of Continuity

Elected medical staff leaders characteristically serve for very few years. One or two years is the usual term for a chief of staff. Typically, by the time he or she has acquired the information and know-how necessary for effective functioning, the term of office is over. The physician then usually returns to his or her neglected practice, rarely surfacing thereafter in the medical staff hierarchy. The physician's administrative expertise and experience are lost, and the successor begins the acquisition process anew.

Information Base

The sheer quantity of information needed to manage the affairs of a medical staff in the hospitals of the eighties and nineties seems to be growing exponentially. In view of the limited terms of office and the demands of their medical practices, elected leaders cannot acquire the information base necessary to effectively carry out the many functions of medical staff leadership.

Lack of Managerial Abilities

Rarely have elected medical staff leaders had significant training or experience in managerial functions, yet these skills are essential for the orderly management of the medical staff. Some leaders seem to have been born with executive skills, and others acquire them over time. But the basic method is "on the job training," not an ideal mechanism given today's enormously complex hospital health care delivery systems.

Potential Conflicts of Interest

As practitioners, medical staff leaders have built-in potential conflicts of interest. Official decisions that they may be called on to make will often impact their practices, their referrals, or their economic interests. The dilemmas are common and will call into question the decision-making processes of the medical staff. In addition, there are frequent instances when the interests of practitioners are opposed to those of the institution.

Authority and Accountability

The derivative authority and the attendant accountability of the medical staff leadership concern the quality and appropriateness of patient care. The various monitoring mechanisms involved in this awesome responsibility include quality improvement or performance improvement, utilization review, and risk management. Also impacting the leadership are the multiple accrediting and regulatory bodies, including the Joint Commission on Accreditation of Healthcare Organizations (JCAHO), the National Committee on Quality Assurance (NCQA), the PROs, relationships with health plans, and state licensing and regulatory agencies. Practicing physicians rarely have the time, the store of information, the skills, or the will needed to fulfill the medical staff's delegated responsibilities regarding quality of patient care.

THE PHYSICIAN EXECUTIVE

The demands of leading the medical staff organization and ensuring that required functions have been fulfilled exceeded the ability of practicing physician volunteers to meet those demands. This led to the emergence, in many hospitals, of the medical director. For purposes of the remainder of this chapter, the title "physician executive" will be used, as this title encompasses the multiple titles currently in use (medical director, vice-president of medical affairs, chief medical officer, senior vice president, and others). Initially, the role of the physician executive was to assist the medical staff leadership by bridging the hospital's clinical and administrative operations. However, as the year 2000 approaches, a new era in health care is rapidly being ushered in—one comprised of new trends, issues and events; one creating new organizations, structures and methods; an era that is changing physician executive roles and careers.

Changes in health care have greatly enlarged the physician executive role in many organizations. Functions that were at one time the focus of a medical director's activities, such as credentialing, are overseen and performed by specialists in those areas (such as medical staff services professionals). As a result, physician executives have a greater role in the overall management of the organization, and are part of the executive management team, and essential players in the strategic planning process.

Depending on the setting in which a physician executive works—such as a hospital or group practice—the title and duties vary. In managed care, the title may be executive vice president for medical management, reflecting the physician executive's expanded managerial role. Many physician executive roles are systemwide positions, and have been elevated to an executive vice presidency within a health care system. The physician executive in any type of organization usually reports directly to the president or CEO and is a member of its executive council.

The physician executive may be a lightning rod for physician anger. The physician executive tends to be "alone on an island" attempting to strike a balance between the management of the organization, the medical or professional staff, and the physicians. It can be a difficult job, one in which the physician executive is perceived to be neither totally part of administration, nor totally part of the medical staff organization.

According to experts, prerequisites to becoming a physician executive include

1. *A physician background.* The American College of Physician Executives (ACPE) recommends that prospective physician executives become board certified clinicians and practice for three to five years, since physician executives must manage physicians, who generally do not like tak-

ing instructions from someone lacking a patient care background. Physician executives who have practiced medicine understand medical care from a provider's perspective.

2. *Ability to handle criticism.* Physician executives must have "thick skins" so they do not personalize the attacks upon their positions or their decisions. They must also recognize that what they—and the organization—value may not be valuable to the individuals whose support they seek.

3. *Good negotiating skills and the ability to compromise.* Despite this, physician executives must always put the quality of patient care above concerns of the organization or individual physicians.

4. *Political skills.* The ability to communicate and plan are both important; however, knowing how to manage competing interests may be the single clearest determinant of a physician executive's success or failure. Physician executives must understand their constituencies, from physicians to patients, or they will have problems in managing those constituencies.

5. *Comfort with change.* Physicians who become physician executives must be able to deal with ambiguity and constant change, two areas that are generally not the strong suit to someone trained in a science.

6. *Management training.* Organizations increasingly want their physician executives to have a degree in management.

7. *Open to promotion.* Physician executives now have the option of becoming the CEO of an organization. Historically, this has not been a common career path for physician executives, because many of them lacked management training. As more physician executives receive advanced management degrees, it is anticipated that their move into the role of CEO will become more common.

Basic Roles and Responsibilities of Physician Executives in Hospitals, Group Practices, and Managed Care Organizations

A physician executive is usually responsible for operation of the medical staff office, primarily supporting medical staff credentialing and privileging, committee structures, and arranging for physician leadership support. The physician executive position has expanded into performance improvement, sometimes limited to the medical staff, although many physician executives are responsible for the departments that support performance improvement throughout the organization.

Departments that commonly report to the physician executive include medical staff services, and at times, the quality management and medical records departments, infection control, and risk management.

Managed care has expanded the physician executive's role to include areas such as contracting, aligning physician groups with the organization, and developing new service lines and sources of revenue.

While physician executives' roles can vary depending upon the type of health care organization in which they work, the ACPE has identified some core elements of the position:

1. Direct utilization review—assess how medical resources are being used to care for patients;

2. Oversee quality assurance—monitor the process of assessing quality of care and setting up systems for improvement where needed;

3. Recruit physicians;

4. Evaluate physician performance;

5. Manage physician performance;

6. Serve as liaison between physicians and administrative personnel;

7. Oversee credentialing and privileging of physicians;

8. Develop provider relations—contracting with physicians, hospitals and other agencies and businesses that will provide some kind of care;

9. Resolve grievances—between patients and physicians or from physicians about the health care organizations' policies, practices, etc;

10. Mediate professional disputes and interdepartmental problems;

11. Serve on the board of directors;

12. Develop staffing plans;

13. Prepare the expense budget for the medical departments;

14. Ensure compliance with the mission statement, corporate policies, and bylaws;

15. Participate in strategic planning;

16. Ensure medical staff efforts meet or exceed standards of various accrediting and regulatory bodies—including JCAHO and NCQA.

In summary, the physician executive will be increasingly important during the coming socioeconomic health care convolutions. The role will continue to be expanded and redefined. Continuing requisites for the job will be broad shoulders, a thick skin, and a sense of humor.

SOURCES

- American College of Physician Executives, (Tampa, Florida).
- *Health Care Competency and Credentialing Report,* "Competency Profiles: Vice President of Medical Affairs," (March, 1998) and "Changing Disciplines: Making Sure Your Physician Executive is Prepared for the Job," (November, 1997).

Chapter 5

The Evolution of the Medical Staff Services Profession

Morgan Brown, MA, CMSC, CPHQ

The Random House *Webster's College Dictionary*[1] has nine definitions for the word *evolution*. The one most applicable to the subject of this chapter reads *"...a process of gradual, progressive change and development...."* Yet another definition states *"...the development of a species, organism, or organ from its original or primitive state to its present or specialized state."* Although the last definition may seem more focused on biology than the medical staff services profession, the words do capture the essence of what this chapter will address: the *development* of the medical staff services profession from its early clerical start to the highly specialized and administratively responsible role in today's health care arena.

HISTORY

Thirty years ago, there was no career designation *medical staff services professional* nor were the individuals who were providing administrative and clerical support to a hospital's medical staff even called *medical staff secretaries*. More often than not, support for the medical staff fell on the shoulders of a secretary in hospital administration or the medical records department. This support to a medical staff was seen only as clerical and not requiring a full-time employee. Typing an occasional letter, taking minutes, keeping a roster, and maintaining background files on physicians were the extent of these responsibilities.

The evolution of the role of that early secretary can be traced back to the first attempts by medical staffs to become *organized* medical staffs. It quickly became apparent to physicians that they needed someone to see to their non-clinical needs, someone to help them *get organized* and *stay organized*. They needed someone to keep the momentum of their organization going while they practiced medicine. The originally designated part-time position quickly became a full-time position called medical staff secretary. In fact, the mere addition of the qualification *medical staff* to the basic title, *secretary,* must be regarded as the first evidence of the beginning of the position, the title, and the evolution of the profession itself.

Early on, medical staff leadership and their medical staff secretaries found that keeping the medical staff roster had become more complicated than the mere mechanics of typing it. At the same time, applications for medical staff membership, which previously asked only for the most cursory summary of a physician's background—perhaps only education history and state medical license—were beginning to become more complicated. Verification of information on the application had been just as cursory as the application itself. Action by the medical staff on these applications was usually a simple *yea* or *nay* vote during a general meeting of the medical staff. The secretary, of course, typed up the list of applicants before the meeting and then the minutes after its adjournment. But the secretary's responsibilities for the credentialing process were about to take a giant leap.

As a result of several precedent-setting legal cases, hospitals found themselves legally responsible for the acts of their medical staffs. That, combined with more stringent credentialing standards from the Joint Commission on Accreditation of Healthcare Organizations (JCAHO) as well as state and federal laws and regulations, made it apparent that improved credentialing methods were necessary. Medical staff secretaries were intricately involved in development and implementation of more sophisticated methods for collecting and verifying information needed for credentialing purposes.

Assigning credentialing responsibilities to the medical staff secretary resulted in the credentialing of health care practitioners becoming the foundation for this new profession. And so it remains today as the core responsibility and skill for which the medical staff services professional can claim unchallenged expertise. The credentialing of practitioners has become so specialized that a certification is now offered that acknowledges an individual's mastery of this process.

Given the increasing administrative responsibilities of the medical staff organization and sensing that it would no longer suffice to assign the administrative and clerical support of its medical staff to just any secretary, hospital administrations began to identify and recruit experienced medical staff secretaries and *coordinators*. Job descriptions for these new positions were often written by the individual hired to fill the position. With identification of an actual description of the duties of these newly identified positions came the first real idea of what a *medical staff office* would actually do. For example, a medical staff coordinator in a one-person office could be expected to

1.   coordinate medical staff organizational activities, acting as a liaison between the medical staff, nursing and hospital administration;

2. maintain a current and thorough knowledge of the JCAHO medical staff standards as well as state and federal regulations;

3. maintain a current master copy and knowledge of the medical staff by-laws and rules and regulations;

4. manage and attend all medical staff committee meetings, including agenda and minute preparation and initiation of appropriate follow-up action as dictated by a committee;

5. maintain on an ongoing basis the financial records of the medical staff;

6. and, provide, upon request, secretarial services to the medical staff.

The coordinator was also responsible, of course, for the credentialing of practitioners and allied health professionals, including

1. acceptance of all applications, reviewing each for completeness and compliance with the medical staff bylaws;

2. initiation of the verification of all information provided by the applicant;

3. assembly of all verified information and preparation of credentials files for presentation to the medical staff's credentials committee;

4. assuring that applications were expeditiously routed through other appropriate medical staff committees, departments and sections and, when appropriate, to the medical executive committee and the hospital's board of directors;

5. maintenance of an ongoing tickler system addressing practitioner and allied health professional reappointments according to a time schedule provided in the medical staff bylaws;

6. and, accepting and processing through the appropriate medical staff committees all requests for additions and/or deletions of clinical privileges and/or changes in staff status.

In addition, many job descriptions included responsibilities for coordinating continuing medical education programs, physician recruitment support, and preparation of various call schedules.

As this evolution progressed, medical staff secretaries and coordinators were joined by credentialing clerks and specialists, credentialing coordinators, medical staff services specialists, medical staff clerks, managers and directors of medical staff services, directors of professional services, administrative and executive directors, and even a few vice-presidents. Medical staff offices became medical staff services departments. Initially, the profession was entirely female, and while it remains predominantly so today, more frequently men are staffing and directing medical staff services departments.

Fast becoming versed in a variety of non-clerical skills and increasingly recognized as a reliable and accurate resource for everything from interpretation of accreditation standards and regulatory requirements to the medical staff bylaws, rules and regulations, these professionals were also becoming the backbone of an organized and effective medical staff organization. And these professionals were assuming leadership roles within the management structure of the hospital itself.

Those early medical staff secretaries paved the way for a profession to emerge. With no identified educational resources on which to rely, they began to self-educate, knowing that to be successful and to survive, they would need to prove themselves invaluable to *both* hospital administration and the medical staff. And faced with what can best be called dual loyalties, they also became consummate diplomats with a political astuteness that often rivaled political operatives seen on the six o'clock news. More frequently, the title *coordinator* was replacing *secretary* as the medical staff services department's role became less clerical support and more focused on administrative and management support.

The medical staff coordinator's acceptance by the medical staff and hospital administration as a trusted aide and confidante was one of the more critical milestones of the profession's evolution. In the role of aide and confidante, the coordinator became more visible to other hospital departments and management personnel. The coordinator became an effective and critical liaison with the medical staff for the majority of the hospital community. If the medical staff's attention needed to be focused on a particular issue, the strategy often included conferring with the coordinator regarding the best approach to the medical staff organization. Although hospital personnel came in contact with physicians daily and interacted with little hesitation, it was in the context of *clinical performance*. When it came to medical staff organizational issues, rules and regulations, policies and procedures, protocols and bylaws, the best person to contact was the medical staff coordinator. And frequently, it was actually the medical staff coordinator who had researched, written or edited those bylaws, rules and regulations for the medical staff organization.

With formalized job descriptions for these new medical staff services positions came the need to identify specific qualifications, competencies, and experience needed by successful candidates for the positions. It was acknowledged that clerical and secretarial skills were intrinsic to the job but these skills were only basic. Accordingly, the profession began to set standards and identify competencies for itself. And the emerging profession began to organize itself.

THE PROFESSIONAL ASSOCIATION

A group of twenty-two women who worked in medical staff offices in Southern California met in 1971 for the purpose of networking. Curious about how the others were coping with the roles they shared in common, the women quickly found that their roles were seemingly similar in concept but varied in actual execution. This first gathering some twenty-six years ago begat the California Association Medical Staff Secretaries, which, in turn, became the catalyst and foundation for the profession's nation-wide association, the National Association Medical Staff Services (NAMSS), which was incorporated in 1976.

Today, NAMSS has over 4,000 members across the U. S. as well as Puerto Rico, Guam, Europe, and the Middle East. NAMSS maintains an executive office in Lombard, Illinois, in close proximity to the headquarters of the JCAHO and other key health care associations such as the American Hospital Association and the American Medical Association (AMA). Supported by a network of state professional associations, NAMSS has forged important relationships with the Joint Commission, the AMA, the National Committee for Quality Assurance (NCQA), and federal agencies such as the National Practitioner Data Bank. NAMSS members and leaders have been invited to participate at AMA meetings and to serve on several JCAHO panels known as PTACs, or *Professional/Technical Advisory Committees* as well as National Practitioner Data Bank committees. Medical staff services professionals have provided an important element to these organizations, a perspective on behalf of the medical staff as an organization without the usual clinical influence.

For additional information, NAMSS can be found on the Internet at the Web site www.namss.org or simply by search, using *NAMSS* as the identifier.

CERTIFICATION

With a mission and vision firmly focused on education, NAMSS administers the two recognized certification programs for the profession. Individuals who wish to be certified as medical staff coordinators and meet the requirements for formal education and experience in the profession are permitted to sit for the 250-question certification examination. Examination content ranges from medical terminology to medical staff law to accreditation requirements as well as practitioner credentialing, managed care and the organizational structure of the contemporary medical staff. Those passing the examination have the right to be identified as *Certified Medical Staff Coordinators* and use the initials *CMSC* following their names.

In 1995, NAMSS recognized the importance of the skills and expertise of those in the profession whose responsibilities are primarily focused on practitioner credentialing, especially those in the managed care arena, and introduced a second certification, *Certified Provider Credentialing Specialist*. As with the coordinator's certification, those meeting both the educational and experience requirements may sit for a written examination. The successful candidate may use the initials *CPCS* as his or her professional credential.

Both certifications are the hallmark of the qualified, experienced, and knowledgeable medical staff services professional. And with such certification, an individual is acknowledged as having highly developed skills and being an expert in medical staff support services.

EDUCATION

As the profession changed over the years, so did the individuals who were drawn to it. An increasing number of both women and men began to seek out the medical staff services profession and regard it as a career and not just a job. Today, there are formal educational programs in community colleges where individuals may earn a degree in medical staff services science. In addition, the NAMSS Institute, the educational arm of the profession's national association, offers an accredited independent study program whose modules are similar in approach and content to college level study programs.

The evolution of this profession has progressed to a point that courses in accounting, marketing, ethics, business, and a variety of computer skills are wise, if not essential. The current listing published by NAMSS of competencies to be maintained by the medical staff services professional runs in excess of five pages and includes a lengthy litany of what an individual must know in order to be effective in the profession.

It is also interesting to note that a recent job classification survey of its membership undertaken by NAMSS reveals that a large percentage of the membership not only have completed two years of college but a sizeable number have bachelor's and master's degrees. Some, though the number is small, have completed doctoral degrees.

TODAY'S MEDICAL STAFF SERVICES PROFESSIONAL

The role and responsibilities of today's medical staff services professional (MSSP) are seemingly light years away from those of the secretaries of 30-some years ago. Today's MSSPs are educators, advocates and advisors, communicators and articulators, authors, and an increasing number are testing their entrepreneurial skills by setting out on their own as health care consultants. Each of these professionals puts his or her own interpretation on the role and each contributes daily to the continuing evolution of the role and the profession.

The MSSP's workdays often pass like a flash of light, finding them organizing an upcoming general meeting of the medical staff one moment, writing a revision of the bylaws the next. They often go from breakfast meetings with the surgeons to lunch meetings with the family practitioners to afternoon meetings with hospital administration and evening meetings of the medical executive committee or a fair hearing proceeding. And the next day, it starts anew...only different.

While the medical staff services profession has evolved over the past thirty some years, so has the health care delivery system. Recent changes in health care have brought about significant change for the profession, specifically, the emergence of *managed care*. As previously noted, the foundation of the medical staff services profession from the very beginning has been practitioner and allied health professional credentialing. It is the major area where MSSPs have had a tremendously positive influence, an area where these professionals have led the way. It is the MSSP who has been responsible for developing new and meaningful credentialing standards, effective and efficient process design, and development. The seasoned MSSP can easily and quickly identify a potential problem with an applicant, often with a brief review of the application.

The emergence of managed care as well as credentials verification organizations (CVOs) has offered opportunities to MSSPs to expand their roles and influence beyond the walls of the acute care hospital setting. Many MSSPs have made the transition from the acute care setting to CVOs and managed care organizations. So valued is the expertise and knowledge of the MSSP that NCQA selected members of NAMSS with the CMSC credential as surveyors for their CVO accreditation survey process.

The evolution of the role of the medical staff services professional as an advisor and confidant to the medical staff and its leadership has been no less important than the evolution of the profession itself. From routine daily work to sentinel events involving a hospital's medical staff, the influence of the MSSP cannot be minimized. Guiding the medical staff through their responsibilities and educating and familiarizing them with the nuances of those responsibilities, the MSSP provides continuity to the medical staff organization.

Medical staff leaders, i.e., the chief of staff, chief of staff-elect, and secretary treasurer, come and go, as frequently as yearly. The physician leader, while respected by his peers and popular enough to win an election, often comes to the leadership role with little or no experience for that role. Faced with today's economic and time constraints upon his or her private practice, the new medical staff officer often has little or no time to educate or prepare for the new responsibilities. Naturally, the newly elected officers come to rely heavily on the MSSP. The role and influence of the MSSP is so important that it is the rare medical executive committee meeting where the chief of staff does not, at some point, turn to the MSSP with a question or asks him or her to address an issue for the committee. Many medical executive committee agendas routinely list a report from the medical staff services director or manager as part of standing business. And while decisions will always remain the responsibility of the medical staff and its leadership, the MSSP has become an integral part of every organizational process that leads to a decision on the part of the leadership. That individual can bring issues into perspective and offer historical precedent, a guarantee for continuity, and the prevention of duplication.

If one takes into consideration the far reaching influence of the MSSP and the dependence of the medical staff on this individual, perhaps it might be time to introduce a variation on those medical staff services job titles already mentioned, to *medical staff executive director*. Although the chief of staff is the elected leader of the medical staff, the MSSP is actually the individual responsible for the daily operation of the medical staff organization. It is he or she who keeps that organization running smoothly and efficiently day after day, year after year. Whether supporting and directing the medical staff committee process, attending a majority of each month's medical staff committee meetings, or interpreting the medical staff bylaws or standards of either the JCAHO or the NCQA in response to a physician's or hospital staff member's question, the MSSP can save the hospital and its medical staff time and resources in his or her role as a knowledgeable and dependable resource for medical staff issues.

THE FUTURE

Coming as far as the profession has, the question of *what* is next for this profession can now be asked. Where will MSSPs be in the twenty-first century? Even though it is certain that the health care delivery system will continue to change, it is also certain that there will be a role for groups of organized physicians (medical and professional staffs) in quality, credentialing, peer review and other activities that require administrative support. MSSPs will be wherever these groups of physicians reside. Just as the skills and expertise required of an MSSP today far exceed the reliance on clerical skills just twenty years ago, it is safe to say requirements for the future will continue to evolve. The skills that MSSPs possess of working effectively with physicians and medical staff organizations in a highly political environment are highly valued in the current rapidly changing health care delivery and payment systems. These skills will prove to be valued as we move into the twenty-first century as well.

An intellectually curious individual will do well in this profession. Looking and thinking "out of the box" is the favorite cliche of management change experts today. It will serve today's MSSP well to do precisely that. To think beyond his or her job description and identify personal career advancement goals will be an invaluable test of a professional's mettle and mark him or her as a survivor. With the rapid pace of changes in health care, it is the wise individual who has a plan. Each MSSP should carefully evaluate the role he or she plays in working with the medical staff and examine the contribution. Is the contribution primarily organizational skills? Is it the ability to attend meetings, prepare minutes, and orchestrate the credentialing process? Or is the contribution more far-reaching, such as influencing leadership and being a catalyst to resolve difficult issues and situations involving conflict? Moving from supporting the team of medical staff organization leadership to being sought after as a member of the team is the hallmark of the seasoned MSSP.

Each MSSP must analyze carefully his or her own contribution and evaluate how his or her skills will be useful to career objectives.

Health care reform in both the acute care setting and managed care creates variations in health care delivery that multiply almost daily. The MSSP can play an important role in many of these. And with NAMSS representatives sitting on regulatory boards, national committees, writing and publishing literature defining the standard of practice, it is certain that the MSSP will have a voice in the continuing evolution of the profession.

NOTES

1. *Webster's College Dictionary* (New York: Random House, 1997): 453.

Chapter 6

Medical Staff Services Professionals and Medical Staff Services Departments

Jodi Schirling, CMSC

THE MEDICAL STAFF SERVICES PROFESSIONAL

The Medical Staff Services Professional (MSSP) plays a vital role in the health care delivery systems of today. Whether in a hospital, ambulatory care center, credentials verification organization or managed care setting, the MSSP brings a variety of knowledge and skills essential for each type of organization. This chapter will focus on the role of the MSSP and the Medical Staff Services Department (MSSD) in the hospital setting.

The MSSP provides coordination for the day-to-day activities of the organized medical (professional) staff. Whether a multi-facility, integrated health care delivery system, or a small rural hospital, the MSSP acts as the link between the medical staff and the administration. This link is facilitated by the access the MSSP has to both the medical staff and members of the administrative team.

In most cases, the MSSP will be one of the first contacts a physician has with the organization. Through the initial credentials verification process and orientation to the organization, the MSSP and MSSD establish a unique relationship with the practitioner. Medical staff members look to the department for interpretation of bylaws, information on hospital policies and procedures, advice on maneuvering through the sometimes complex administrative structure, and basic support for the activities of the organized medical staff.

The MSSP also provides a unique service to the hospital administration. Due to the relationships that develop between the MSSD staff members and physicians, MSSPs are sometimes first to know of an underlying issue within the medical staff organization. The issues can be as minor as changes in the physician parking lot or as major as a controversy over new hospital ventures. This information can then be transmitted to the appropriate administrative staff member for attention or resolution.

The MSSP's role is one that engenders trust—from both the medical staff and the hospital administration. Medical staff members need to trust that the MSSP and MSSD maintain confidential information, provide accurate, timely information, and respect the confidences of the physicians. The administration needs to trust that the MSSP and the MSSD will maintain accurate records, follow established procedures and practices in all activities, maintain activities which meet accreditation standards, and apprise them of major issues within the medical staff organization.

KNOWLEDGE

In order to be effective, the MSSP must have thorough knowledge in several key areas.

The U.S. health care delivery system is extremely complex. Emphasis on health care in both the political and legal arenas results in an ever-changing system. The medical staff and the hospital deal with the complexity of the various payment systems daily. The MSSP should understand the various components of the delivery system. An understanding of the legal system and how the law shapes the delivery system is helpful. There is also a need to understand how the political system impacts the health care environment. An example of this would be the 1993 "Jackson Hole Group," established by President Clinton, which had an overwhelming impact on health care by virtue of its discussion of health care reform. Even though many of the group's efforts did not go forward in the government sector, the private sector embraced many of the reform efforts.[1] An MSSP's knowledge of current political topics that have potential impact on health care is valuable to the hospital and medical staff.

Health Care Financing

An appreciation of the financial components of the health care system is required. At a minimum, a basic understanding of utilization management is essential. The MSSP should be familiar with basic terms used in managed care. The difference between a health maintenance organization, preferred provider organization, or independent practice association should be understood. The role of the Health Care Financing Agency (HCFA) should be known. The MSSP must be familiar with the various reimbursement systems with a special focus on how the physician is impacted. One of the many criteria that may be used during the reappraisal and reappointment period is utilization information. Efficiency of physician practice is becoming more and more important to hospitals. The MSSP must assure that appropriate information is provided while maintaining a balance between clinical and economic criteria for reappointment.

Medical Staff Organization

The MSSP also needs to understand the basic concepts of medical staff organization, for example, whether or not the medical staff organization accomplishes its functions in a departmentalized or non-departmentalized structure.

Accreditation Knowledge

Perhaps the most important aspect of the knowledge that an MSSP brings to the hospital is that of accreditation standards. As mentioned in Chapter 2, there are many accrediting agencies with which the MSSP should be familiar, including Joint Commission on Accreditation of Health Care Organizations (JCAHO), National Committee on Quality Assurance (NCQA), American Accreditation Healthcare Commission/Utilization Review Accreditation Commission (AAHCC/URAC), HCFA, and Commission on Accreditation of Rehabilitation Facilities (CARF). Some additional accrediting bodies include the American College of Surgeons–Commission on Cancer and Committee on Trauma certification programs, institutional review boards, and continuing medical education (see Chapter 11). The MSSP must maintain current knowledge of the accreditation standards applicable to his or her facility.

Understanding the standards is not enough, however; the MSSP must also be able to interpret the standards and implement systems to comply with them. For example, the MSSP may need to assist the medical staff in policy development or expansion of their quality improvement process as the standards change. The MSSP must be familiar with all JCAHO standards, not just the section containing medical staff standards. Currently, many standards that affect the medical staff are noted throughout the JCAHO manual. In larger facilities, the JCAHO network standards or the ambulatory care standards may also apply and the MSSP will need to have a working knowledge of those standards as well.

The Law

Knowledge and understanding of state laws related to licensure and peer review is also required. Since the MSSP may serve as a resource for physicians applying for a state medical license, there must be understanding of the requirements for licensure. The MSSP should also know the differences between the various medical training—is an MD equivalent to a DO? In addition to laws and statutes that regulate the practice of medicine, the MSSP must be aware of other state laws that have an impact on the medical

staff or hospital. Examples of such laws would be those related to organ dona-
tion or use of advance directives.

The MSSP also needs to have knowledge of medical staff laws, particularly those relating to medical staff issues such as credentialing, privilege restriction, medical staff membership, restraint of trade, and peer review. Knowledge of the various laws and legal precedents will help the MSSP understand
what has to be done and *why*. The MSSP can then communicate information
on legal implications of peer review to the medical staff. Although the MSSP
is not a substitute for legal counsel, he or she can be instrumental in advising
the staff when legal counsel should be sought.

The Credentials Process

The MSSP must also have a complete understanding of the credentialing
process—from initial appointment to privilege delineation to on-going monitoring to reappointment. Not just what to do, but why it is important, and how
to establish systems for assuring that the processes are carried out correctly.

Ethical Issues

Understanding ethical issues surrounding medical staff activities is also
an important part of the body of knowledge an MSSP brings to the job. Professional ethics, such as maintaining professional relationships and confidentiality, must be practiced by the MSSP. The MSSD may be instrumental is
assisting the medical staff in establishing an ethics committee. Therefore, the
MSSP must understand medical ethics such as patients' rights and responsibilities as well as requests for treatment withdrawal.

Quality and Resource Management

The MSSP should understand the basics of utilization management, quality assurance, and continuous quality improvement. This understanding can
be obtained by working collaboratively with the hospital departments of quality and utilization management. MSSPs should take advantage of continuing
education programs on these topics. Another way to obtain information on
these subjects is to read current literature.

Management

Finally, the MSSP must be a competent manager. Regardless of the size
of the facility or the medical staff organization, the MSSP acts as a manager

for many functions and may also manage staff. The knowledge of basic management theory will be useful to the MSSP.

Understanding Process

Many functions are the responsibility of the MSSD. The MSSP must understand and be able to break down a process into distinct tasks and develop procedures for the staff to follow. This type of assembly-line thinking is a critical skill for the MSSP serving at the coordinator or director level. Multiple staff members must perform the specific function in a consistent manner. A basic principle of continuous quality improvement is to understand causes of variation in a process. Having clearly defined procedures to follow helps to reduce the variation. Understanding process makes it easier to develop the necessary procedures.

Budgeting and Finance

The MSSP working in a single person office or in a supervisor or director role must have a basic understanding of budgeting process as well as financial management. The MSSP must be able to calculate staffing needs and forecast expenses for the department. Most medical staff departments are not revenue producing. Therefore, the MSSP needs to manage resources prudently. During the fiscal year, the MSSP must be able to review monthly financial reports to determine areas that are out of line with the budget. The MSSP should develop strategies for managing the department's resources, such as having the hospital library purchase key journals rather than purchasing them with department funds. Other strategies can include placing controls on ordering office supplies, sharing high cost resources (such as fax machines) with other departments, or providing video-taped educational programs for staff rather than higher cost travel to seminars.

Medical Terminology

MSSPs use knowledge of medical terminology in many ways, most specifically in delineating clinical privileges. Additionally, a good understanding of basic terminology is required for those in the department who support specific committees. Although the MSSP may never be asked to identify the root of a specific medical term, the knowledge and correct use of medical terminology will enable the professional to communicate more effectively with the medical staff.

SKILLS

In addition to the requisite knowledge outlined above, the MSSP must possess the work skills that will enable him or her to run an efficient MSSD. He or she must establish policies and procedures, define processes for work completion, write job descriptions, interview, hire, discipline, terminate staff, facilitate meetings, manage multiple projects, and implement quality control mechanisms.

Organization

Good organizational skills are required as the MSSP must maintain important records of the activities of the organized medical staff. Filing systems, credentials files, meeting minutes and other activities must be easily accessed and maintained in an orderly manner. In larger offices where numerous staff may perform the work, the director must be able to establish processes for assuring that records are maintained appropriately and that each staff member follows the same process. In an MSSD with more than one staff member, the department director or supervisor must not only manage his or her own work, but must manage the work of subordinates. This is made easier if the office is well organized.

Time Management

The MSSP must be able to manage multiple projects at the same time. Time management skills are essential. The knowledge of the use of project management tools such as Gant Charts or other computerized project management programs will be a bonus.

Attention to Detail

Attention to detail will allow the MSSP and the department to fulfill the requirements for medical staff documentation and credentials verification, to name just a few. Challenges to medical staff peer review process, credentialing decisions, or bylaws interpretations can be addressed more easily if the MSSP has maintained detailed, organized documentation that supports the medical staff's actions.

Work Independently

While there are clear-cut reporting hierarchies within the hospital setting, the MSSP must be able to perform required functions independently. The MSSP at the coordinator and director levels must use their own judgment in prioritizing work, delegating tasks, managing projects, and setting their own deadlines. The chief of staff, vice president of medical affairs, or hospital administrator needs to trust that the MSSP will be able to perform the job with minimal direction or supervision. The typical MSSP will be faced with many challenges to meet deadlines. It is not unusual to have interruptions throughout the day, or to have sudden shifts in priorities. The MSSP must be able to adapt to changing priorities, re-establish deadlines, and get the work done!

Judgment

The knowledge of when to ask for feedback or direction from a supervisor is a skill that will develop over time as the MSSP and his or her supervisor become more comfortable with each other's style. The MSSP must also use judgment in relaying information to hospital administration that becomes available to him or her through interaction with the medical staff. Is the information vital to the chief executive officer? Will it keep the administration from being caught unaware in a meeting? Does the administration need the information to better prepare for new programs, services, or respond to issues raised by the medical staff? This is not to imply that the MSSP's goal is to gather intelligence for the hospital. Rather, it is to enforce the role of the MSSP and the MSSD to facilitate open, effective communication between the medical staff and the hospital administration. The hospital and medical staff should be working toward a common goal—providing excellent patient care. The MSSP plays a large role in facilitating the medical staff's achievement of that goal.

Maintaining Confidentiality

During the performance of their duties, MSSPs have access to sensitive information that must be maintained in confidence. Types of information received may include physician-specific professional liability claims histories, details of previous disciplinary actions or license sanctions imposed on physicians. Other sensitive information is received from the quality department related to the clinical work of the physician, including peer review actions. Trended data on patient care outcomes such as mortality rates, infection rates, or surgical complication rates is also available. The utilization management department may provide information to the department regarding resource utilization and practice efficiency of individual physicians. All of these data elements are necessary in the preparation of the reappointment profile for each staff member. The MSSP must assure that the confidentiality of this information is maintained. Care must be taken to store such information in secure, locked areas. Information on computerized systems should have limited access with password protection. Policies should be in place that define who has access to such information. In addition, the MSSP must always refrain from discussing sensitive information with staff who are not otherwise privy to that information.

Communication Skills

One of the most important skills required of the MSSP is the ability to communicate effectively. Whether in written or oral formats, clear, concise communication is necessary in this role. The MSSP must be able to communicate to a variety of audiences as well. These audiences may include physicians, board members, representatives from accrediting agencies, and peers within the hospital, to name a few. The MSSP must be able to interpret standards, governing body directives, policies, and so on, and communicate them effectively to the medical staff.

Delegation

MSSPs, especially those working in a leadership capacity in a department with more than one staff member, must be able to delegate effectively. Delegation does not simply mean giving the job or task to another person to perform. Delegation includes providing clear, concise instructions to follow, establishing time lines, and determining the frequency of progress reports that are needed. For some staff members, the MSSP may simply delegate the function and request a report when the work is done. For others, the MSSP may need to provide directions and request status reports at various steps in the project. The MSSP in the coordinator or director role will need to be able to evaluate the work style of his or her employees to determine the delegation style that will be effective for each.

Interpersonal Skills

The hospital medical staff is a diverse organization. Many types of personalities and cultures are represented by its members. The MSSP must be able to work effectively with many kinds of people. The ability to work professionally with administrators and physicians is a must. To be most effective the MSSP must be able to maintain emotional balance even in the most stressful situations. Relationships should be kept on a professional level. The MSSP must be able to facilitate discussions between physicians and administrators (without their knowing it). The MSSP must be able to give feedback as well as receive it. For the MSSP who serves as a supervisor of staff, the ability to provide positive or negative feedback to employees is an essential skill.

Computer Literacy

Good computer skills are essential for the MSSP. In today's work environment, the use of word processing, databases, and spreadsheets as management tools is critical for anyone in a supervisory level. The ability to use statistical analysis tools is also required—particularly as they relate to interpreting quality outcomes during the reappointment process. The MSSP should also keep abreast of industry trends related to use of electronic media. Many facilities use electronic mail for internal communication. What types of safeguards for confidential information should be in place? The MSSP should play a key role in the development of guidelines for electronic transmittal of confidential, medical staff peer review information.

Knowledge of information systems is valuable when working to automate the data collection required for physician profiling. Hospitals typically have more than one computer system. For example, there may be a billing system, a registration system, and an electronic patient charting system. The ability to identify which data elements are necessary for profiling and where they reside in the many hospital computer systems is important. The MSSP with information systems knowledge will be able to work with the appropriate information systems staff to link the databases and generate physician profiles.

Having a working knowledge of the hospital financial system will assist the MSSPs in determining the efficiency of a physician's practice. Efficiency data is one criterion that should be taken into consideration at the time of reappointment in addition to quality and peer review data.

JOB TITLES

The MSSD within a hospital will have a designated leader or supervisor. This person could have the title of director, medical staff services; administrative director, medical staff services; or coordinator, medical staff services. The title should clearly identify the administrative responsibility of the role.

Depending on the size of the organization, the MSSD may include one or more staff who function at different levels of responsibility.

Medical Staff Services Clerk

An employee at the clerk level performs basic tasks that may or may not require previous experience in the medical staff services field. For example, a clerk may be utilized to update a computer database or file licenses and other documents in credentials files as they are received. The skills necessary for the clerk include organization, the ability to follow directions, understanding filing systems, and knowledge of computer systems.

Medical Staff Secretary

Staff functioning at the medical staff secretary level should have the same skills as that of the clerk. In addition, the medical staff secretary should have a basic understanding of committee support functions such as agenda planning, taking minutes, preparing minutes, and completing follow-up after the meeting is concluded. The medical staff secretary should have effective interpersonal and communication skills, as this level of staff has many more opportunities for interaction with physicians and other hospital staff.

Medical Staff Assistant

The medical staff assistant needs to have the skill sets of both the medical staff secretary and the clerk. In a small to medium size facility, the medical staff assistant may perform all the required functions in a one-person office. The assistant then should have knowledge of the credentials process, accreditation standards and compliance, and medical staff laws. In a larger facility, the medical staff assistant may have job functions that deal primarily with committee support and medical staff liaison activities such as orientation.

Credentials Specialist

In a large MSSD, it is conceivable that the duties and responsibilities are assigned according to functions. For example, one staff member manages meetings while still another is assigned to accomplish the credentials verification process. The credentials specialist is responsible for following established procedures for verifying physicians' credentials and preparing the application for review by the appropriate clinical department chairs and committees. A person in the credentials specialist role should have a basic knowledge of the credentials process, including the rationale for performing verification, sources for verification, and medical staff law as it pertains to credentialing. Professional certification as a Certified Medical Staff Coordinator (CMSC) or a Certified Professional Credentialing Specialist (CPCS) may be required. Such certifications are available through the National Association Medical Staff Services. This employee should have the ability to work independently, while following set procedures. Many challenges faced by the medical staff are those that result from credentialing decisions. The credentials specialist must assure that the procedures are followed meticulously and consistently for each applicant. A credentials specialist must have strong documentation skills and be organized. Depending on the size of the organization, the credentials specialist may also provide support to the credentials committee. The credentials specialist should understand the hospital policies, procedures, and bylaws as they relate to credentialing procedures. The specialist will also need to understand relevant state law. In this role, the credentials specialist is in a position to guide the credentials committee and department chairmen in decisions related to credentials verification.

Medical Staff Coordinator

In many mid-size hospitals, the title of the MSSP is medical staff coordinator. The coordinator has responsibility for "coordinating" the activities of the organized staff. These can include all aspects of the services provided by the department, including accreditation compliance, credentials verification, medical staff committee support, policy and procedure, and bylaws development. If the MSSD consists of more than one staff member, the coordinator may be responsible for interviewing and hiring employees, initiating disciplinary actions, conducting evaluations, and coaching staff. In addition, the coordinator prepares the budget, writes departmental policies and procedures, and manages the day-to-day activities of the department.

Director, Medical Staff Services

The director of medical staff services is typically the title of the department head in a large, multi-person department. The director is responsible for hiring, coaching, disciplining, and terminating employees. The director must provide orientation and training to enable staff to perform the functions to which they are assigned. The director must also be financially astute. Developing budgets and maintaining fiscal accountability are major roles for the department director. The director must understand the processes involved in performing the department's work. These processes must then be translated into procedures to be followed by all staff. The director, working with the facility's human resources department, will write job descriptions and perform evaluations of the work done by subordinates. The director will also establish work standards and quality controls.

Other Staff Members

Depending upon the size of the facility, the MSSD could also include a continuing medical education coordinator and graduate education coordinator. It is not unusual for the medical library function or the institutional review board function to rest with the MSSD in small and large facilities. Regardless of the functions residing in the department, there should be strong direction, organization, and established policies and procedures for performing the work.

THE MEDICAL STAFF SERVICES DEPARTMENT

Regardless of the size of the organization and the number of staff in the department, the MSSD functions as the administrative center for the organized medical staff. The office is the "home base" for the elected officers of the medical staff. In many facilities, the decision is made to locate the department in close proximity to the medical staff lounge. The physical location encourages interaction between the MSSD staff and the physicians. Services provided by the MSSD almost always include management and coordination of activities related to credentialing and medical staff organization committees and departments. In addition, many MSSDs support the medical staff organization's continuing medical education program, the medical staff library, the institutional review board, and play a role in the residency training programs if the organization is an academic facility or is affiliated with one. Other activities that are sporadic, but time consuming, include accreditation preparation activities and support for corrective actions, investigations, and fair hearings.

Organizational Structure

The MSSD typically reports to the hospital administrator or to a vice president of medical affairs. In addition to the formal reporting structure for the MSSP and his or her supervisor, there is an informal reporting structure for the MSSP and the elected officers of the medical staff organization. Figure 6-1 depicts how the typical MSSD is positioned in the hospital organizational structure.

Figure 6-1. The Medical Staff Services Department in Relationship to the Hospital and Medical Staff Organization.

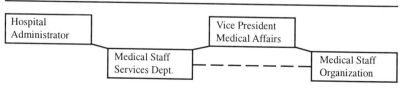

Relationship With Other Hospital Departments

The MSSD does not stand alone in the organization. Due to the relationships that are established between the medical staff members and the MSSD staff, many hospital departments rely on the MSSD to facilitate communication with the physicians.

Administration

The MSSD interacts with various members of the administrative team. The MSSD communicates hospital policies and procedures to the medical staff. The MSSD assists the administration in meeting accreditation standards and appraises the various leaders of key medical staff issues.

Director of Nursing

The director of nursing as well as various nursing units rely on the MSSD for notification of new staff members. The MSSD maintains the official medical staff roster and records related to clinical privileges. The MSSD must establish a mechanism for assuring that nursing staff has access to current privileges information. The department must also establish systems to notify nursing units when physicians join or leave the staff, when privileges are suspended or revoked, and when temporary privileges are granted.

Medical Records Department

Accurate and timely completion of medical records is an important function that the medical staff must perform. This function is performed in conjunction with the medical records department. The medical records department will enlist the assistance of the MSSD in enforcing policies for completion of records. As medical record suspensions may be one of the criteria for reappointment, suspension of clinical privileges for failure to complete records must be done in coordination with the MSSD. The MSSD relies upon the medical records department for accurate reports on the number of suspensions for each physician. The MSSD also relies upon the medical records department for accurate volume data for each physician. The volume data (number of admissions, discharges, consultations, surgical procedures, and so on) comprise the denominator for many of the reappointment criteria.

Quality Assurance or Improvement Department

The MSSD works collaboratively with the quality department, which also plays a key role in support of medical staff organization functions. The data collected by the quality department is the most important information used in the reappointment process. The clinical department chair, prior to making a decision to reappoint a physician must review surgical complication rates, mortality rates, and other outcome data. Timely sharing of this data between departments is necessary. The quality department also gathers data that may trigger the medical staff peer review process. The MSSD and the quality department must work closely together and should identify procedures for information sharing. While the MSSD relies upon the data collected by the quality department, that department depends upon notification by the MSSD of new staff physicians, changes in clinical privileges, new or changes to procedures, clinical pathways, or changes in accreditation standards that have an impact on the medical staff quality program. Monthly meetings between the two departments helps to facilitate communication and sharing of data.

Utilization Management

As mentioned previously, the utilization management department (case management department in some hospitals) maintains information on the efficiency of the physicians' practice. This data is also necessary during the reappointment process. The same type of cooperative relationship that exists between the quality department and the MSSD must also exist between the MSSD and the utilization department.

Social Services

The social services or social work department (sometimes part of the case management department) interacts with physicians on a daily basis. There is a need for social work staff to know about new physicians and changes to medical staff status and privileges. The medical staff may develop policies and procedures that impact the work of the social services department. The MSSD can facilitate policy and procedure development in a collaborative way. There should be a mechanism in place within the MSSD so that those departments that may be impacted can review proposed medical staff policies. The social work department also identifies issues related to community resources for various patient types. The MSSD may be instrumental in enlisting the medical staff organization's assistance in working with community organizations to address these needs.

Emergency Services

In many hospitals, the MSSD is the keeper of the "call schedules," which provide for specialty physician back-up coverage for emergency patients. These schedules are necessary for the functioning of the emergency services department. The MSSD must share this information in a timely fashion. The emergency services department also needs to know about new physician members of the medical staff, changes in status or privileges, and suspensions from the medical staff.

Patient Relations

The patient relations department is responsible for addressing the concerns and complaints lodged by patients. The MSSD should be aware of this department's policies and procedures. The MSSD may be asked to respond to complaints related to physicians. At the very least, the MSSD must communicate with the appropriate medical staff clinical department chair to seek resolution of the complaint. The patient relations department can provide aggregate data to the MSSD regarding complaints filed for each physician, which are another criterion for reappointment evaluation.

Marketing and Business Development

If the hospital has a separate department for marketing and business development, the MSSD will interact with the department regularly. The business development department may produce announcements for new staff and so will rely on the MSSD for notification of new medical staff members. In many organization, a professional "sales staff" of physician relations liaisons are part of the marketing department. These liaisons have the potential for recruiting physicians to join the medical staff. It is necessary for the MSSD to understand the role of the physician relations staff—just as it is important for the physician relations staff to understand basic medical staff procedures, such as how to apply for medical staff privileges.

Another function performed by the marketing and business development office may be that of contract negotiation or recruitment of new physician employees. Recruitment efforts should always be done in conjunction with the MSSD. Close cooperation is necessary to assure that all licensing and credentialing standards are met. In the area of contracting, the MSSD director should have the opportunity to review contract language that relates to delegated credentialing, for example.

Public Relations (PR)

The PR department can provide many services for the MSSD. Editorial services for the medical staff newsletter, continuing education series for physicians and their office staffs, announcements of new staff, and print advertisements for new physicians and services are just a few areas where collaboration is possible. The MSSD can utilize the expertise of the PR staff in the areas of editing and writing.

Physician-Hospital Organization (PHO)

In larger facilities, the presence of a PHO will require clear definition of the roles of the MSSD. Will the MSSD serve as an internal credentials verification body for the PHO? Will the MSSD share information regarding licensing and credentialing? The MSSD will need to understand the type of relationship desired by the organization and establish clear policies and procedures to be followed. If the relationships are not clear, the MSSD should ask for clarification so that the organizational intent can be supported.

Admissions Department

The hospital admissions department depends upon the medical staff services office for an accurate, up-to-date medical staff roster. Most MSSDs control the input of physician data into the hospital registration systems. The admissions department is a primary customer of the department. There should be a cooperative relationship between admissions and medical staff services; the admissions department should contact the MSSD anytime there is a question about a physician's ability to admit and care for patients.

Risk Management

There should be a strong link between the risk management department and the MSSD. The MSSD will rely on the legal expertise of hospital counsel or risk manager for issues related to bylaws and policy development. In addition, the risk management department is an important source of claims information necessary for physician reappointment. The MSSD should have in place a system for communicating potential liability or risk issues to the risk management department.

The MSSP and the Medical Staff Attorney

MSSPs are often the conduit through which medical staff leaders have access to legal counsel for medical staff organization activities. Ideally, the MSSP will develop a close working relationship with an attorney who specializes in medical staff organization legal issues. The MSSP may work with the attorney on medical staff bylaws, policies and procedures, credentialing issues, and related correspondence. In addition, when corrective action is contemplated or actually occurs (e.g., summary suspension, limitation of privileges, and so on) or investigations occur that result in reports to the National Practitioner Data Bank and triggering of fair hearing processes, it is critical that the MSSP seek legal guidance and assistance on behalf of the medical staff organization.

STAFFING AND STAFFING ANALYSIS

The medical staff services industry has sought a benchmark for the number of staff needed for MSSDs. In response to this need, some MSSPs have used formulas, ratios, and other approaches to determine the number of staff required to perform specific activities. Because of wide variations in the scope of services provided to the medical staff organizations MSSDs support, plus the use of technology to accomplish certain functions, an industry benchmark standard for staffing MSSDs does not exist. An example in credentialing is that some medical staff applications are seven pages long and others are 15 pages. The time required for data entry in these two cases varies widely. Some MSSDs use electronic methods for querying verification organizations, while others rely soley on manual methods. The latter can increase the resources required to complete the task by tenfold or more. Therefore, it is essential to clearly define the methods that will be used to deliver services before any attempt is made to derive the staffing standard for the department. It is more important for MSSPs to focus efforts on developing a sound approach for analyzing staffing needs as opposed to searching the literature for a magic number.

In order to determine the number of employees needed to accomplish the many functions of the office, the department director must be able to perform a detailed staffing analysis. Each function should be broken down into the number of hours required to complete the process. For example, committee support should take into consideration pre-meeting activities such as agenda planning meetings, agenda preparation, committee packet preparation (copying and distribution). It should also include attendance at the actual meeting, minute preparation, and preparation of committee follow-up of action items. An example of staffing analysis of support needed for one committee meeting includes the steps outlined in Table 6-1.

Table 6-1. Example of Staffing Analysis For One Committee.

Task	Time Frame (in hours)
Number of hours spent with the Chair to set the agenda	1
Number of hours spent typing the agenda and photocopying agenda for distribution	1
Number of hours spent preparing and actually mailing the packet	.5
Number of hours spent in the actual meeting	1.5
Number of hours spent following the meeting preparing minutes and follow-up	2
Estimated number of staff hours to support one committee	6

The following formula is then used to determine the number of FTEs needed to support one committee. (Each committee requires analysis of its support. This illustration cannot be used as a benchmark standard for all medical staff meetings.)

$$
\begin{array}{lll}
 & \text{6 hours of staff time is used} & \\
\text{x} & \underline{\text{12 months}} & \text{(the committee meets monthly)} \\
\equiv & \underline{\text{72 hours}} & \text{(total hours per year needed to support the committee)} \\
\div & 1800 & \text{(the number of hours one full time person actually works/year)} \\
 & = \mathbf{0.4} & \text{FTE needed to support the committee.}
\end{array}
$$

FUNCTIONS

The MSSD performs many functions for the hospital and medical staff. A brief description of several key functions follows.

Committee Support

Many medical staff organizations have established a committee structure to assist them in meeting the many accreditation requirements. The MSSD must have a good understanding of the committee structure. It is typical within a medical staff organization to allow only the medical executive committee (MEC) to take actions; other committees of the medical staff make recommendations for action to the MEC. Some medical staff organizations delegate some decision-making authority. It is imperative that the MSSD personnel assist the medical staff in maneuvering through the committee structure. The MSSD should develop a system for transmitting agenda items and recommendations from committees and departments up to the MEC. Systems should also be in place to demonstrate when actions were taken. The department also maintains a follow-up system to assure that the actions agreed upon are completed in a timely fashion (see Chapter 15).

In addition, the MSSD should have a good understanding of group process. Committees can be effective tools if the members work toward a common goal, if the members understand and agree on the purpose of the committee. The ability to recognize a committee that has become dysfunctional is a valuable skill. Medical staff services personnel can then assist the chair in bringing the group back to common ground.

The MSSD staff is the resource for the various accreditation standards related to medical staff. The department's understanding of accreditation standards requiring documentation of specific medical staff functions is critical. Accreditation agencies rely on documentation to demonstrate that the various functions are being performed.

The MSSD maintains the minutes and follow-up materials for medical staff organization groups. The ability to summarize and document committee proceedings is an acquired skill. It takes practice to learn how to discern what is important to the meeting documentation. MSSPs are able to identify the issue being discussed, why it is being discussed, important aspects of the discussion, conclusions drawn by the committee, and any actions taken.

The key to an effective committee meeting is good preparation and agenda planning. The MSSP serves to assist the chairs in agenda development and follow-up. Effective agenda planning includes reason for presentation, any supporting documentation, and an understanding of the desired outcome.

Medical Staff Liaison

The MSSD acts as the liaison to the medical staff. MSSD staff have daily contact with many members of the medical staff and can assist them in various ways. Issues brought up by physicians are routed to the appropriate committee or administrator via the MSSD. Members of the medical staff should be able to rely on the MSSD for information about the hospital and its services as well as information about policies and procedures that may affect patient care. Additionally, the MSSD may provide special services for the physicians such as use of fax machines, copy machines, and so on.

Orientation

The MSSD is often responsible for assuring that the newly appointed physician receives an orientation to the hospital and the medical staff organization. In conjunction with the medical staff organization, the MSSD will establish orientation objectives and identify what information is necessary for a physician prior to caring for patients in the hospital. Working with many other departments, such as human resources, the MSSD develops and implements the orientation program. Recognizing that the physician's time is valuable, many MSSDs have developed orientation programs using the latest technologies. A video-taped orientation program that can be viewed by the physician in his or her office or at home is one way to assure the information is provided in a useful format. Another method is putting the information on a computer disc that is mailed to the physician's office. Innovative MSSDs are also using Internet or Intranet Web sites as a mechanism for providing information to new physicians.

Credentials Verification

One of the most important functions of the department is to complete the verification of physician and other licensed independent practitioner credentials for initial appointment and reappointment. Working in the framework established in the medical staff bylaws, the department will establish complementary policies and procedures to assure a consistent approach to the process. The procedures include reviewing the application for completeness when received, determining the source of verification for the credentials elements, outlining how the application is prepared for clinical department review and committee review, and so on. Procedures will also address how the MSSP responds to "red flags" in the credentials process (see Chapter 7).

Procedures related to the reappointment process outline the time frame for distributing the reappointment application, determining the source of verification for the credentials elements, identifying the sources for the profiling information (utilization management, quality and peer review, risk management, and so on), and procedures for updating medical staff databases. It is critical that the procedures established for the credentials verification function be followed consistently. It is also critical that the staff member(s) in the department responsible for carrying out the process is trained as to how the procedures are carried out and why.

Accreditation Support

Regardless of the accreditation held by the hospital, the MSSD and MSSP play a key role in the survey process. The MSSD assists the medical staff organization in their compliance with relevant standards. The documentation from the various medical staff committees and departments is maintained in the department. The department also maintains all of the credentials files. By virtue of the information under its control, MSSD personnel should be included in the survey preparation efforts as well as the actual survey. An effective role for the department director is as a member of the accreditation preparation task force. This task force usually consists of key administrative personnel

(CEO, director of nursing, administrator responsible for ambulatory services, quality director, and the medical director) and the MSSP. The task force's duties include communicating changes in standards to the hospital departments as well as for all survey preparation activities. Survey preparation activities can include mock surveys and in-service education for hospital and medical staff members. During the actual survey, the MSSP should accompany the physician member of the survey team.

Support of Medical Staff Leadership

In many hospitals, the medical staff leaders are elected to their positions and must accomplish the responsibilities of their offices while maintaining heavy patient care loads. The MSSD can assist the leaders in fulfilling their duties in a variety of ways. The MSSD can prepare correspondence for the review and signature of the leader, arrange meetings on behalf of the leadership, establish a quiet space within the department for the leaders to use for meetings, committee follow-up, and so on. The MSSP can also assist in keeping the leaders up-to-date on the activities of the medical staff. Reports on the number of times temporary privileges have been granted or the failure of a committee to adequately perform its functions will assist the leaders in identifying opportunities for improvement in the medical staff organization structure. In addition, the MSSD should appraise the leadership of any issue raised in committee or by an individual medical staff member that may be controversial and require a joint medical staff and administrative response. This enables the leader to gather additional information and prepare his or her response to the issue.

In that most medical staff leaders are elected and serve limited terms, the MSSP plays a valuable role in continuity of medical staff organization activities.

Policy and Procedure Development

The MSSD can also assist the medical staff leaders in identifying topics for policy and procedure development. Policies and procedures (or rules and regulations depending on the specific medical staff structure) should be limited to issues which may lead to a credentialing action (such as failure to complete medical records documentation) or that outline how a particular standard is to be met. The MSSD is in a position to identify the need for a new policy or procedure. Review by the MSSD of trends in complaints or issues raised by other departments can trigger the development of a policy. The MSSD staff may draft policies for consideration of the medical staff leadership. Once policies are developed, the MSSD will establish a mechanism for periodic policy review and revision.

Resource Center

The MSSD should establish a resource center for the medical staff leaders and hospital administrators. The information contained in this center should focus on medical staff issues. Some examples of documents that should be available include

1. JCAHO Standards Manual,
2. Current Medical Staff Bylaws,
3. Current Medical Staff Policies/Rules/Regulations,
4. Hospital Policies and Procedures,
5. Current State Statutes—licensure, peer review.

PERFORMANCE IMPROVEMENT IN THE MSSD

A management philosophy adopted by many health care organizations is one of continuous quality improvement. The MSSD should participate in the hospital quality improvement program by establishing a department specific plan. A simple process can be followed to establish a performance improvement process for the MSSD.

1. Identify the department's customers: physicians, patients, insurers, other hospital departments. What are their expectations of the department? Do they expect committee support, timely processing of their application for membership, an accurate medical staff roster?
2. Identify the department's major services. These might include credentials verification, committee support, accreditation coordination, serving as medical staff liaison, or maintaining the medical staff database.
3. Identify any standards that have to be met by the department. These can be external such as accreditation standards or internal departmental standards. Examples of internal standards are turn-around-time for application processing or response time for requests for verification of staff membership. Internal standards should be established by the department staff in a collaborative manner.
4. Determine how department staff knows if the customer's needs and expectations are being met. What is being measured to determine compliance?
5. Establish measurement systems. What is going to be measured? Then identify frequency of data collection. How often is the data going to be collected? Is it going to be collected continuously or by a sampling method? Who is going to collect it? What tools are going to be used?

An example of a simple measurement tool is a run chart that documents process time for each application completed. A telephone log can be used to document that calls are returned within whatever time standard has been set by the department. Once these decisions have been made and the data collected, it must be analyzed. The department must determine who is going to analyze the data and how it is going to be reported. Keep in mind the end user of the data. Who is going to see the report—the medical director? credentials committee? administrator? Or is the report for internal use of the department director only? A sample department performance improvement plan is shown in Table 6-2.

EXPANDED ROLES

In today's changing health care environment there may be opportunities for MSSDs and professionals to assume expanded roles within the organization. These roles may offer a chance to assume greater responsibility within the organization or may provide the department an avenue for revenue generation. The department director should approach each opportunity carefully and prepare well thought-out business plans for consideration by the organization's leaders.

Table 6-2. Sample Performance Improvement Plan.

Customer	Need/Expectation	Standard	Measurement	Who Collects Data	Frequency of Reporting	Report Format
Physician	Prompt Processing of application	Verification complete w/in 90 days	Process time from receipt of application to presentation at Credentials Committee	Credentials Clerk	Quarterly	Run chart
Nursing Staff	Accurate Medical Staff roster	Rosters updated quarterly and when changes in privileges occur	Number of updates performed quarterly	Medical Staff Secretary	Quarterly	Run chart
Administrator/ VPMA	Credentials verification process performed consistently	Medical Staff Policy bylaws	# times temporary privileges are granted	Credentials Clerk	Quarterly	Run chart

Integrated Delivery Systems

The MSSD currently has procedures in place to perform credentials verification. In an integrated delivery system, the MSSP may have the opportunity to centralize certain functions for the organization. These functions might include credentials verification, maintenance of credentials files, or managing the enrollment of physicians in managed care plans.

Delegated Credentialing

When a managed care company enters into an agreement with a hospital or group practice, part of the standard contract language includes the manner in which physicians will be credentialed to be enrolled in the plan. The concept of delegated credentialing is recognized by managed care companies as a way to avoid duplication of processes. The managed care company can delegate the credentialing of a group practice or select faculty members to the hospital. This means that the managed care company will accept the credentials verification work already done by the hospital. This saves the physician and managed care plan considerable time and avoids duplication of efforts. When entering into a delegated credentialing agreement, the managed care company will do a pre-agreement site visit. At that visit, select credentials files will be reviewed, the application forms will be reviewed, and medical staff bylaws and medical staff services policies and procedures for the performance of the credentials process will be evaluated. It is important to note that the managed care company is evaluating the processes to assure compliance with National Committee for Quality Assurance standards. Once it is determined that the procedures meet the standards, a delegation agreement may be executed. Once the delegation agreement is in place, the managed care company must show oversight of the process. This is accomplished by the performance of an on-site audit each year. This audit will entail review of a select number of credentials files and policies and procedures. If standards continue to be met, the delegation can continue. If the standards are not being met, an action plan may be required from the MSSD outlining how the department will change procedures to meet the standards.

A delegated credentialing arrangement can be very effective. It reduces the paperwork required from physicians and can expedite the enrollment process. The hospital MSSD should establish procedures on how to deal with requests for delegation, from contract language review, to scheduling of on-site audits, to providing updates to the managed care company as needed. With the appropriate policies in place, delegation compliance can be accomplished in an efficient manner. For more details, see Chapter 8.

Credentials Verification Organization

In some health systems or integrated delivery networks, there may be several facilities that duplicate credentials verification for the same practitioners. The MSSD has long experience with the credentials verification process and has established procedures in place. There is logic in centralizing the credentials verification procedures performed at all facilities under the existing MSSD. By establishing an organization-wide CVO, the MSSD can save the organization the costs associated with staffing an office at each location. For more details, see Chapter 9.

Physician Referral Service

Some hospitals have established physician referral services. These telephone services offer patients the opportunity to find a physician affiliated with the hospital and to schedule appointments. This strategy is an effective way to build physician loyalty to the hospital. Many MSSDs take a leading role in managing this service.

Quality Improvement

As hospitals look toward reengineering or continuous quality improvement strategies, opportunities may arise to consolidate departments. The consolidation of the medical staff department and the quality department is a reasonable one. The medical staff services and quality departments have been working closely for years in assuring that physician peer review is accomplished and reported for reappointment. As the emphasis in quality improvement is shifting toward process improvement and away from traditional peer review, the MSSD can assume the responsibilities for medical staff peer review. It is not necessary to have a clinical background in order to manage a quality department. Quality departments typically consist of nurses and other clinicians who can provide the non-clinician director with necessary input. Additionally, the hospital usually identifies a physician liaison who works closely with the quality department and assists with clinical matters. The knowledge and skills held by an MSSP will permit him or her to provide effective leadership of additional hospital departments.

Physician Relations

The use of physician relations representatives to market the hospital and its services to physicians has proven to be an effective strategy. By virtue of their knowledge of the health care system and the way the hospital functions, the role of physician relations representative can easily be assumed by a MSSP. The MSSP demonstrates two key skills for this position—good interpersonal skills and the ability to communicate effectively with a diverse audience.

CONCLUSION

The activities of the MSSP are as diverse as today's health care environment. The MSSP provides essential services to the health care facility. His or her unique role as resource person and facilitator enables the hospital and medical staff organization to work toward a common goal – providing quality care for patients. The responsibilities of the MSSP and MSSD are numerous. The provision of quality patient care can be directly linked to the work performed in the department. In order to fulfill its responsibilities the MSSD must have strong leadership, established policies and procedures, and a clear reporting relationship within the administrative structure. Medical staff services can be a challenging and rewarding field.

NOTES

1. Helen L. Smits, MD, "Quality Management and Consumer Protection Under the President's Health Reform Plan," *The Quality Letter for Healthcare Leaders* 5 (December 1993- January 1994): 2-6.

Chapter 7

The Hospital Credentials Process

Vicki L. Searcy

The author acknowledges F. C. Dimond, Jr., MD, (now deceased) who wrote the chapter entitled "The Credentials Process" in the previous edition of this book.

WHY CREDENTIAL?

The primary purpose of the credentials process is to ensure that any individual who wishes to provide patient care services within a hospital or other health care facility is qualified and competent to exercise the clinical privileges that have been granted to the individual. There are many reasons why hospitals perform credentialing, many of them having to do with the fact that it is a mandated and heavily regulated process.

It Is Required

One reason that hospitals perform credentialing is because it is required by regulatory and accreditation bodies, including hospital licensing requirements (each state has specific requirements), Medicare Conditions of Participation (for those hospitals that receive federal funds for providing care to Medicare and Medicaid patients) and the Joint Commission on Accreditation of Healthcare Organizations (JCAHO) for those hospitals that seek accreditation. In addition, many hospitals have relationships with payers who require a credentialing process as a condition of contracting. Insurance companies often require that hospitals have a credentialing process as a condition of being insured.

Risk Management

If an individual always performed only what he or she was qualified to do and did it well, there would theoretically be no need for a credentialing process. In the real world, however, this process is critical, with the burden on the medical staff and governing body to ensure a careful matching of credentials to privileges.

If practitioners are credentialed in a haphazard manner, not only can patients be harmed, but the health care organization may find itself paying out large sums of money in response to lawsuits because of negligent credentialing. When a patient or family is unhappy with the care received in a hospital, the credentialing and privileging of the practitioner who provided the care will almost inevitably be examined.

Doubters of the necessity for credentialing have but to review any number of significant court cases noting the impact on hospitals. Chapter 17, Current Legal Issues, Significant Case Law Summary, describes significant credentialing cases.

Protect Patients

Credentialing is essentially a patient-protective activity. As the courts have stated, hospitals and their governing bodies have a duty to the public to ensure that only qualified, competent practitioners are allowed to provide care in health care organizations. Physicians and other independent practitioners must be licensed, of course, but hospitals cannot rely on the fact that a practitioner has a license, because licensing agencies do not establish competency to perform specific clinical privileges. That is what hospitals, through their medical staff organizations and governing bodies, do as part of the privilege delineation process.

Credentialing is the foundation of the quality program for the medical staff organization. Quality care begins with making sure that care is directed and provided by practitioners who have the appropriate training, experience, and who are determined to be currently competent to exercise specific clinical privileges.

KEY DEFINITIONS

The term "credentialing" is commonly used to describe a variety of processes or activities, including the initial medical staff appointment, the initial delineation of clinical privileges, and the periodic reappraisal and reappointment of medical staff members. Within credentialing, two processes which must be separated are as follows:

Membership on the Medical Staff

Some licensed independent practitioners are granted membership with no clinical privileges. For example, a physician in an administrative role with a hospital (e.g., Vice President, Medical Affairs) may be a member of the medical staff, but have no clinical privileges. Many medical staff organizations have an "honorary" medical staff membership category for those practitioners who no longer practice (and therefore have no clinical privileges) but wish to retain their membership. There should be criteria for membership which can be separated from the criteria for clinical privileges.

Granting of Clinical Privileges

Some licensed independent practitioners may have clinical privileges but not be granted membership on the medical staff organization. Usually when a practitioner is granted temporary privileges, for example, he or she is granted only those privileges requested and not temporary membership. In addition, many hospitals grant privileges to some allied health professional staff who practice without supervision but these allied health professional staff are not granted medical staff membership. Again, the criteria for clinical privileges should be distinct from the criteria for membership.

Since most hospitals seek JCAHO accreditation, the following definitions are provided. The source is the *Consolidated Accreditation Manual for Hospitals* published by the Joint Commission which was in effect in July, 1998.

Credentialing

The process of obtaining, verifying, and assessing the qualifications of a health care practitioner to provide patient care services in or for a health care organization.

Clinical Privileges

Authorization granted by the appropriate authority (for example, a governing body) to a practitioner to provide specific care services in a organization within well-defined limits, based on the following factors, as applicable: license, education, training, experience, competence, health status and judgment.

Licensed Independent Practitioner

Any individual permitted by law and by the organization to provide care and services without direction or supervision, within the scope of the individual's license and consistent with individually granted clinical privileges.

Current Clinical Competency (Source: JCAHO Lexikon)

Capacity equal to requirement, as in the competence of a medical or professional staff member to meet the requirement of the task assigned.

KEY PLAYERS AND THEIR ROLES

The critical steps in the credentialing and privileging processes are as follows:

1. **Establish the credentialing and privileging processes.** This involves making decisions related to what types of licensed independent practitioners will be eligible to be credentialed and receive privileges (i.e., physicians, dentists, podiatrists), basic standards that must be met by all licensed independent practitioners (e.g., current licensure, professional liability insurance in the required amount, board certification). Establishing the processes is usually a collaborative effort by medical staff leaders and the governing body. Documentation of these decisions can be found in the medical staff bylaws and policies and procedures.

2. **Data collection.** Data is collected from applicants through the use of applications, privilege delineation forms, and so on.

3. **Data verification.** Data is verified in accordance with approved policies and procedures.

4. **Data evaluation.** Throughout the credentialing and privileging process, data is constantly evaluated. Is the data complete? Does data indicate that there may be a problem? What data requires more investigation? When an application is sent through the medical staff organization for recommendation to the governing body, the accumulated data is evaluated so that an appropriate recommendation can be made.

5. **Decision-making.** The governing body makes credentialing and privileging decisions, based upon pre-determined standards which have been established and recommendations made by the medical executive committee.

6. **Data management.** Once an individual has been credentialed and been granted clinical privileges, data about the practitioner must be maintained in a retrievable fashion and updated as information becomes outdated or expires.

Key players in the credentials process include the medical staff services department staff, medical staff leaders, and the governing body. The roles of each follow.

Medical Staff Services Department

The Medical Staff Services Department (MSSD) plays several critical roles in the credentialing and privileging processes. One role is to make sure that the medical staff bylaws clearly define the credentialing and privileging processes and that what is in the bylaws is in compliance with applicable regulatory licensing and accreditation standards.

Policies and procedures should then be written to describe specifically how the process will be implemented. For example, medical staff bylaws commonly require that those licensed independent practitioners who are credentialed and granted clinical privileges must have professional liability insurance. Credentials policies and procedures will be more specific, identifying the amount that must be carried, the type of insurance, what type of evidence will be required to prove that the licensed independent practitioner actually has the required coverage, and how often this information will be updated (e.g., at the time of expiration of the current policy, or annually, or at the time of reappointment). The credentials policy and procedure manual will include the application forms to be used (initial application form, reappointment application form, application form for temporary privilege, and so on), privilege delineation forms for all specialties, and forms used to verify information. The MSSD must make sure that appropriate policies and procedures are developed in order to assure that the credentialing and privileging processes are adequately described and carried out consistently for all licensed independent practitioners.

The MSSD then plays a supporting role in the credentialing and privileging processes by implementing the appropriate policies and procedures. For example, in an initial application process, the MSSD will usually perform the following services:

1. Initial screening of a potential applicant, to assure that the applicant meets the standards to apply for membership and/or clinical privileges;

2. Send out application materials, including application, medical staff bylaws and related documents, privilege delineation form(s), and any other required documents;

3. Review the returned application to assure that the application meets standards to begin the verification process;

4. Implement the verification process, following established policies and procedures;

5. Prepare the credentials file for medical staff leaders and committee members who will review and evaluate the file. This step often includes preparing a summary of the file and identification of potential adverse or problematic information ("red flags") to assist in the decision-making process;

6. Route the file through the review, evaluation, and decision-making process (usually beginning with a department chair, credentials committee, medical executive committee, and the governing body). Provide documentation of the committee recommendation process in the minutes of the committees;

7. Prepare a transmittal to the governing body related to the medical executive committee's recommendation;

8. Communicate with the applicant during and at the conclusion of the application process, informing the applicant of the governing body's decision;

9. Notify hospital departments (if the applicant was approved by the governing body) of essential information related to the applicant, his or her new status at the hospital, clinical privileges, and other necessary information.

The MSSD also plays a key role in data management, and is almost always the department responsible for maintaining an accurate database of all licensed independent practitioners.

Medical Staff Leaders

Medical staff leaders are responsible for collaborating on design of credentialing and privileging processes, particularly in the area of establishing standards for membership and clinical privileges and then assuring that standards are uniformly and consistently applied to all licensed independent practitioners.

Governing Body

The governing body makes credentialing and privileging-related decisions.

APPLICABLE STANDARDS

The JCAHO is the accreditation body most likely to provide accreditation services in the hospital environment, although a number of hospitals seek accreditation from additional sources (see Chapter 2).

At the time that this chapter was written, the JCAHO standards related to credentialing in hospitals were contained in the JCAHO *Accreditation Manual for Hospitals* in the chapter entitled "Medical Staff." These standards should be carefully reviewed by all individuals who have a significant role in credentialing and privileging. The standards define the type of information to be documented in bylaws, policies and procedures; roles and responsibilities in the credentialing and privileging process; elements of current clinical competency; and other requirements related to the credentials process.

Other JCAHO accreditation programs (e.g., ambulatory care, health care networks) have similar credentialing and privileging requirements, but standards related to credentialing and privileging are located in chapters entitled "Management of Human Resources" because there is no requirement for an organized medical staff in these other accreditation programs. The only accreditation program that requires an organized medical staff is the accreditation program for hospitals.

It should also be noted that the JCAHO credentialing standards related to health care networks are consistent with credentialing standards for hospitals with one significant exception: the health care network may have licensed independent practitioners who provide services within the network but not in a network "component." A component would be an ambulatory care facility, hospital, or other facility that would be surveyed under standards specific to the setting. The health care network must be in the process of developing a process to grant clinical privileges to licensed independent practitioners who practice outside of network components. This means that health care networks must begin to develop clinical privileging systems for licensed independent practitioners in the office setting.

CREDENTIALING DOCUMENTS

Credentialing requirements are described in documents including medical staff bylaws, rules and regulations, departmental rules and regulations, policies and procedures, and delineation of privileges forms.

Medical Staff Bylaws

Medical staff bylaws usually describe the following:

1. types of licensed independent practitioners eligible for medical staff membership and clinical privileges;

2. basic criteria for membership and clinical privileges (e.g., current licensure, professional liability insurance, and any other requirements for membership);

3. medical staff membership categories (e.g., active, associate, courtesy, consulting), including requirements for each category and prerogatives (e.g., voting at meetings, attendance requirements, if any; ability to hold elected office);

4. information that applicants for membership and clinical privileges must provide;

5. initial appointment and reappointment processes;

6. elements of a complete application;

7. evaluation and decision-making process;

8. circumstances under which temporary privileges may be applied for and granted;

9. "provisional" period for new applicants (which may or may not include requirements for proctoring);

10. fair hearing plan.

Many organizations are streamlining the medical staff bylaws and the bylaws contain only a bare description of the credentialing and privileging processes, with most of the above information contained in a "Credentialing Plan" which supplements the medical staff bylaws.

Rules and Regulations

Medical staff general rules and regulations may contain more specific information related to the credentialing and privileging processes. For example, the medical staff bylaws might require professional liability insurance and the rules and regulations may contain the specific required amount (e.g., $1 million/$3 million). Or the bylaws may state that an applicant must live close enough to the hospital to provide continuous care to his or her patients and the rules and regulations might define the specific parameters (e.g., must be able to get to hospital within 20 minutes).

Alternatively, the above information could be included in a credentialing plan or in a credentialing policy and procedure.

Department-specific Rules and Regulations

Department-specific rules and regulations often contain criteria specific to the privileging recommended by each department. For example, the rules and regulations for the department of obstetrics and gynecology might require that applicants to the department provide documentation of having completed residency training in obstetrics and gynecology or board certification by the American Board of Obstetrics and Gynecology.

Privilege Delineation Forms

The privilege delineation forms are critical documents because they describe the services that can be provided by a specific specialty. Current methods used to describe or delineate clinical privileges include

1. an exhaustive, detailed laundry list,
2. categories or levels,
3. core and special privileges.

The laundry list is a lengthy list usually consisting of surgical or other invasive procedures that may be performed. The disadvantages of the laundry list are that it is cumbersome and difficult to keep up to date. If a specific procedure is not included in the list, the implication is that the practitioner is not privileged to perform the procedure. Laundry lists also tend to focus on procedures and ignore the cognitive privileges that all physicians exercise (e.g., treatment of conditions and illnesses).

Categories or levels describe privileges in terms of a hierarchy of levels based either on treatment groupings or the level of training and experience. An example of categories based on treatment levels follows:

1. **Category I**—Privileges for the treatment of uncomplicated illnesses, injuries, or conditions that have lower risk for the patient and represent no apparent serious threat to life.

2. **Category II**—Privileges for the treatment of major illnesses, injuries, or conditions posing no significant risk to life and requiring skills usually acquired after one year of residency training.

3. **Category III**—Privileges for the treatment of severe life-threatening or potentially life- threatening illnesses, injuries, or conditions usually requiring skills acquired after residency training sufficient to qualify the applicant for board certification.

At the present time, many organizations use the laundry list approach but want to move to the core privileges approach. Core privileges encompass treatment of medical conditions or performance of procedures for which the applicant has been trained in the residency or fellowship program. Special privileges include procedures or treatment of conditions for which training is obtained over and above the residency training program.

Credentials Policies and Procedures

Credentials policies and procedures contain detailed information on precisely how credentialing is to be implemented. Policies and procedures are critical to assuring that credentialing activities are conducted in a fair and uniform manner. These policies and procedures should be developed by the medical staff organization and approved by the governing body. The medical staff services department is usually responsible for supporting policy and procedure development, and may even instigate the development of appropriate policies and procedures. Forms used to conduct the credentialing and privileging processes should be incorporated into the appropriate policy and procedure (e.g., forms used to verify education, training, experience, peer references, and so on).

Exhibit 7-1 is a sample policy and procedure for the initial apppointment.

Exhibit 7-1. Sample Policy and Procedure - Processing a Medical Staff Application.

SAMPLE POLICY AND PROCEDURE
PROCESSING A MEDICAL STAFF APPLICATION

POLICY

It is the policy of _____ Hospital/Medical Center to verify information on a medical staff application so the medical staff can properly evaluate the applicant's qualifications for medical staff appointment and delineation of clinical privileges.

PROCEDURE

1. Date stamp application in upper right hand corner upon receipt. IF APPLICATION REQUEST PROCESS IS IMPLEMENTED: Pull pre-application request file and place with application.

2. Check application for completeness. All blanks should be filled in, all questions answered, all supporting documents attached. All time must be accounted for from time of graduation from medical school to time of receipt of application. Application and appropriate privilege form(s) must be signed by the applicant. If incomplete, obtain missing information (FORM __). Obtain required application fee, unless fee has been waived. No application should be processed until the required fee has been received or waived by someone authorized to do so.

3. Within ____ days of receipt of application enter data in computer (if computerized) and generate letters to verify the following, using standard form letters for each or other method of verification. Enclose a copy of the applicant's statement releasing information and a copy of the privilege request form(s) as appropriate, as well as a return envelope.

    • Medical, dental or podiatric school - Address to registrar, include year of issuance of MD, DO, DPM, or DDS degree, date of birth of applicant and social security number if available. (FORM __)

Exhibit 7-1. Sample Policy and Procedure - Processing a Medical Staff Application. *(continued)*

- Licensure(s) - Include license number of practitioner. Assure that letter(s) are sent to appropriate licensure board: MD/DO, DDS, DPM. (FORM __)

- Internship/Residency Training - Address to chairman of training program at affiliated university. Include dates of training. Send separate letters if training is completed at different facilities.

  Include copy of privilege form(s) to residency training program if completed within past 5 years. (FORM __)

- Fellowship - Address to chairman of training program. Include dates of training. This letter should be separate from internship/residency letter. Include copy of privilege form(s) if completed within past 5 years. (FORM __)

- Peer References - Relatives and/or peers who have not directly observed the clinical work of the applicant are not acceptable references. Include copy of privilege form(s). (FORM __)

- Professional liability insurance coverage and claims history. (FORM __)

- Board Certification (if applicable). (FORM __)

- Hospital Affiliations - Address to chief of staff or chair of credentials committee in care of medical staff office of hospital. Verify all current and previous affiliations. (FORM __)

- Request Physician Profile Data from the American Medical Association Physician Masterfile or the AOA File. (FORM __)

- Verify ECFMG, if applicable. (FORM __)

- Request data from National Practitioner Databank.

4. Prepare checklist of receipt of requested information. (FORM __)

5. Set up credentials file. (Identify how credentials file to be set up and what goes in each section in this part of the procedure.)

6. Monitor return of letters and note date of receipt on checklist. (FORM __) Date stamp all letters as received and place in applicant's credentials file. Discuss questionable references with the appropriate department chair. When reference letters make vague reference to professional problems or contain significant omissions, telephone calls should be initiated to peer references or previous/present hospital affiliations. These calls should be made by the department chair or credentials committee chair. Notes (memos to the credentials file) summarizing content of the discussion are made and placed in the applicant's file. (FORM __).

Exhibit 7-1. Sample Policy and Procedure - Processing a Medical Staff Application. *(continued)*

In all cases, references who have given verbal references should be encouraged to put the comments in writing.

When it is obvious there is some sort of professional problem with an applicant, ask for names of additional references to contact. Either write or telephone these additional references. Information should be gathered to the degree that no one is uncomfortable recommending an applicant for membership and privileges or everyone is uncomfortable doing so.

7. Send second requests if answers are not received within _____ weeks. Notify the applicant of the status of his/her application.   (FORM __)
    If there is still no response after _____ weeks, notify the applicant. The burden of proof is on the applicant.

8. When all information on the application is verified, notify department chair to review. Prepare summary of file for use by department chair, credentials and executive committee meetings. (FORM __)

9. Schedule any required interviews with the applicant.

10. After the appropriate department chairman has reviewed the file and made a written recommendation, route the application through the credentials committee, medical executive committee and governing body, with appropriate recommendations. (FORM __)

11. Notify the applicant and all concerned hospital departments when the appointment is approved. (FORM __)

    (If application and/or request(s) for clinical privileges are denied by the medical executive committee, contact attorney and follow the medical staff bylaws fair hearing procedures carefully.)

    Copy privilege form(s) and forward to appropriate hospital departments where required, i.e., surgical privilege forms to surgery, obstetrical privileges to labor and delivery, invasive procedures to the intensive care unit, etc.

12. Add physician information to hospital computer database, rosters, mailing lists, and so on, if not computerized in MSSD.

THE PRE-APPLICATION PROCESS

Many hospitals across the country have adopted a pre-application process in which a candidate for medical staff membership and clinical privileges is sent a list of the hospital's membership criteria that has been approved by the governing body. If the candidate does not meet these criteria, an application form is not sent. This saves time in processing applications, as it screens out candidates obviously not qualified for staff membership (e.g., candidates lacking the required amount of professional liability insurance coverage and not intending to obtain it).

In order to expedite the application process, many hospitals are conducting this process by telephone with the applicant, discussing the criteria by telephone and sending the application only upon assurance by the applicant that he or she meets all qualifications. If the application is received and it is apparent the applicant does not meet applicable criteria, the application is not processed.

Criteria for Membership

The requirements for medical staff membership and privileges are stated in the medical staff bylaws. They usually include

1. type of practitioner (e.g., physician, dentist, podiatrist),
2. appropriate professional licensure,
3. appropriate educational and training credentials,
4. practice in one of the clinical services provided for the community by the hospital or into which the hospital is expanding,
5. professional liability insurance coverage in the amount required by the governing body.

Occasionally medical staff bylaws require the applicant to agree to reside and maintain an office within a stated distance from the facility. This requirement is made to ensure the practitioner's availability to care for patients in a timely manner, including emergencies. However, the distances or described boundaries have sometimes been drawn or changed to reduce or eliminate competition. Hence, when setting up such a requirement, the hospital should seek legal counsel.

More and more frequently, the medical staff asks about specialty board certification as a criterion for medical staff membership. Although there is limited court support for this, requiring certification is both reasonable and desirable. However, it probably is not acceptable to most medical staffs at this time. The two main requirements are very clear. First, the requirement for board certification must be clearly related to quality of care. Otherwise it may be construed by some as an attempt to freeze out competition for patients. Second, the requirement must be consistent with state law, determination of which may require a legal opinion.

Other considerations related to board certification as a medical staff membership requirement include the following:

1. The requirement must start on the date the governing body approves the medical staff bylaws change. At the same time the decision must be made as to whether all non-board-certified staff members are to be automatically "grandfathered" in.

2. If the "grandfathering" occurs, is it to be permanent or is there to be a reasonable period during which these individuals must become board certified?

3. How will a specialty board requirement for periodic recertification be factored in?

4. If there is a practice requirement between the completion of a physician's formal training and when he or she can sit for the board exams, would this prevent the facility taking in a highly qualified physician pending his or her taking the board exams? And if the physician does not become certified, will he or she have to leave the staff?

5. To help ensure the same level (standard) of certification, would physicians have to be certified only by boards approved by the American Board of Medical Specialties? Would another board certification system for physicians be considered?

6. What would be the certification system used for all the different categories of non-physician medical staff applicants or members?

7. Although some hospitals may like to advertise the number of board-certified specialists on staff, this must be done carefully in order not to suggest guaranteeing a higher standard of care than other neighboring facilities. If this is interpreted by patients as a guarantee of better care, they may be more prone to sue when their higher expectations are not met.

APPLICATION FOR MEMBERSHIP AND PRIVILEGES

Application Form

The first serious dialogue between the applicant and the medical staff and governing board is the filing of a completed, signed application form (with any required attachments). The form requests all routine background and current information and, in addition, poses some critical questions. Routine information includes the following:

1. full name of applicant, date and location of birth, current home and office address and telephone numbers, date of application, and professional (practice) affiliation;

2. undergraduate education information including name of school, location, dates attended, and degree received;

3. postgraduate education information including name of school, location, dates attended, and degree received;

4. residency (includes internship if not a recent trainee) or fellowship information such as hospital, location, dates of training, and specialty;

5. previous and current hospital and other health care affiliations including names, locations, dates;

6. membership in professional associations, societies, academies, colleges, and faculty or training appointments;

7. specialty board certification status including name of board and date of board certificate (if not certified, whether or not a current candidate for examination should be indicated). Terms such as board qualified or board eligible should not be used on the application form, which should be stated on the form so that these terms are not written in;

8. list of all state licenses, with the expiration date of each;

9. federal Drug Enforcement Administration (DEA) registration certificate number and date of expiration (similarly, any state narcotics certificate number and expiration date should be indicated when the state has such a requirement; a hard copy should also be required);

10. professional references who have personal knowledge of the applicant's recent professional performance and experience (peers who have not personally observed the clinical work of the applicant, as well as relatives and business associates, are not acceptable. Most hospitals require two to four professional references);

11. all previous practice information such as solo practice, partnerships, locations, and dates;

12. list of continuing medical education for the past two years;

13. professional liability coverage information including carrier, amounts, and dates of coverage;

14. past and present professional litigation and liability history, including any open cases;

15. staff categories (list categories per medical staff bylaws);

16. clinical privileges requested (this information will be contained in a privilege request form appended to the application and consistent with the specialty in which the applicant proposes to practice);

17. Optional items such as

- a list of publications and major speeches given, with subjects, locations, and dates;

- a small recent photo, attached in the designated place on the application (the bylaws should state that the photo will help identify the applicant at the time of any required interview or to any training or education program requested to comment on the applicant; the photo is an excellent requirement, but must be used properly);

- a list of a specified number of patients treated or procedures performed, and any related records;

- Any required fee for processing the application, and whether or not it is applied toward annual medical staff dues for successful staff applicants.

Critical Questions for the Applicant

The following are critical questions that must be included in the application for the purpose of detecting previous professional problems:

1. Have you ever been requested to appear before any licensing or regulatory agency (e.g., the State Board of Medical Examiners, the Drug Enforcement Administration, the Professional Review Organization (PRO), or the Inspector General) for a hearing or complaint of any nature?

2. Has any professional license of yours ever been denied (on application), suspended, revoked limited, or otherwise acted against?

3. Have you ever been denied (on application) or surrendered a narcotics tax stamp?

4. Has any (professional/medical) license of yours ever been denied (on application), suspended, revoked, or limited?

5. Has your DEA Registration ever been denied (on application), suspended, revoked or limited?

6. Have your clinical privileges (including admitting, consulting, and assisting) or staff membership at any health care facility ever been denied, suspended, limited, revoked, not renewed, or otherwise acted against?

7. Have you ever been denied membership, or renewal thereof, or had your membership revoked or otherwise acted against, or been subject to disciplinary action, in any medical or professional organization or by any licensing agency of any state, district, territorial possession, or country?

8. Have you ever been convicted of a felony or misdemeanor (other than minor traffic offenses)?

9. Has any liability insurance carrier canceled, refused coverage, or increased rates because of unusual risk?

10. Are any actions pending for items 1-9 above?

11. Have any judgments or settlements been obtained against or from you in professional liability cases?

12. Are any professional liability cases pending against you?

13. Have you ever been under treatment for drug addiction or alcoholism? (If so, list any rehabilitation program(s), with dates.)

14. Have you ever received psychiatric treatment or care? (If so, list any treatment program(s) with dates).

15. Are you currently under care for a continuing health problem?

16. Have you ever discontinued practice for any reason (other than for routine vacation or formal education/training) for one month or more?

If any of the answers to the questions above are yes, the applicant should be asked to furnish details.

A health status question such as the following should be included:

> Do you feel that your health status is adequate enough to permit you to provide the patient care services for which you are requesting clinical privileges with or without reasonable accommodation? Yes___ No___

If the answer is no, the applicant should be asked to furnish details. The applicant could also be asked to enclose a copy of his or her most recent comprehensive physical examination report or include authorization for release by the examining physician.

The application usually includes an "Immunity from Liability" section as well as a series of pledges by the applicant to

1. adhere to generally recognized standards of professional ethics of his or her profession;

2. not participate in fee-splitting or "ghost" surgical or medical care;

3. participate, as required, in peer evaluation activities;

4. provide continuous care for his or her patients and delegate the responsibility for diagnosis or care of patients only to a practitioner who is qualified to undertake that responsibility;

5. obtain appropriate informed consent as required for the intervention contemplated;

6. abide by the medical staff bylaws, rules and regulations and hospital policies affecting the medical staff;

7. complete adequately, and in a timely fashion, the medical and any other required records for all patients he or she admits or in any way provides care for in the hospital;

8. seek consultation whenever necessary;

9. maintain the required amount of professional liability insurance coverage;

10. reasonably assist the hospital in fulfilling its uncompensated or partially compensated patient care obligations within the areas of his or her professional competence and credentials; and,

11. reasonably cooperate with the hospital in its efforts to comply with accreditation, reimbursement, and legal or other regulatory requirements.

The application should conclude by indicating that one or more interviews may be required and asking if the applicant would be willing to be interviewed at the hospital if requested. The applicant should sign the form. Somewhere on the application form, perhaps below the signature area, should be a highlighted note to the effect that failure to complete any part of the form or the inclusion of false information will delay the application processing and may render the applicant ineligible for staff membership. The bylaws should support this.

A copy of the current medical staff bylaws, rules, and regulations and a *relevant* privilege request form should accompany the application form for staff membership.

PROCESSING THE APPLICATION

Once the application form is received and the applicant is seriously pursuing staff membership and clinical privileges, a new applicant processing checklist should be started, which permits the medical staff services professional to know at a glance what information is already captured and what is missing. If the hospital uses credentialing software, the software program will be able to generate the checklist.

The processing checklist automatically includes and focuses on application items that require written *source* verification. These include state licenses, postgraduate degrees (medical, dental, podiatric), residency and fellowship training, specialty board status (to verify any statement made by the applicant as to certification or candidacy for examination), professional liability insurance coverage, and other hospital affiliations. The references provided by the applicant should be sent a letter asking specific questions about the applicant's qualifications.

RED FLAGS

Some points need to be specifically considered in reviewing the completed application form and in relation to source verification. Look for "red-flag" items, such as are listed below:

1. Any incomplete item that is pertinent to the application requires a letter telling the applicant his or her application is on hold. This is particularly true regarding the critical questions section, particularly with regard to liability and health issues. Telephone calls to the applicant usually are not productive and there is no hard copy record of the information exchange. If a second letter is needed, it should be sent by certified mail to document arrival and ensure a signed receipt. The second letter should also indicate a final date by which the information must be received if the application is not to be placed in the "incomplete" file.

2. When the application reveals an unexplained time gap in the training or practice sequence since graduation from (e.g., medical school) this gap requires serious attention. The applicant must explain why there was a long period of inactivity or the application cannot be processed.

3. Any indication of a voluntary or involuntary loss of one or more privileges at another hospital or a restriction or loss of a license or DEA registration certificate, past or present, is another red flag that requires clarification before further processing of the application. If both the other facility or agency and the applicant refuse to cooperate in providing the needed information, then the application should go into the incomplete file and the practitioner be so notified.

The medical staff bylaws should define what constitutes a completed application and also include language specifying that unresolved questions about an applicant make an application incomplete.

4. Since it takes time to build a practice, frequent changes in location in a short span of time requires investigation of the applicant. Practitioners may have a sound reason for moving from one state to another. On the other hand, a move may be related to problems with the state licensing agency, litigation problems, felony convictions, or health problems, none of which were mentioned on the application form. The health problems may relate to impaired physician status that has not been resolved.

5. The practitioner who has a number of lawsuits pending or settled requires additional investigation. Professional liability claims are not necessarily an indication of a problem, but extra checking should be undertaken to determine that a pattern of substandard practice was not the cause. Obtaining source information on the applicant's professional liability coverage may require the applicant's written permission unless the bylaws or the application form or the cover letters accompanying it provide otherwise. The insurer, however, can still insist on written permission, however, to release the information.

6. The practitioner previously impaired by alcohol or drug abuse may apply for membership and privileges. Documentation of rehabilitation and a period of monitoring helps to verify recovery and provide evidence that the problem has been corrected (see Exhibit 7-2 entitled "Some Credentialing Red Flags" and also Chapter 13).

Exhibit 7-2. Some Credentialing Red Flags.*

SOME CREDENTIALING "RED FLAGS" AND RESPONSES TO THEM

The Problem	Recommended Approach
1. Failure by any hospital, medical staff organization, training program, or professional society with which the applicant has been affiliated to respond completely to any written or oral reference inquiry.	This is the most common indication that a problem may exist. If a complete reference response is not forthcoming from any such entity, the Hospital Credentialing Committee should inform the applicant that the application will be deemed incomplete until a complete reference is obtained, and that failure to provide the reference within a set period of time will be considered a withdrawal of the application.
2. Equivocal or incomplete response to a written or oral reference request.	The Hospital Credentialing Committee should inform the applicant that it will be necessary for him or her to authorize the reference individual to provide a full and complete explanation of any equivocal or incomplete response and that the application will be deemed incomplete until that explanation is received. If the applicant fails to produce the full explanation required by the Committee within a set period of time, the application should be deemed withdrawn.
3. "Off the record" (but credible) reports of "problems" relating in any way to an applicant's professional practice.	This is the second most common form of evidence that a problem exists. Individuals may report investigations, concerns or disciplinary actions taken at other facilities (or of other problems) of which they are aware. The reporting individuals may be known to Membership Committee members and may be credible. But, the reporting individuals may be unwilling to provide information on the record.

---

*Source: Lowell C. Brown, Esq., Foley & Lardner, 2029 Century Park East, Suite 3500, Los Angeles, California 90067. Reprinted with permission.

Exhibit 7-2. Some Credentialing Red Flags. *(continued)*

The Problem	Recommended Approach
3. *(continued)*	The Hospital Credentialing Committee should never base its recommendation on unconfirmed, "off the record" information. Such information may turn out to be unreliable or may not result in any usable information at a subsequent hearing. Instead, the Hospital Credentialing Committee should get as much detail as possible about the reported problem, even if that detail is off the record. Then, the Committee should require the applicant to furnish specific documentary evidence relating to whatever problems were reported off the record. For example, the Committee may require the applicant to produce all correspondence with another hospital or medical staff organization, or to authorize another medical staff organization to provide a verified statement including copies of all peer review reports and minutes reflecting an evaluation of the applicant's practice. Likewise, the Committee may require the applicant to provide a verified statement transmitting copies of particular office or hospital patient records (with names expunged) or other documents which may confirm information received off the record. The application should be considered incomplete until all such information is received and should be considered to be withdrawn if the information is not *produced by a particular date.*
4. Difficulty in verifying nature and volume of recent hospital practice.	The applicant should be informed that the application is incomplete until documentation of such information in whatever form the Hospital Credentialing Committee requires is received. If the information is not received within a set period of time, the application should be deemed withdrawn.
5. Difficulty in verifying compliance with general requirements, such as professional liability insurance coverage, patient coverage arrangements, and establishment of office practice in the Hospital's service area.	The applicant should be informed that the application is incomplete until documentation of such information in whatever form the Hospital Credentialing Committee requires is received. If the information is not received within a set period of time, the application should be deemed withdrawn.
6. Any resignation or withdrawal of an application for appointment or reappointment from any hospital, medical staff or professional society at any time in an applicant's career.	This is another strong sign of a potential problem. The Hospital Credentialing Committee should require the applicant to produce a signed verification from the facility or organization involved, transmitting copies of all correspondence, committee minutes, memoranda, reports, or other documents relating in any way to the withdrawal or any pending investigations or disciplinary actions.
7. Past "disciplinary actions" by another hospital, medical staff, professional society or practice arrangement.	This is the type of information that the Hospital Credentialing Committee is required to obtain and evaluate carefully. The Hospital Credentialing Committee should inform the applicant that it will be necessary for him or her to produce a signed verification from the facility or organization transmitting all correspondence, memoranda, reports, committee minutes, transcripts, statements of charges, exhibits, and other documentation in any way relating the disciplinary action. The application should be deemed incomplete until that information is provided. Failure to provide the information within a set period of time should be deemed *a withdrawal of the application.*
8. Pending investigation by any hospital, medical staff organization or professional society.	This is also the type of information which the Hospital Credentialing Committee is required to obtain and evaluate carefully. As with past disciplinary actions, the Hospital Credentialing Committee should inform the applicant that it will be necessary for him or her to produce a signed verification from the facility or organization transmitting all correspondence, memoranda, reports, committee minutes, transcripts, statements of charges, exhibits, and other documentation in any way relating the disciplinary action. The application should be deemed incomplete until that information is provided. Failure to provide the information within a set period of time should be deemed *a withdrawal of the application.*
9. Pending recommendation of "disciplinary action" by any hospital, medical staff organization, professional society or practice affiliation.	As with items 7 and 8 above, the Hospital Credentialing Committee should inform the applicant that it will be necessary for him or her to produce a signed verification from the facility or organization transmitting all correspondence, memoranda, reports, committee minutes, transcripts, statements of charges, exhibits and other documentation in any way relating the disciplinary action. The application should be deemed incomplete until that information is provided. Failure to provide the information within a set period of time should be deemed a withdrawal of the application.

Exhibit 7-2. Some Credentialing Red Flags. *(continued)*

The Problem	Recommended Approach
10. Past or present investigation by the Medical Board of California (formerly, Board of Medical Quality Assurance).	The Hospital Credentialing Committee should inform the applicant that he or she must provide a signed verification from the Medical Board transmitting all correspondence, memoranda, investigative reports, witness statements, expert evaluations and other investigative material relating to the investigation. In addition, if that material discloses any disciplinary actions at other facilities, the applicant should be required to produce a signed verification from that facility transmitting all relevant documentation. If this information is not received within a set period of time, the application should be deemed withdrawn.
11. Disciplinary action by the Medical Board of California.	As with Item 10 above, the Hospital Credentialing Committee should inform the applicant that he or she must provide a signed verification from the Medical Board transmitting all correspondence, memoranda, investigative reports, witness statements, expert evaluations and other investigative material relating to the investigation. In addition, if that material discloses any disciplinary actions at other facilities, the applicant should be required to produce a signed verification from that facility transmitting all relevant documentation. If this information is not received *within a set period* of time, *the application should be* deemed withdrawn.
12. Pending Medical Board of California accusation (regardless of whether an administrative hearing has been completed or whether the applicant is appealing the administrative determination in court).	Again, the Hospital Credentialing Committee should inform the applicant that he or she must provide a signed verification from the Medical Board transmitting all correspondence, memoranda, investigative reports, witness statements, expert evaluations and other investigative material relating to the investigation. In addition, if that material discloses any disciplinary actions at other facilities, the applicant should be required to produce a signed verification from that facility transmitting all relevant documentation. If this information is not received within a set period of time, the application should be deemed withdrawn.
13. Settlement of any professional liability claims (whether or not they resulted in litigation) within the past five (5) years.	The applicant should be asked to provide a signed verification from an individual, other than himself or herself, who is knowledgeable about the settlement transmitting copies of all settlement agreements, documentation, court pleadings, deposition transcripts, expert opinion reports, correspondence or other documents relating to the terms of the settlement or the charges upon which the claim was based. The application should be deemed incomplete until this information is received and if the information is not received within a set period of time, the application should be deemed withdrawn.
14. Adverse judgment in any professional liability action during the past five (5) years.	The applicant should be required to produce signed verifications transmitting copies of the judgment, court papers demonstrating the specific charges upon which the claim was based. In appropriate cases, the information requested might include deposition transcripts, expert opinion reports, correspondence, and other documents relating to the claim, as well as patient records, office records, hospital investigation reports, and documents relating to disciplinary actions by any other facilities. Until all such documentation is received, the application should be deemed incomplete.
15. Pending professional liability actions.	This is one of the most important pieces of information that may come to the Hospital's attention, and one which the Hospital is probably legally required to review. The applicant should be required to produce signed verifications transmitting the materials generally described in item 14 above.
16. Other civil litigation relating to the applicant's professional practice or qualifications. (This may include, for example, claims of sexual misconduct with patients or claims of insurance fraud or investigations by a professional review organization.) Such information would probably not come to the Hospital's attention as a result of the applicant's completion of the Hospital Application. It would probably come to light through news reports or other unofficial means.	The applicant should be required to produce signed verifications transmitting copies of court documents sufficient to explain the nature of charges against him or her and the status of the litigation (including any settlement thereof). In addition, the applicant should be required to produce signed verifications transmitting copies of correspondence, reports, committee minutes, and any other documents relating to the underlying charges or any investigation or disciplinary actions relating to those charges. Again, the application should be deemed incomplete until that information is produced and should be deemed withdrawn if the information is not produced within a set period of time.
17. Investigations or disciplinary actions by a professional review organization, or any third-party payer (including Medicare, Medi-Cal, or private insurance).	The applicant should be required to provide a signed verification transmitting copies of all investigative reports, correspondence, related disciplinary actions or administrative investigations relating to this matter. Again, the application should be deemed incomplete until such information is received and should be deemed withdrawn if the information is not received within a set period of time.

Exhibit 7-2. Some Credentialing Red Flags. *(continued)*

The Problem	Recommended Approach
18. Participation, in the last five (5) years, in any treatment or diversion program relating to drug use, alcohol dependency or psychiatric problems.	The applicant should be required to provide signed verifications transmitting copies of all documents relating to the terms and conditions of participation, correspondence relating to such participation and all evaluations of the applicant's physical, mental or emotional condition. The application should be deemed incomplete until all such information is received and should be deemed withdrawn unless all such information is received within a certain period of time.
19. Evidence of any criminal charges brought against the applicant with the past five (5) years.	The applicant should be required to provide signed verifications from public authorities transmitting copies of charges and of any court documents demonstrating the resolution or status of such actions. The applicant should also be required to produce signed verifications transmitting such documents as the Committee deems necessary relating to the underlying conduct reflected in the criminal accusations. The application should be deemed incomplete until such information is furnished and should be deemed withdrawn unless the information is produced within a set period of time.
20. Pending criminal charges.	In many cases, the criminal charges, if proven, would disqualify the applicant from the Hospital membership. Accordingly, the applicant should be required to produce signed verifications of court documents as well as such related documentation as the Hospital Credentialing Committee requires. Generally, it will be impossible for the Committee to resolve the issues presented by a criminal charge relating to the applicant's professional practice or qualifications until after the criminal proceeding is completed. Accordingly, the Committee, in appropriate circumstances, may consider the application incomplete until the criminal matter is fully resolved.
21. Criminal convictions during the past five (5) years.	Again in many cases, the criminal charges, if proven, would disqualify the applicant from the Hospital membership. The Hospital Credentialing Committee should require the same information from the applicant as recommended in Item 20 above.

Telephone Calls Concerning Applicants

Occasionally insight about the above problems can be gained through an administrator-to-administrator (or physician-to-physician) phone call, but unless a dated memo of the conversation is made, there will be no hard information on which to help base a decision. When phone calls are made to discuss an application problem or a negative reference letter, specific questions should be asked of the physician or administrator contacted. Included might be questions about the receipt of reports of poor medical practice; poor relationships with peers or hospital staff that have been detrimental to patient care or hospital operations; and mental or physical illness or substance abuse problems that have interfered with ability to practice quality medicine. Names of other informants who might be contacted can be obtained at the time these phone calls are made to a previous hospitals and peer references.

Verifying Information on the Application

In seeking information from other hospitals, training programs, and peer references, it is important that needed information be requested correctly. The best chance of obtaining the needed information is through use of a form that requires a minimum of writing on the respondent's part. When developing a form keep these points in mind:

1. When indicating that the individual is requesting procedural privileges, include a list of the specific privileges requested by the applicant and ask if he or she has performed them and how satisfactorily. It is not at all uncommon, especially in the case of training program graduates, to learn that certain procedures for which privileges are being requested were never performed by the individual in the program or else that the necessary training was not provided in the program.

2. Inquire about the individual's health status to determine if there is a known health problem that might prevent the applicant from exercising the privileges being requested.

3. Ask if the applicant has the ability to work and cooperate well with other members of the health care and hospital team. As with other items on the form, a simple grading of three or more levels of performance can be provided in order to make it easier for the respondent.

Additional Sources of Information on Applicants

Other potential sources of information on physician applicants that should be used are the Federation of State Medical Boards (which is a data bank containing disciplinary action information as reported by all state boards of medical examiners and other sources) and the National Practitioner Data Bank. This data bank should eventually contain a wealth of information, especially information concerning licensure and inadequate performance. For completeness of information sources, the American Medical Association Physician Masterfile should be obtained for physician applicants.

The Credentials File

Once the application has been received and processing starts, a segmented credentials file should be instituted. How it is set up is an individual choice. However, some basic advice may help to make the use of the file more efficient. It takes two and a half times longer to file documents in a clipped fashion. Consider using files that allow for drop filing.

Place in one section all one-time items, such as the application form, the letters of reference, and so on. In another section, include the recurring date-related documents that need to be immediately accessible, such as state licenses, the DEA registration, and professional liability coverage documents. For these items, there is usually a tickler file in the computer for renewal purposes. In another section, place staff reappointment information, usually with the most current on top. A separate section should be reserved for clinical privileges. Some hospitals use an additional separate section for peer review information (both good and bad) and related actions.

Some hospitals are interested in "paperless" files and are using scanning technology to achieve a paperless credentials file. Documents that are scanned into the system can be printed out, if necessary. Data security issues must be addressed if a hospital wishes to pursue a paperless system.

DELINEATION OF CLINICAL PRIVILEGES

Privilege delineation, properly performed and monitored, continues to be the most important function performed by the medical staff and governing body. As noted previously, privilege delineation is basically performed in three ways: (1) using a laundry list approach, (2) using a category or levels approach, or (3) using a core privilege approach. In addition, sometimes combinations of these methods are used. When the category approach to clinical privilege delineation is used, care must be taken to ensure that the privileges are actually delineated in a way that makes the limits of practice very clear. Some specialty organizations have published sample categories but when read carefully, it is obvious that within each category level, the physician actually delineates what his or her practice will be.

Although determination of staff membership and the delineation of clinical privileges are two separate processes, they are interrelated and simultaneously culminate in a governing board decision. Probably the only exceptions are when a staff member requests a change in privileges following satisfactory completion of the required training or when a staff member involuntarily suffers a reduction in privileges.

The credentials file should not be cluttered with excessive privilege delineation forms. This most frequently happens with two types of laundry privilege lists: the bound booklet type and the loose-leaf multipage type. In both cases, the entire set of forms is sent to each staff applicant for completion on the assumption that some practitioners will request procedures under more than one specialty area. In both cases, the credentials files bulge with many unused pages of privilege delineation forms. There are at least three ways to prevent this situation:

1. Only the specialty privileges ordinarily associated with the type of practice of the applicant should be provided.

2. In addition to the specialty-specific privileges listed, there should be a supplemental procedure list that covers all procedures that are not absolutely peculiar to one type of practice. This list should be given to all

applicants and to all staff members at time of reappointment. This system offers multiple advantages in that it indicates who is doing what procedures in the hospital; helps identify procedures that need evaluation or practitioners who need monitoring; identifies procedures for which no standards of care have been set; and, best of all, only requires revision of one form when some procedural privilege has to be deleted from or added to the list. It is not uncommon to find physicians performing procedures (e.g., endoscopy) that they have been performing in the hospital for years without having ever been granted privileges to do so.

3. The privilege lists sent out to applicants or used for practitioners seeking reappointment should be limited to hospital-specific privileges. For example, privileges for obstetrics, radiation therapy, or cardiac surgery should not be listed if these services are not offered by the hospital.

Other concerns relating to privilege delineation forms include the following:

1. For each privilege, the applicant must clearly indicate whether the privilege is or is not being requested. This is a further reason for not sending out the bulky forms described in the previous section. Blanks are dangerous because it can't be determined whether or not the physician has requested a certain privilege or procedure, and if so, whether or not the privilege or procedure has been approved.

2. Reviewing, recommending or approving groups must indicate whether the requested privileges are individually recommended or approved. Again, blanks are dangerous and challenge the credibility of the process.

3. It must be made clear whether an assistant or a consultation is required for any particular privilege. The better forms add columns for checking these requirements.

Criteria for Granting Privileges

The medical staff is required by JCAHO to establish an objective framework for determining what privileges will be granted to an applicant. Criteria must be established that describe minimum training or direct experience that must be documented or demonstrated before privileges are granted.

As mentioned earlier, the medical staff bylaws usually describe broad membership criteria which include licensure, training, experience, current competence, and health status. More specific criteria must also be developed to determine what precise training or experience an applicant must have obtained to be approved for specific procedures or treatment of a particular diagnosis. These criteria must also be developed for new procedures that evolve as a result of new or improved technology.

Criteria for granting privileges may include

1. minimal formal training, such as an approved residency training program;
2. required previous experience, such as performance of 50 major surgical procedures within the last two years or treatment of a minimum of 50 patients within the last two years;
3. a certificate of attendance at an approved formal training course, accompanied by the course outline;
4. completion of a specified number of proctored cases.

Exhibit 7-3 demonstrates an example of core and special privileges for the specialty of anesthesiology as well as the criteria for granting privileges.

When an applicant applies for specific clinical privileges, his or her training and experience are compared to the criteria established. If the applicant does not meet established criteria, the privileges cannot be granted. If this occurs, the applicant should be informed of the training or experience needed in order to qualify for the requested privilege.

Sometimes physicians attempt to keep otherwise qualified physicians from performing certain procedures based on economic considerations. When developing criteria for granting privileges, care should be taken to ensure that all qualified groups have input into the criteria and that requirements are reasonable.

PROVISIONAL STATUS

The provisional period is usually defined by the medical staff bylaws as the first six to 12 months of staff appointment. Some medical staffs have formalized this period by establishing a "provisional staff" category. This period is necessary because the applicant has been accepted for staff membership and has been granted specific privileges based on paper credentials. The period of observation is needed to confirm that the decision was justified. From a fairness standpoint, it is necessary that the initial provisional period be equal for all newly appointed staff members. The bylaws may, however, provide for extension of the period for two reasons: (1) the provisional member has not used the hospital enough during the initial period to permit review of performance, or (2) the member's performance is questionable and additional review is needed prior to rendering a final decision.

Although the initial provisional period is the same length for all new staff members, the number of cases or procedures to be proctored during the period may vary depending on the individual's previous experience and on the opinion of the proctors. The word "proctoring" sometimes bothers the medical staff, and other terms may be used, such as observing, monitoring, sponsor-

Exhibit 7-3. Clinical Privilege Delineation Description.*

CLINICAL PRIVILEGE DELINEATION DESCRIPTION

Anesthesiologist

Practice Specialty:

Required Qualifications for privileges as an anesthesiologist:
In order to be eligible for privileges as an anesthesiologist, the applicant must have completed an ACGME-approved residency training program in anesthesiology and be board certified by the American Board of Anesthesiology or have completed an AOA-approved residency training program in anesthesiology and be board certified by the American Osteopathic Board of Anesthesiology.

Privilege Description	Criteria For Privileges			Privileges may be exercised	
	Education/ Training	Clinical Activity	Outcomes	In the Following Settings:	To the Following Age Groups:
Basic General Anesthesia: Provide assessment of, consultation for and preparation of patients for anesthesia; provide insensibility to pain during surgical, obstetric, therapeutic and diagnostic procedures and management of patients so affected; provide monitoring and restoration of homeostasis during the perioperative period, as well as homeostasis in the critically ill or injured patient; provide clinical management of cardiac and pulmonary resuscitation, as well as respiratory function. **Excludes:** Privileges to admit for inpatient care.	See *Required Qualifications*	NOTE: Medical staff organization (via departments or sections) to determine if clinical activity requirement for these privileges should be established, and if so, the required activity level.	NOTE: Medical staff organization (via departments or sections) to determine if outcomes for these privileges should be established for purposes of evaluating performance. If outcomes are to be established, those would be defined here and then show up on a profile. The profile would be used for ongoing performance evaluation purposes, as well as at the time of reappointment.	Ambulatory Surgery Center Birthing Center Inpatient Services	All, excluding neonates
Participate in residency training program by supervising residents	See *Required Qualifications*			Ambulatory Surgery Center Birthing Center Inpatient Services	All, excluding neonates
Supervise allied health professionals (CRNAs)	See *Required Qualifications*			Ambulatory Surgery Center Birthing Center Inpatient Services	All, excluding neonates
General Anesthesia Procedures: Inhalation; Intravenous; Deliberate hypotension: Deliberate hypothermia: Cardiopulmonary bypass; Monitored anesthesia care; Complicated airway management, including fiberoptic bronchoscopy, retrograde intubation, transtracheal jet-ventilation.	See *Required Qualifications*			Ambulatory Surgery Center Inpatient Services	All, excluding neonates
Conductive Anesthesia Procedures: Central axis neural blockade including spinals, epidurals, caudals; IV regional blocks; Sensory and motor nerve blocks; other nerve blocks, spinal and epidural narcotics; Airway management associated with conductive anesthesia procedures.	See *Required Qualifications*			Ambulatory Surgery Center Birthing Center Inpatient Services	All, excluding neonates
Invasive Monitoring Procedures: Placement of central venous, pulmonary or peripheral artery catheters.	See *Required Qualifications*			Ambulatory Surgery Center Inpatient Services	All, excluding neonates
Pain Management: Diagnosis and management of painful syndromes. Includes privilege to admit for inpatient care and perform the history and physical examination.				Ambulatory Surgery Center Inpatient Services	All, excluding neonates and pediatric patients
Transesophageal Echocardiography (TEE)	SAMPLE: Have satisfactorily completed an accredited course in TEE (must be verifiable from course provider), which includes hands-on training. Course must be acceptable to the Chair of the Anesthesiology Department. OR Have had hands-on TEE training during residency training, and competency is verified by the Residency Program Director.			Inpatient Services	All, excluding neonates and pediatric patients

---

*Source: "Health Care Competency and Credentialing Report," vol. 1, no. 2, April 1997. Reprinted with permission.

ing, and so on. Whatever it's called, several rules apply and the whole process itself should be spelled out in the medical staff bylaws or in a policy approved by the executive committee of the medical staff.

To begin with, the bylaws or policy should define how proctors are selected (the selection is ordinarily done by the department chair in a departmentalized medical staff and by the chief of staff in a non-departmentalized medical staff). Among the rules should be the following:

1. The proctor must not be a relative or a practice partner or associate of the practitioner being proctored.

2. Proctoring shall include both direct observation and review of the related records for both non-surgical and surgical types of practice.

3. Proctoring will include the most sophisticated type of procedures that have been granted and will cover the full scope of privileges granted. For instance, performing varicose vein surgery, varicocelectomies, and hemorrhoidectomies does not equate with surgery for aortic aneurysm or femoropopliteal bypass surgery when proctoring a physician granted vascular surgery privileges. Similarly, an inguinal hernioplasty and appendectomy do not equate with surgery of the common bile duct for general surgery proctoring purposes.

4. A written report should be submitted promptly for each case or procedure proctored. The report form should not require a lot of writing and should be easy to complete. Reports should be placed in the appropriate credentials file after review by the department chair or designee.

5. Reports should be reviewed in an ongoing manner rather than waiting until the end of the provisional period. This is to assure that any patient care performance problem is detected as soon as possible. When a problem is detected, the physician being proctored should be notified immediately and steps should be taken to rectify the problem.

6. As an alternative, when the practitioner being proctored does not admit or treat enough "sophisticated" cases in the hospital, cases from another hospital may be substituted, provided the proctor has privileges in both hospitals.

At the end of the initial proctoring period, one of several actions should be taken, the practitioner should be notified, and the information placed in the credentials file. Possible actions include the following:

1. The practitioner's performance has been satisfactory and he or she is advanced to the appropriate non-provisional staff category (e.g., active, courtesy, consulting).

2. The practitioner's caseload or procedure load has been inadequate at the facility or acceptable alternative facilities for rendering a judgment as the acceptability of performance, and additional provisional time is required. The bylaws should specify a time limit (e.g., 12 months) beyond which the provisional period may not be extended. At that point, a decision will have to be rendered as to staff membership and privileges. If the practitioner has failed to comply with the caseload requirement, particularly over a long period (e.g., two years), he or she should be dropped from the staff (as provided in the bylaws) and notified of this in writing. The practitioner is entitled to any procedural rights specified by the bylaws.

3. If the practitioner has adequate cases for review, yet patient care has been deemed not to meet standards, whether in the initial or an extended provisional period, he or she should be suspended or dropped from the staff (as provided in the bylaws) and notified of this in writing. The practitioner is entitled to any procedural rights as specified by the bylaws. When a practitioner is dropped for failing to meet the quality of care standards, it should be ensured that he or she has had more than one proctor, that the proctors agree on the level of care provided, and that, to the degree possible, the proctors are not in obvious competition for the same patients. When competition exists, it is preferable to arrange for a respected peer practitioner from outside the economic competitive area to review the cases.

During the provisional period, the practitioner being evaluated should also be monitored for compliance with other staff and hospital requirements (e.g. timely completion of medical records, adequacy of medical records, meeting attendance, and so forth). These requirements should be essentially the same for all staff members with provisional status and should be indicated in the bylaws or a policy. The information acquired through monitoring will be collected by the medical staff services department and should be compiled at the end of the provisional period and forwarded to the department chair for evaluation.

TEMPORARY PRIVILEGES

In the absence of a rule prohibiting the use of temporary privileges, the medical staff should be quite strict in recommending or approving such privileges. In fact, temporary privileges should be given for only three reasons as indicated in the medical staff bylaws:

1. governing body approval is pending, but *all* required information has been verified and a positive response is anticipated from the medical staff executive committee and the hospital governing body;

2. a non-transportable patient requires the skill and expertise of a physician specialist who is not a member of the staff.

3. there are inadequate numbers of certain specialists on the medical staff or general practitioners cannot find in-house replacement. It would be wise to specify that a *locum tenens* must be at least as qualified as the physician he or she is temporarily replacing and will not exercise privileges granted other than those granted to the staff member.

Temporary privileges should not be granted to just anyone only for a limited number of visits. They should never be granted solely for patient desire or convenience (in such cases, the involved practitioner may have only recently been suspended or dropped from the hospital medical staff of another local hospital for quality or legal reasons).

When temporary privileges are granted to a medical staff applicant, all of the required verification should be complete in the applicant's file and the department chair should have reviewed it and approved the application. The chief of staff should also review the completed file and make a recommendation. The hospital chief executive officer or his or her designee is the additional person who will review and make the decision regarding approval of temporary privileges.

STAFF REAPPOINTMENT

Credentials

The credentials process also involves staff reappointment. Reappointment is necessary for multiple reasons, including the updating of information relating to claims and litigation, health, and changes in outside affiliations; and additional training, education, certification. It is also mandatory to assess the practitioner's performance profile since the last staff appointment to ensure that the practitioner is currently competent to exercise the clinical privileges that he or she has been granted.

One frequently overlooked medical staff and governing body responsibility is the obligation to ensure that the practitioner has met any requirements for privileges the exercise of which requires evidence of continued proficiency. If a procedure has not been done enough to give reasonable assurance of proficiency, the privilege should be withdrawn or the practitioner proctored. Consideration should be given, of course, for documented cases done at another facility. Another check at time of reappointment should be made to assure that all clinical privileges are still hospital-specific. A practitioner may have different privileges in each of three different hospitals based on the specific patient services offered by each hospital. Thus professional qualifications are not the only determinant of privilege delineation.

During the period between staff appointments, a staff member's credentials are established through the medical staff quality and peer review system. The medical staff committees and departments review performance data and may also review specific patient care cases. Ongoing practitioner performance data is maintained and includes the findings of the hospital's performance improvement program (see Chapter 10). Findings should be included from procedure evaluation, drug therapy evaluation, blood therapy evaluation, medical record documentation review, utilization review, hospital risk management, and other monitoring and evaluation programs. These numerator findings should be included on a profile that also notes denominator information (i.e., the number of admissions, procedures performed and consultations). The denominator information is important as it helps to put into perspective any negative data generated. A practitioner who has admitted only three patients and had quality problems with the treatment of all three patients is in a different category from a practitioner who has admitted dozens of patients but experienced quality problems with only three. Additionally, each practitioner's data should be compared to data for other practitioners within the same specialty as well as to data from an external source. Exhibit 7-4 is a sample performance profile that provides for the display of comparative data.

It is important, especially for a large medical staff, to have a staggered system of reappointment. That is, the entire staff is not reappointed at the same time but is divided by department, by birth date, by appointment date, or alphabetically, so that large numbers are not reappointed at the same time. This permits a more in-depth evaluation of each candidate for reappointment and of the concomitant clinical privilege delineation.

The Reappointment Form

A reappointment form should be sent to each staff member for completion along with a copy of his or her current privilege form. The reappointment form should require the following:

1. confirmation of all required demographic information;
2. confirmation of current licenses, DEA registration, and professional liability coverage (this information should be updated at the time of expiration and therefore, it may not be necessary to query the applicant regarding current information that is already on file). Because states vary with respect to licensure date requirements and hospital medical staffs vary with respect to reappointment dates, it may be necessary to verify the state licensure twice—once at expiration date and once at time of

Exhibit 7-4. Consolidated Performance Profile.*

SAMPLE HEALTH CARE SYSTEM
Consolidated Performance Profile

Performance Profile Goals:
- *To positively influence practice patterns when necessary to decrease cost of care while maintaining or improving outcomes.*
- *To provide data which supports competency of practitioners.*
- *To meet credentialing-related requirements of JCAHO and NCQA*
- *To provide data to credentialing decision-makers in a format which makes it difficult to ignore significant variations*

PRACTITIONER: _____
SPECIALTY: _____
TIME PERIOD: From __/__/__ To __/__/__

_____ PRIVILEGES: Y or N
_____ PRIVILEGES: Y or N
_____ PRIVILEGES: Y or N

NOTE:
This profile to be used for primary care practitioners who have inpatient privileges as well as primary care network practitioners.

PERFORMANCE PARAMETER	PRACTITIONER-SPECIFIC DATA				INTERNAL COMPARATIVE DATA	EXTERNAL COMPARATIVE DATA
	NPH	CHS	SMH	TOTAL		
INPATIENT ACTIVITY						
• Inpatient Discharges						
• Total Patient Days						
• Average Length of Stay						
• Outpatients						
• Consultations Performed						
• Total Procedures Performed						
STAFF REQUIREMENTS						
• Number of Medical Record Suspensions						
INPATIENT-SPECIFIC INDICATORS						
• Readmission Rate (unplanned)						
• Unexpected Mortality Rate						
• Unplanned Returns to Special Care Unit						
• Crossmatch/Transfusion Rate						
• Pharmacy intervention rate						
• Indicator related to patient /family satisfaction						
MEDICAL RECORD REVIEWS						
• Indicator(s) related to documentation quality and timeliness						
	NPH	CHS	SMH	TOTAL		
UTILIZATION MANAGEMENT						
• Indicator(s) related to resource utilization						
CASE-SPECIFIC REVIEW						
• Total # of cases reviewed						
• # of cases receiving scores of "3" or "4"						
ACTIVITY: MEDICAL GROUP						
• Panel Size						
• # of Specialty Referrals						
• Average # of patient encounters per month						
LITIGATION						
• Number of Cases Pending*						
• Number of Judgments*						
• Number of Settlements*						
MEDICAL GROUP-SPECIFIC INDICATORS						
• Successful Site Visit	Y or N				N/A	N/A
• Indicator related to member satisfaction						
• Indicator related to member complaints						

*Source: Vicki L. Searcy, © BDO Seidman. Reprinted with permission.

reappointment. This has become more important in recent years as medical staffs have wisely shifted to staggered reappointment systems.

3. confirmation of the attainment of specialty board certification since appointment or last reappointment;

4. an indication as to whether a privilege change is being requested, and, if so whether specific additional privileges are the issue (if additional privileges are requested, the staff member must state, in terms of training and so on, why he or she is qualified to exercise the additional privileges). A practitioner may also wish to drop privileges due to a change in the pattern of practice. For example, an older obstetrician/gynecologist may want to discontinue practicing obstetrics and limit his or her practice to gynecology. It is important that this change be noted on the clinical privilege form;

5. the answers to critical questions relating to status *since the previous appointment*, including these:

    •   Has your membership in another health care facility been denied, revoked, or otherwise acted against, or been subjected to disciplinary action?

    •   Have any privileges been voluntarily or involuntarily withdrawn in another health care facility?

    •   Are you currently under charges that, if upheld, could lead to conviction for a felony or misdemeanor (other than minor traffic offenses)?

    •   Have any judgments been made against or settlements been obtained from you in professional liability cases?

    •   Are any professional liability cases pending against you?

    •   Have you been under treatment for drug addiction or alcoholism?

    •   Have you been under psychiatric treatment or care?

    •   Are you currently under care for a continuing health problem? (Note: If the answers to a through h are "yes," please include details.)

    •   Do you feel that your health status is adequate enough to permit you to provide the patient care services for which you are requesting clinical privileges? (Note: If the answer is no, please include details.)

6. description of continuing education since last appointment;

7. any other requirement of the medical staff bylaws, rules, and regulations;

8. the signature of the individual seeking reappointment;

9. the reappointment fee (if any).

The completed application will be routed through the evaluation process accompanied by the profile information supplied through the quality improvement program and the medical staff services department. This information usually includes both administrative aspects of staff membership (e.g., meeting attendance statistics - if attendance is required, medical record delinquency status, committee appointments, and hospital practice statistics) and clinical performance data (e.g., clinical outcome statistics, committee and department citations, governing board sanctions, and peer review and quality improvement reviews and actions). All hospitals are required to check with the National Practitioner Data Bank to determine whether any adverse information has been reported during the past period of appointment.

Reappointment of Practitioners with Low Activity

Some hospitals have large numbers of staff members whose primary practices are centered at other area facilities. It is difficult to obtain adequate performance data for these practitioners at the time of reappointment. In each such case, the facilities at which the practitioner most actively practices must be contacted to obtain the information needed for reappointment. As with reference letters used to obtain information for the initial appointment, these should be carefully worded to elicit the precise information needed. The value of the information obtained is also dependent on the quality and scope of the quality and peer review programs at the other facilities. However, some attempt should be made to determine whether the practitioner has experienced professional problems at these facilities. Some hospitals are attempting to reduce the number of staff members who mainly practice elsewhere by requiring (as provided in the bylaws) a minimum number of admissions, procedures, or consultations for maintenance of staff membership and privileges.

Routing Reappointments through Channels

The completed reappointment form and profile information should be evaluated by the following, with an indication of approval, approval with stated exceptions (e.g., denial of certain privileges), or disapproval and the reasons therefor:

1. the medical staff clinical department chair. This individual should indicate that he or she has (a) reviewed the application and profile information and found it in satisfactory order, (b) has no knowledge of any health problem that would prevent the individual seeking reappointment from exercising the privileges requested, and (c) has made a recommendation (e.g., approval). (This statement may have to be made by the chief of staff in a hospital that is still not departmentalized);

Exhibit 7-5. Steps in the Reappointment Process.

1. Ninety days prior to the membership expiration date, the medical staff services department sends a reappointment application to the practitioner, including the deadline for receipt; notifies the quality department of the need for a practitioner clinical profile and the date needed; submits the name of the practitioner being reappointed to the National Practitioner Data Bank and requests information

2. Sixty days prior to the expiration date, the practitioner returns the completed application form. The quality department forwards the profile to medical staff services.

3. Medical staff services verifies the information on the completed application and sends the application, administrative data, National Practitioner Data Bank information, clinical profile, privilege delineation request form, and verification from other facilities (in the case of a practitioner relatively inactive at the hospital) to the department chair for review.

4. The department chair reviews the profile and all supporting information, comments on the practitioner's health status, and sends a written recommendation for privilege delineation and reappointment to the credentials committee.

5. The credentials committee reviews all information and the department chair's recommendation, submits its recommendation to the executive committee.

6. The executive committee reviews the previous recommendations, makes its own recommendation, and then forwards it to the governing body. (If an adverse recommendation is made, the applicant must be offered due process.)

7. The governing body takes final action.

8. The applicant is notified of the governing body's decision.

2. the credentials committee or the body performing the credentialing function;

3. the medical staff executive committee;

4. the governing body, which has final decision-making authority.

Any person required to evaluate the reappointment request can request further relevant information before making a recommendation or decision. However, if the process is performed properly, this type of delay will rarely occur.

If a medical staff member voluntarily relinquishes certain privileges (e.g., because of age, a desire to cut back practice, or poor results), it is critical that the change be formalized through the medical staff and governing body system. Otherwise, the staff member may decide after several years of inactivity to exercise the same privileges again. This could be catastrophic. Before formalizing the voluntary relinquishment of privileges, check state or federal reporting requirements relating to privilege changes.

ALLIED HEALTH PROFESSIONALS

Allied health professionals (AHPs) are entering health care organizations in greater numbers than ever before. Historically, AHPs were usually brought into a hospital because they were employed by a physician member of the medical staff organization who wished to use the services of his or her employee while attending to patients. Because of this link between the physician and his or her employee, AHPs were credentialed through the medical staff organization. The credentialing and privileging systems that were used for physicians were adapted for AHPs. These AHPs were often nurses from physician offices, who assisted as scrub nurses in the operating room or accompanied the physician on patient rounds, providing patient teaching, and so on.

Now a wide array of AHPs provide services in hospitals and related ambulatory care settings. And AHPs are being used to extend the services of the physician. AHPs may be hospital or physician employees or they may have a contract with the organization to provide services. They may be granted privileges or the authority to provide designated patient services. There appears to be no limit to the number of possible titles; for example, certified registered nurse anesthetists, physician assistants, nurse practitioners, perfusionists, registered nurse-midwives, speech pathologists, as well as acupuncturists and other alternative care providers. The hospital and medical staff determine who these individuals are, and the procedure for appointment and the scope of practice should be defined in the organization-wide documents, not the medical staff bylaws.

Factors common to allied health professionals include the following:

1. The source of employment has absolutely no bearing on their need to be authorized to provide services. In other words, a hospital-employed nurse anesthetist, a physician assistant employed by a medical staff member, or a speech pathologist under contract with the hospital must be credentialed through the regular medical staff channels.

2. They usually provide direct care to patients, that is, "lay hands on" or are in close verbal contact with patients.

3. Some may render judgments on their own.

4. Some may practice independently.

Some allied health professionals must have a license, certification, or registration and are regulated or guided by state requirements. However, the hospital has the final say as to the extent of services the individual may provide within the hospital's jurisdiction. This is defined in a task list or privilege list of allowable services.

Unsupervised allied health professionals must apply, on a designated form, to provide patient care services in the hospital. Their performance must be evaluated regularly and objectively. And they must be evaluated regularly on the basis of a performance record. AHPs who practice in an unsupervised manner are considered to be licensed independent practitioners and should be credentialed in the same manner as other licensed independent practitioners, for example, physicians and dentists. AHPs who function in a supervised capacity should not have delineated clinical privileges and, according to JCAHO, can function under a job description. Supervised or dependent AHPs may be authorized to provide services in the hospital through a variety of mechanisms. One mechanism could be through the medical staff organization's credentialing process. Alternatively, the process could be administered by human resources.

An application form for an allied health professional who functions in an unsupervised manner should include the following:

1. name, home and office address, telephone numbers, citizenship, marital status, and professional affiliations;

2. licensure, certification, and registration, with expiration dates;

3. education and training (high school, college, nursing school, other graduate education or training);

4. current hospital affiliations;

5. military service and any specialized training;

6. membership in professional organizations;

7. previous experience in hospitals or other health care facilities;

8. references (three individuals with personal knowledge of professional ability, ethics, character);

9. evidence of professional liability insurance (carrier, policy number, dates, and limits);

10. type of practice anticipated if granted privileges would be
    * self-employed (free-lance);
    * employed by medical staff member part time;
    * employed by medical staff members full time;
    * member of, or affiliated with, a group practicing this specialty;
    * other (specify).

11. distance from office or home to hospital (in miles);

12. answers to these questions; if the answer to any of the following questions is yes, please give full details on a separate sheet of paper. All questions must be answered. (One possible answer is "not applicable.")

    - Has your license to practice in any jurisdiction ever been limited, suspended, placed on probation, or revoked?

    - Has your certification or registration status ever been revoked?

    - Have your privileges at any hospital or other health care facility ever been revoked, suspended, reduced, subject to observation (beyond what is normal) or not renewed?

    - Have you ever been denied membership (or renewal thereof) or been subject to disciplinary action in any professional organization?

    - Have you ever been a defendant in a professional liability or negligence case?

    - Is there any professional liability claim pending against you?

    - Has a settlement of any professional liability claim involving you ever been made?

    - Is there any health status problem that could prevent you from performing the privileges requested?

13. continuing education information (list on a separate sheet of paper all continuing education courses attended and for which you have received credit in the past two years);

14. duties you desire to perform in the hospital; (Be specific. If the hospital is to employ you and a current job description covers all areas of practice, so state.)

15. liability coverage information; if you are the employee of a member of this hospital's medical staff, have your employer answer the following two questions:

    - Is this applicant covered by your liability carrier? List carrier name, amount of coverage, and expiration date.

    - Is this applicant covered by his or her own liability insurance? List carrier name, amount of coverage, and expiration date.

The applicant should sign a statement authorizing the inspection of records and documents that may be pertinent to the evaluation of professional, moral, and ethical qualifications and competence to carry out the clinical privileges requested.

The AHP applicant should also sign a statement agreeing to

1. never engage in the practice of medicine as defined by the State Medical Practice Act, the State Board of Medical Examiners, or other statutory or regulatory provisions;

2. adhere to the medical staff bylaws, rules and regulations and hospital or facility policies as they apply to actions or duties;

3. comply with all relevant requirements of the Joint Commission on Accreditation of Healthcare Organizations as interpreted by the hospital;

4. wear proper identification indicating name and title whenever in the hospital; and

5. maintain adequate liability insurance coverage at all times.

Reappointment of Allied Health Professionals

Licensed independent allied health professionals should also be reappointed at least every two years in the same manner as medical staff members. The reappointment form should include the following:

1. confirmation of current license, registration or certification;

2. confirmation of the current liability carrier, address, policy number and amount of coverage;

3. a list of any liability litigation, claims, or settlements since the previous reappraisal or now pending;

4. any change in employment status;

5. any change desired in privileges or patient services allowed in the hospital (if additional privileges are requested, supporting information on education and training should be included);

6. any health status problems that would keep the professional from performing the privileges or tasks requested;

7. relevant continuing education programs completed since the previous appraisal.

The reappointment should be routed through the department, credentials and executive committees for recommendations, and to the governing body for final action in the same manner as a medical staff reappointment. Performance data with regard to the practitioner in question must be included.

Figure 7-1. Steps in Routing an Application.

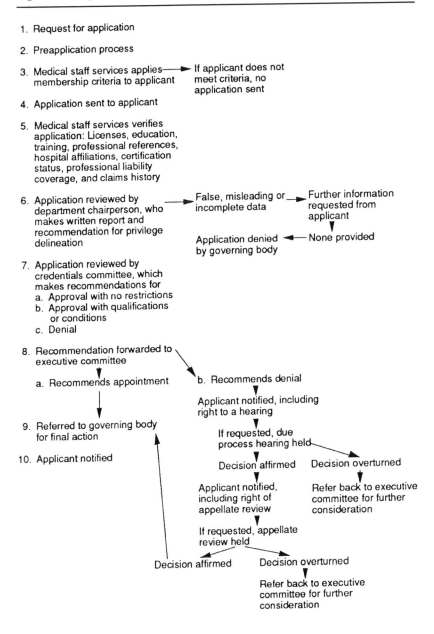

1. Request for application

2. Preapplication process

3. Medical staff services applies ⟶ If applicant does not membership criteria to applicant meet criteria, no application sent

4. Application sent to applicant

5. Medical staff services verifies application: Licenses, education, training, professional references, hospital affiliations, certification status, professional liability coverage, and claims history

6. Application reviewed by ⟶ False, misleading or ⟶ Further information department chairperson, who incomplete data requested from makes written report and applicant recommendation for privilege delineation Application denied ⟵ None provided by governing body

7. Application reviewed by credentials committee, which makes recommendations for
   a. Approval with no restrictions
   b. Approval with qualifications or conditions
   c. Denial

8. Recommendation forwarded to executive committee

   a. Recommends appointment   b. Recommends denial

   Applicant notified, including right to a hearing

9. Referred to governing body for final action   If requested, due process hearing held

10. Applicant notified   Decision affirmed   Decision overturned

   Applicant notified, including right of appellate review   Refer back to executive committee for further consideration

   If requested, appellate review held

Decision affirmed   Decision overturned

   Refer back to executive committee for further consideration

CONCLUSION

Whereas it is the responsibility of the medical staff organization to evaluate the information on applicants for medical staff membership and privileges, it is the responsibility of the medical staff services professional (MSSP) to gather the information. Credentialing policies and procedures in place in the hospital must be applied objectively and equally by the MSSP to each applicant. The MSSP must be alert to potential problems and initiate further investigation whenever there is questionable, equivocal or negative information on an applicant.

The vast majority of applicants for medical staff privileges will be well-trained and well-qualified practitioners. It is the unqualified or substandard few whom the MSSP needs to keep a watch for. When verifying information returned to the hospital is incomplete, vague, or negative, the MSSP must take the initiative to start the process of further checking. Medical staff leaders are frequently inexperienced in these matters and will look to the MSSP for guidance.

As mentioned earlier, medical staff leaders should be asked by the MSSP in these cases to make telephone calls to peer references, training program directors, or past hospital affiliations in an effort to clarify vague or incomplete information or confirm (or disconfirm) negative information. Respondents will frequently be willing to discuss physician-to-physician or administrator-to-administrator sensitive information they do not want to put in writing. An effort should be made to obtain names of additional references for the purpose of checking further into reports of professional problems. All persons contacted should be encouraged to put the information in writing to the hospital, but should they be unwilling, the person making the call should prepare a memo to the file that contains a summary of the conversation.

For each applicant, the information gathered should be sufficient to dispel any discomfort in recommending appointment and clinical privileges or be sufficient to demonstrate the unreasonableness in doing so (in which case the appointment should be denied).

When the credentials file is completed, the MSSP is responsible for routing it through the appropriate medical staff channels to the governing body (see Figure 7-1). Supporting the credentials process is one of the most critical responsibilities of the MSSP. In providing support, medical staff bylaws and credentialing policies should be followed to the letter. Accurate, thorough, and complete documentation should be obtained on each applicant. Legal counsel should be consulted when there is a question as to whether the hospital is carrying out the process appropriately. Medical staff and hospital leaders will look to the MSSP to guide the process skillfully and diligently.

Chapter 8

The Managed Care Credentials Process

Madeline Schneikart, CMSC

ADVENT OF CREDENTIALING IN MANAGED CARE ORGANIZATIONS

Managed care began as early as 1945 in California with Kaiser Permanente forming a hospital-based staff model health maintenance organization. As the Joint Commission on Accreditation of Hospitals formed and began accrediting hospitals in the early 1950s, Kaiser Permanente, along with other acute care facilities, addressed credentialing standards in a somewhat unified manner. There was virtually no "ambulatory care credentialing" being performed by the provider groups or in managed care health plans. This was true until case law began to move into the managed care arena in the late 1980s and began to hold managed care organizations to the same standards for credentialing imposed on hospitals by case law beginning as early as 1965.

In these early days of corporate managed care, health plans were still operating under the assumption that they were merely third-party payers and not health care institutions. The rule was to serve their corporate accounts with rapidly pulled-together networks of practitioners for geographic areas, focusing on formulated ratios of primary care practitioners and specialists as determined to be needed to serve a specified number of insured lives. Health plans were making assumptions that they had no public duty to ensure the quality of the practitioners being contracted and expected the hospitals to perform that piece of work for them if they were under contract.

There were also some managed care attorneys advising health plans to operate under the theory that "what they didn't know about the practitioners could not harm them." The operative push to put networks into place very quickly generally disallowed the effort to be cautious about the quality of all the practitioners in the networks.

In the early days of managed care, especially in metropolitan areas, most of the well-established and high-quality practitioners had busy practices of full-pay patients still insured by indemnity plans and also supported by much more liberal Medicare benefits. Many of the practitioners rushing to join the newly formed managed care networks were the younger, less experienced, less well-established, and in some cases, less well-trained of the available practitioners. There is a general perception that the consequences of this trend resulted in a steady decline of the quality of care being provided in the managed care networks in some parts of the country.

Typically the recruiting of network practitioners consisted of initially contracting with a given hospital and subsequently sending invitations to medical staff members of the contracted facility to join the network. These invitations were often based on the number of specialists and primary care practitioners needed in a particular geographic area. The first practitioners to apply were generally accepted "de facto," based on their hospital credentialing and medical staff membership. Typically, the only criteria of the health plans for contracting with hospitals were that the hospitals be Medicare providers and Joint Commission on Accreditation of Healthcare Organizations (JCAHO)-accredited.

This was, unfortunately, also during the period when JCAHO was suffering its own problems of being accused of not providing such an excellent survey process. In October, 1988, the *Wall Street Journal*[1] published a scathing report about the poor quality conditions found in some hospitals which had recently been accredited by JCAHO. The result of this public scrutiny of the JCAHO accreditation process led to increased federal oversight and subsequent federal sanctions against hospitals.

CASE LAW FOR MANAGED CARE CREDENTIALING

A precedent-setting court case against a health plan in 1989 clearly spelled out a shocking interpretation of culpability for health plans for the quality of practitioners contracted into managed care settings (see Chapter 17). The health plan was held liable for negligent credentialing based upon "ostensible agency" just as hospitals have been held liable for many years. The parallel was clear to the courts. Practitioners were typically not employees of either hospitals or health plans. Health plans published lists of practitioners from which patients could select their primary care practitioners. The primary care practitioner would serve as the "gate keeper" for access to specialty care. Therefore, insured patients had limited choice of practitioners and were at the mercy of the health plan's selection of practitioners. Yes, patients could "go out of network" according to the health plans, but doing so resulted in limited or greatly decreased insurance coverage. This was not considered a real choice by the courts. The final interpretation of the courts indicated that publication of network practitioner lists was in itself de facto evidence of the duty owed to the unsuspecting insured public for the quality of health care plan practitioners offered by the health plan.

The larger health plans realized it would be beneficial to have industry standards. JCAHO was not an option as a potential accreditation organization and definer of standards because they had backed out of the managed care accreditation market by this point in time. The National Committee for Quality Assurance (NCQA) accepted the challenge to develop and implement universal accreditation standards for health plans and managed care organizations.

HISTORY OF NCQA STANDARDS FOR MANAGED CARE CREDENTIALING

The NCQA accreditation process for managed care organizations was initiated in 1991. The process has evolved with annual refinements to the standards. The Standards Interpretation Group has also implemented over time, through published surveyor guidelines, a more objective survey process. NCQA considered credentialing a critical function and heavily weighted the credentialing standards. Other surveyed areas include quality improvement, members' rights and responsibilities, preventive health services, utilization management, and medical records.

HISTORY OF DELEGATED CREDENTIALING

Health plans began to credential practitioners with whom they contracted for services. Many provider organizations were unwilling to sign contracts if it meant each of their practitioners would have to make individual application to multiple MCOs. It became clear that a compromise was needed. This resulted in the practice of "delegating" the credentialing process to organizations such as hospitals which were believed to have access to the knowledge and expertise to manage this process. This was overseen by a system of health plan audits to ensure that the organizations did, in fact, have sound credentialing processes in place. If, upon on-site audit, these organizations were deemed to have processes that met NCQA credentialing standards, the various health plans "delegated" the process on an annual basis to the organizations with periodic re-visits and audits. While the health plans were not really relieved of the responsibility of the outcomes with the process, delegation of credentialing served two important purposes. The cost of individually credentialing each contracted practitioner fell back on the provider groups and out of the cost centers of health plans, and there were better relationships with the contracted groups. Upstream liability to the health plans was still a risk, but most of the plans considered it a business risk worth taking to gain relief from an otherwise nettling problem.

NCQA addresses delegated credentialing in its MCO standards. Delegation can be partial (verification only) or full (verification and decision-making authority). Organizations that have received any delegation from MCOs are randomly selected to be surveyed by NCQA to assure that the MCO has provided appropriate oversight of the delegated functions.

Delegation can take on a new dimension when credentials verification is "outsourced" to a credentials verification organization (CVO). In 1996, NCQA began certifying CVOs. Oversight of outsourced credentials verification is obviated when an MCO contracts with a certified CVO (see Chapter 9).

Some health plans have made their own delegation programs more stringent than the minimum NCQA standards. Provider groups that want to receive delegated status from multiple health plans must carefully review delegation requirements of each health plan, because requirements can vary widely. It is critical that the extent of the delegation (partial or full) is clearly defined and understood by all parties. The lowest common denominator becomes the rule rather than the exception as no two health plans seem to have exactly the same set of delegation rules. Most provider groups contract with up to 30 or 40 health plans. Careful review is necessary to determine what process to put into place in order to meet the credentialing requirements of all contracted health plans. It is definitely to the provider group's advantage to receive full (rather than partial) delegation for this activity by as many contracted health plans as possible. Full delegation will eliminate the necessity for duplicative (and costly) credentialing and, more importantly, expedite activation of contracts.

NCQA CREDENTIALING STANDARDS

The NCQA credentialing standards are quite prescriptive and attempt to be precise on what is expected to be verified and what is considered to be appropriate sources as well as allowable time frames. This set of requirements has also evolved over time and continues to be refined. The 1998 NCQA *Surveyor Guidelines for the Accreditation of Managed Care Organizations,*[2] Credentialing Standards 1 to 13 contain the following elements.

Standards CR 1.0 through CR 1.9 address the requirements for documenting who will be credentialed and how that will be done. MCOs usually meet these standards by writing policies and procedures or a credentialing plan. These documents must address all of the following:

1. scope of practitioners covered (must include all practitioners except hospital based physicians who have no independent contract with the MCO and physicians practicing in free-standing facilities, e.g., mammography centers, urgent care centers and surgicenters);

2. criteria and primary source verification of information used to meet criteria;

3. process used to make decisions;

4. the extent of delegated arrangements for credentialing;

5. practitioner rights to review information submitted support of credentialing applications (peer review protected documents are excluded from review);

6. the process for notification of practitioners of any information which varies substantially from information rendered by the physician on application;

7. the practitioner's right to correct erroneous information;

8. the medical director or other designated health care professional's direct responsibility and participation in the credentialing program;

9. the process used to ensure the confidentiality of all information obtained in the credentialing process.

Standard CR 2 requires the managed care organization to designate a credentialing committee that makes recommendations regarding credentialing decisions.

Standard CR 3 provides the minimum list of mandated information that must be verified from primary sources or other sources as indicated as well as specific exceptions and advice of approved sources for each when multiple sources are available. They include licensure, clinical privileges at a primary admitting facility, Drug Enforcement Administration (DEA) registration as applicable, education and training for dentists and physicians (unless board certified panel members), board certification with the exception of chiropractors, work history (review only), malpractice insurance coverage, and history of liability claims resulting in settlements or judgments.

Standard CR 4 discusses several mandated pieces of information that must be included on the practitioner application form regarding Americans with Disabilities Act (ADA) issues concerning inability to perform essential functions of the position with or without accommodation, lack of present illegal drug use, history of loss of license and felony convictions, history of loss or limitation of privileges, and attestation to correctness and completeness of the application information, as completed.

Standard CR 5 lists additional information that must be received by the managed care organization prior to making a final credentials decision. That list includes a National Practitioner Data Bank (NPDB) query, a state licensing query, and information on Medicare and Medicaid sanctions activity.

The standards include the following about elements for primary source verification and a discussion of how the elements are surveyed: licensure validation as well as sanctions activity or limitations from the various approved licensing boards, e.g., the State Board of Medical Examiners, (or the Federation of State Medical Boards), the Podiatric Licensing Board, the State Board of Chiropractic Examiners, the State Board of Dental Examiners; DEA registration; liability insurance coverage in limits as determined adequate by the managed care organization; NPDB query (includes professional liability insurance claims history for five years, and as the Medicare and Medicaid sanctions list has now been added to the NPDB as of March of 1997, it is provided that the NPDB query will address this item); board certification or highest level of training; a review of the practitioner's employment history for chronological gaps; and hospital privileges in good standing at the practitioner's primary admitting facility.

The standards are explicit as to the acceptable variations of obtaining "primary source" verifications for both initial credentialing as well as recredentialing. The DEA registration, for instance, may be considered "verified" by producing a current and valid copy of the DEA certificate. The National Technical Information Systems (NTIS) tapes or NTIS-CD ROM also may be used for this verification. The face sheet of a current professional liability insurance policy will suffice for verification of currently valid insurance coverage. The NPDB may be used to verify both the professional liability claims history for five years and the Medicare or Medicaid sanctions (since March of 1997). The American Medical Association (AMA) Masterfile may be substituted for verification of training and education rather than writing to the actual training institution. The American Board of Medical Specialties or the American Osteopathic Association may be used for verification of board certification. Several rationales are included in the standards regarding credentials verification for dentists, chiropractors and podiatrists. As these interpretations are continuing to evolve, this general discussion is not intended to be an adequate substitute for purchasing and studying the current set of standards and surveyor guidelines.

The standards specify a strict time frame in which verifications must be accomplished. The managed care organization has 180 days from the date of the practitioner's signature on the application in which all required information must be verified and the decision made. This is referred to as the "180 day rule."

Standard CR 6 describes the mandated initial office site visit to all primary care practitioners and all Obstetricians/Gynecologists. There follows rationale and required content of the site visit. It basically covers physical accessibility, appearance, adequacy of waiting and examining room space, availability of appointments, and adequacy of medical record-keeping.

A medical record review sheet is found in the standards as an Appendix entitled, "Guidelines for Medical Record Review" and is strongly recommended for use. The guidelines contain 21 points of review and NCQA considers six of them to be critical. The medical records review standard is not found in the credentialing standards but in the medical records standards. It is mentioned here as this review is frequently performed concomitantly with the administrative office site visits at initial and recredentialing intervals.

Both the office site visits and the medical records reviews may be delegated to another agency with the same responsibilities for oversight for the quality of the contract performance as for delegated credentials verification. CVOs are not currently certified for the site review or medical records process, but can contract to perform these services with oversight by the managed care organization.

NCQA RECREDENTIALING STANDARDS

Standards CR 7 through 10—recredentialing standards—mirror those of the JCAHO by insisting on a formal recredentialing review and reverification of certain elements at least every two years after initial credentialing. The elements to be reverified for recredentialing include: licensure, status of clinical privileges at the practitioner's primary admitting facility, DEA and state narcotics registrations, board certification, malpractice insurance coverage and history of malpractice claims, a current signed attestation statement with prescribed questions relating to illegal drug usage, ADA issues concerning accommodation for disabilities, NPDB query, sanctions or limitation on licensure, Medicare or Medicaid sanctions activity, and a series of quality of care review data on primary care practitioners including member complaints, information from quality improvement activities, member satisfaction, and site visits as previously discussed.

CR 10 mandates a revisit to practitioners' offices at recredentialing to verify any changes in the facility, equipment, staffing or medical record-keeping practices that might affect quality of care or service provided to the MCO member/patients, since the initial or previous visit. 1999 Standards require that primary care practitioners who have more than 50 MCO members have office site visits at recredentialing every two years after initial credentialing. This standard applies to chiropractors and podiatrists only if they are designated as primary care practitioners. No site review tool is prescribed but guidelines are provided for the types of administrative systems to be reviewed.

Standard CR 11 describes the managed care organization's policies for altering the conditions of the practitioner's participation based on issues of service and quality of care. These policies must define the range of actions the organization may take to improve performance prior to termination. There is also a standard relating to a formal appeal process for practitioners (see Chapter 17). This is a fairly new standard, as previously, most practitioner managed care contracts were styled "termination for no cause." There has been new case law taking this issue into the traditional interpretation of the courts for hospitals, i.e., practitioners must be afforded due process. Policies must include corrective action steps that may be taken to improve performance prior to termination.

Standard CR 12 provides for credentialing standards relating to the initial and ongoing assessment of organizational providers, e.g., hospitals, surgical centers, and other institutions with whom the organization contracts. These standards relate to the organization being in good standing with state and federal regulatory bodies, holding an accrediting body's status of accreditation, and the requirement to review and ascertain these good standing statuses at least every three years.

Standard CR 13 is the final credentialing standard and relates to an MCO delegating any credentialing or recredentialing activity and the oversight required for such delegations. A delegation document is required and the standards address specific components of what information should be contained therein including outlining specific responsibilities of the delegated agency, the delegated activities, the process for evaluation of the contract, and the remedies for non-performance of the delegation contract. The reference to waiver of oversight is not described in the managed care standards, but is described in the Introduction[3] to the NCQA CVO standards, which states:

> CVO Certification reduces duplicative oversight and inefficient gathering of information by managed care organizations and CVOs. For managed care organizations seeking to be accredited by NCQA, CVO Certification takes the place of health plan reviews of a CVO's structure and performance in verifying practitioner credentials. Accordingly, MCOs that contract for credentials verification with an organization that has been certified by NCQA will be exempt from the due-diligence oversight requirements specified in NCQA Credentialing Standard 13.0 for all verification services for which the organization has been certified.

CR 13 also addresses the right of the MCO to approve and terminate individual practitioners and the requirement for evidence that the MCO evaluates the agency's capacity to perform the delegated activities in accordance with NCQA standards prior to delegation, and annually. There is a discussion of the need for the MCO to continuously monitor the quality of the delegation contract and provide for an annual on-site oversight review of the delegate's operations. The major exception to this is that, if a CVO is certified by NCQA, the MCO can assume that the delegate is carrying out responsibilities in accordance with NCQA standards. In these cases the MCO does not need to conduct an annual audit or evaluation and the reports required may contain only the information necessary for the MCO to ensure that the delegate is meeting the MCO's needs.

CATEGORIES OF PRACTITIONERS

The NCQA credentialing and recredentialing standards address five categories of practitioners: physicians (MDs and DOs), dentists, podiatrists, and chiropractors. Even though the standard also addresses "other licensed independent practitioners with whom it [the managed care organization] contracts or employs who treat members outside the inpatient setting and who fall within its scope of authority and action,"[4] NCQA is officially silent about who these other practitioners are. Physician specialties specifically excluded from the credentialing requirement include all exclusively hospital-based practitioners who do not independently contract with the MCO or otherwise attend patients outside of a hospital setting (pathologists, radiologists, anesthesiologists, and emergency medicine physicians). The rationale for excluding these specialties is that these groups are under contract with the hospital and have no independent relationship with the MCO. Also excluded are any specialists who work exclusively in outpatient facilities. Only dentists who provide care under the MCO's medical benefits are required to be credentialed by the MCO. As of the 1997 edition of the standards, dentists providing normal dental care under a dental plan are excluded. As mentioned earlier, each MCO must identify the categories of practitioners covered by their credentialing and recredentialing policies and have written criteria for evaluation of applicants.

COMPARISON OF NCQA AND JCAHO STANDARDS

The primary difference between NCQA and JCAHO standards for hospitals is that JCAHO hospital standards require delineated clinical privileges and NCQA does not. Therefore, NCQA does not have requirements which relate to current clinical competence. JCAHO has many requirements (such as peer recommendations) that focus on obtaining information which relates to a practitioner's current clinical competence to exercise specific delineated privileges. In addition, NCQA standards define specific elements for which verification is required. These requirements are generally consistent with the JCAHO standards for hospitals with the notable exception that the JCAHO standards tend to be more general. For example, NCQA requires that the practitioner's highest level of training be verified and identifies approved sources for this verification. JCAHO requires verification of education and training from "primary sources."

NCQA STANDARDS FOR BEHAVIORAL HEALTH NETWORKS

Managed Behavioral Health Organization (MBHO) standards appeared in 1997 as a separate set of standards specific to mental health networks.[5] They are approximately the same as the MCO standards with regard to credentialing and recredentialing. One additional element requires review of specialized training for non-traditional behavioral health care practitioners. Exceptions for primary source verification are identical and include DEA (a copy of the paper certificate will constitute verification) and work history (a review of chronological history with attention to gaps will suffice for this review). All other elements must be verified independently and include valid licensure, clinical privileges in good standing at a primary facility, graduation from an accredited professional school and/or highest training program applicable to the academic degree or licensure, board certification, if applicable, insurance coverage, NPDB query and claims history. As in MCO standards, the 180 day rule for verifications is required. Recredentialing is also required every two years and includes reverification of all elements with the exception of static information relative to education and training. The recredentialing process also includes current attestation statements by the applicant relative to current ability to perform with or without accommodation and absence of present illegal drug usage.

NCQA STANDARDS FOR PHYSICIAN ORGANIZATIONS

In 1997 NCQA issued standards relating to Physician Organizations. The credentialing and recredentialing standards do not vary from the MCO or the MBHO standards except when citing appropriate primary sources necessary for certain categories of allied health professionals.

EVOLUTION OF STANDARDS AND STANDARDS INTERPRETATION

Due to the youth of the NCQA organization relative to older accrediting bodies, evolution of standards seems to be accelerated to stay in touch with the industry's issues through field trials. Interpretations of appropriateness of primary sources for various categories of practitioners are evolving.

Some differences exist in standards for MCOs, Physician Organizations and MBHOs. The differing standards tend to address the various ways in which these organizations do business rather than any real differences among the various sets of credentialing standards.

ACCREDITATION SURVEY PROCESS FOR HEALTH PLANS

The NCQA survey for MCO accreditation covers a much broader area than just credentials issues and because of delegation usage by the health plans, a survey usually entails a multi-site audit of the delegation process as well. A survey of a health plan that delegates credentials verification to physician organizations or medical groups will generally include a few delegated group sites and conduct of an audit at the delegated groups' site to test the oversight of the delegating health plans. Health plans also experience an internal audit for those credentials processes and procedures that the health plan performs internally for non-delegated contracted practitioners.

JCAHO'S ROLE

JCAHO rejoined the managed care accreditation process and now accredits networks including Health Maintenance Organizations, Independent Delivery Networks, Preferred Provider Organizations, Independent Practice Associations, Physician Service Organizations and others under their Healthcare Network and Managed Care Plans Standards. A network is defined by JCAHO as "an entity that provides or provides for integrated health care services to a defined population of individuals. A network offers comprehensive or specialty services and is characterized by a centralized structure that coordinates and integrates services provided by component organizations and practitioners practicing in the network."[6] Eligibility criteria for networks include quality processes, applicable standards, geographic limitations, and identified scopes of service. All network component entities must be eligible under one of the many other sets of accreditation standards. After a network survey, a category of accreditation status is awarded to the overall network if all entities were found to be in compliance with the applicable standards.

JCAHO NETWORK STANDARDS

A helpful "Crosswalk" document published by JCAHO compares the 1997 NCQA standards with the 1998 JCAHO Network standards.[7] The JCAHO network standards are similar to the hospital standards in that they are less prescriptive than those of NCQA and provide more generic guidance in the areas of concern with a heavy emphasis on quality of care processes.

NCQA limits the scope of a credentialing program to five types of practitioners. JCAHO, on the other hand, reviews for all categories permitted by law and the network to practice independently in the network. JCAHO suggests that the defined process, at a minimum, includes an appeals procedure for practitioners. JCAHO does define certain elements for primary source verification including current licensure, relevant education, insurance, if required by the network, and NPDB query at the time of initial and reappointments. Unlike NCQA, JCAHO requires that clinical privileges be reviewed against training and education. Office practice evaluations are required for all primary care practitioners. Appointment periods must be no longer than two years. Clinical records must be evaluated for all primary care practitioners prior to initial appointment and at reappointment. The privileges must be component specific, or in other words, specific to the facility within the network in which numerous facilities are under an umbrella corporation or network. This concept harks back to the JCAHO hospital standard that addresses delineated clinical privileges being specific to the scope of services offered by the hospital.

URAC ACCREDITATION

The American Accreditation HealthCare Commission, formerly the Utilization Review Accreditation Commission (URAC), is a not-for-profit entity fairly recently founded in 1990 which joined the accreditation industry for managed health care. URAC initially focused on the accreditation of utilization review programs, but has since expanded its activities to include other accreditation programs in managed care, specifically with the focus on Preferred Provider Organizations (PPOs) and now CVOs.

URAC approaches its accreditation programs on a flexible modular approach in which managed care organizations can seek accreditation under several different sets of standards which best address that organization's range of services to their purchasers and consumers.

Standards are developed by a group of experts identified from across the country who determine which standards are appropriate for a particular aspect of managed care. Accreditation programs are available in the areas of utilization management, provider networks, health care practitioner credentialing, workers' compensation, utilization management, and workers' compensation networks. URAC began accrediting PPOs and similar networks in July of 1997. As of August, 1997, 15 states and the District of Colombia had utilization management organizations either mandated or deemed accredited by URAC.[8]

URAC's member organizations include the American Association of Health Plans, American Health Quality Association, American Hospital Association, American Medical Association, American Nurses Association, American Psychiatric Association, American Society of Internal Medicine, Association of Managed Health Care Organizations, Blue Cross Blue Shield Association, Health Insurance Association of America, National Association of Insurance Commissioners, National Association of Manufacturers, United Auto Workers International Union, and the Washington Business Group on Health.

CONCLUSION

The primary agencies providing accreditation options in managed care include NCQA, URAC and JCAHO. NCQA addresses health plans, physician organizations, managed behavioral health organizations and CVOs. URAC accredits CVOs, PPOs and Utilization Review Programs. JCAHO accredits networks and health care systems.

As we have seen in this chapter, there are variations in the accreditation standards of acute health care facilities and managed care organizations. The variations are principally due to differences in the business management of managed and acute care delivery systems. Variations are also due to the relative difference in the age of two industries. Managed care is much newer to the health care scene than acute care and is, in many cases, just now "coming of age" in some of the processes to quantify and improve quality. The standards will continue to evolve as the accrediting organizations mature.

NOTES

1. Walt Bogdanich, "Small Comfort: Prized by Hospitals as Seal of Approval, Accreditation Often Masks Substandard Patient Care," *The Wall Street Journal*, October 12, 1988.
2. National Committee for Quality Assurance, *1998 Surveyor Guidelines for the Accreditation of Managed Care Organizations* (Washington, DC: National Committee for Quality Assurance, 1998).
3. National Committee on Quality Assurance, "Introduction" in *1997 Standards for Certification of Credentials Verification Organizations* (Washington, DC: National Committee on Quality Assurance, 1997): 1.
4. National Committee for Quality Assurance, *1998 Surveyor Guidelines for Accreditation of Managed Care Organizations,* 141.
5. National Committee for Quality Assurance, *1997 Standards for Certification of Credentials Verification Organizations,* 61-71.
6. Joint Commission on Accreditation of Healthcare Organizations, "Introduction" in *1998-2000 Comprehensive Accreditation Manual for Health Care Networks* (Oakbrook Terrace, IL: Joint Commission on Accreditation of Healthcare Organizations, 1998): 1.
7. Joint Commission on Accreditation of Healthcare Organizations, "Crosswalk of 1997-National Committee for Quality Assurance (NCQA) Standards to 1998 Joint Commission Health Care Network Standards" (Oakbrook Terrace, IL: Joint Commission on Accreditation of Healthcare Organizations, 1997) 79 pages.
8. The American Accreditation HealthCare Commission/URAC, "About URAC" (Washington, DC: The American Accreditation HealthCare Commission/URAC Web site). Available at: http:\\www.urac.org. Accessed April 30, 1998.

Chapter 9

Credentials Verification Organizations

Madeline Schneikart, CMSC

HISTORY OF CREDENTIALS VERIFICATION ORGANIZATIONS

The first Credentials Verification Organizations (CVOs) were started by local medical societies to provide centralized credentialing services to hospitals within a limited geographic area. These early CVOs were usually started because of demand by physicians who were burdened by the duplication of credentialing that occurred at each hospital in which they held membership and privileges. In addition, many hospitals welcomed the opportunity to participate in centralized credentialing to reduce labor intensive, costly, and redundant services.

The growth of centralized credentialing services was limited by several factors. One problem was the perception that the use of a centralized service would jeopardize the hospital's accreditation status. The Joint Commission on Accreditation of Healthcare Organizations (JCAHO) has been silent on whether information collected by a third party would be acceptable as primary source documentation. In addition, some medical staff services professionals perceived these services as a threat to their job security. A third factor relates to concerns about confidentiality of sensitive credentialing documents.

When managed care organizations that sought National Committee for Quality Assurance (NCQA) accreditation began credentialing their practitioners, the need for centralized credentialing services exploded, and commercial CVOs entered the market to compete with existing medical society and health care association-sponsored verification services.

In addition, CVOs have been created by many health care systems and networks to provide credentialing services to components of their organization. For example, a health care system that includes multiple hospitals, a provider network, an ambulatory care center, a surgicenter and a home health agency, may find it more cost effective to create its own proprietary CVO which provides services only within the health system.

A large opportunity remains for improvement in true centralization. Thousands of hospitals and managed care organizations continue to duplicate requests for information on practitioners. But there are so many players that it becomes very difficult to obtain the broad level of cooperation needed to agree on processes, forms, and cycles to achieve an optimum level of centralization.

WHAT IS A CVO?

The acronym, CVO, initially was loosely interpreted as "centralized verification organization" and more recently became defined by NCQA as "credentials verification organizations" when NCQA introduced a certification process for CVOs in 1996.

A CVO provides verification of practitioners' credentials to a wide variety of customers. Customers include hospitals, health plans, medical groups, ambulatory care facilities, insurance companies, and others.

CVOs provide verification services to their customers, but because of the use of technology, particularly by commercial CVOs (as opposed to those sponsored by professional groups), today's CVOs are not restricted to providing services in a limited geographic area. Technology available today includes the use of electronic databases which can be queried using Internets as well as databases (such as the American Medical Association's Physician Masterful) that can be purchased by CVOs that have the capital to invest. Current limitations on growth and use of CVOs are related to the inability to get potential customers of CVOs to agree on credentialing cycles (e.g., recredentialing dates for practitioners), verification methods, and the credentialing product (i.e., will the customer receive the original verified documents, copies of verified documents or a transmittal report which confirms information that was verified).

Some CVOs consider their true customer to be the practitioners for whom verified information is continuously maintained. This verified information is sold to health plans, hospitals, and others. Costs are reduced for health plans and hospitals when the verified information can be resold numerous times. Therefore, the practitioners benefit because they avoid having to complete numerous applications and provide duplicative documentation to multiple entities, and health care organizations benefit because their costs are lowered, and typically, they receive verified information in an expedited manner.

SERVICES PROVIDED BY CVOS

A wide variety of services is offered by CVOs, including primary source verifications for initial and recredentialing, application management services, maintenance of information subject to expiration, allied health professional credentialing, physician office site surveys, software sales and service, evaluation of files, and consulting services.

The services that follow are often provided by commercial CVOs as well as CVOs which are proprietary to a health system.

Primary Source Verifications

Primary source verification describes the verification of information submitted by the applicant from the sources that produced the information. For example, if an applicant indicates that he attended a certain medical school for the years of "X to Y" and graduated on a certain date, then the medical school(s) indicated constitute the appropriate "primary source" with whom one should verify the information. There are, however, some allowances made as to which sources are considered appropriate. These variances are described in the respective standards of the various accreditation entities.

NCQA defines these sources in the most detail and frequently gives a list of choices to be made in the selection of sources based on the category of practitioner. In some cases the rationale is given in the *Surveyor Guidelines* published by NCQA.[1]

The JCAHO is considerably looser in its language on primary source verification, but in fact, tends to survey this area with the heavier hand. For example, JCAHO does not specifically state in their standards that peer references must be queried at the time of reappointment. But the use of peer references by hospitals is widespread to document that the practitioner has been evaluated by peers and, therefore, found to be currently competent. NCQA does not focus attention on current competence as most managed care operations do not attempt to delineate clinical privileges. Therefore, most managed care organizations do not query peers as part of their credentialing process for either initial credentialing or recredentialing.

NCQA, on the other hand, has imposed the requirement for verification that practitioners have not been sanctioned by the Health Care Financing Administration for misuse of the Medicare or Medicaid insurance programs. This check can be conducted via the Internet sanctions list or by querying the Federation of State Medical Boards (for MDs or DOs). The JCAHO has never addressed checking this sanctions list.

It is therefore incumbent on a commercial CVO to be very aware of the variations in the standards that might affect the client's accreditation status (whether through NCQA, JCAHO or both) if the CVO is being called upon to assist the client with development of a primary source verification program.

Application Management Services

Application management services refers to initial application or reapplication distribution, and collection and tracking of these documents prior to performance of the verification process. This means that the CVO mails applications to practitioners and tracks their return, rather than this process being performed by the hospital or health plan. This service is generally more sought after by managed care clients as they tend to perform credentialing activities for large networks all at once rather than spacing them out as is more the standard in acute care settings. Hospitals that use this service often rely on the CVO to manage reappointment applications, rather than initial applications, as they are generally not in the business of heavy recruiting for initial staff membership in the same volume as managed care groups "pulling up" new networks in geographic areas. Hospitals also prefer to manage the initial contact with new applicants.

Management of Information Subject to Expiration

Many CVO customers find it beneficial to contract with a CVO to maintain information that can expire in the intervals between credentialing decisions. For example, malpractice insurance, licensure, DEA registration, and other critical information is subject to expiration, but health care organizations obviously have an interest (either because of accreditation requirements or liability) in making sure that current information is continuously maintained.

Allied Health Credentialing

There is no uniform national definition of what types of health care professionals are classified as allied health professionals (AHPs). In the managed care setting, a practitioner who is not a physician is generally classified as an AHP. (In most hospitals, dentists and podiatrists are considered potential members of the medical staff and not AHPs. In some states, psychologists also qualify under state statutes for medical staff membership.)

Not all CVOs have experience with the nuances between credentialing physicians and AHPs. NCQA began to require credentialing of certain non-physician health care professionals in 1997. There is a reference in the 1997 MCO standards to "other independently contracted providers,"[2] but NCQA's official interpretation is that it does not specifically review files of practitioners other than physicians (MDs and DOs), dentists, chiropractors and podiatrists. The 1998 NCQA Managed Care Standards refer to AHPs required to be credentialed only as chiropractors, dentists and podiatrists, and other licensed independent practitioners with whom it contracts or employs who treat members outside the inpatient setting and who fall within its scope of authority and action. Documentation must, at least, address the scope of practitioners covered, criteria, and primary source verification of information used to meet the criteria, the process used to make decisions, and the extent of any delegated credentialing or recredentialing arrangements. The 1998 NCQA Managed Behavioral Health Standards mention psychologists and other types of mental health providers.[3]

If a health care organization chooses to use a CVO to verify the credentials of its practitioners, there should be confirmation that the CVO selected understands how to perform verifications on all the types of health care professionals that the organization needs to have credentialed.

Physician Office Site Surveys

NCQA standards for managed care organizations require a physician office site survey covering administrative systems and facilities as well as medical record review. JCAHO standards for networks are similar. Office site reviews must be conducted at initial credentialing for all primary care practitioners, obstetrician/gynecologists and "other high volume specialists" as determined by the managed care organization. At the time of recredentialing, primary care practitioners who have more than 50 MCO members must have an office site resurvey. In some cases, a CVO may contract to perform these services for a managed care organization. There is currently no NCQA standard for certification for this component of services offered by CVOs.

Software Sales/Service

Certain CVOs have developed proprietary credentialing software and have chosen to make it available for sale and service to clients. Some of the software is integrated to provide for both hospital and managed care data needs, but it is more frequently specific to either hospitals or managed care organizations. There are upsides as well as down sides to purchasing such proprietary software. Any type of software is subject to technological advances, and in order to run subsequent editions and enjoy continuing maintenance contracts with the developers, there is frequently a need to have the capital to stay current with hardware and software technology. This can be a very expensive proposition if a facility is not backed by sophisticated technology support. There also may be some disadvantages to the inability to extract ad hoc reporting with ease from such canned systems by unsophisticated computer users.

Evaluation of Files

Some CVOs contract to perform evaluation of files for clients. Many CVOs are unwilling to assume the potential liability associated with file evaluation because the CVO customer may make decisions solely based upon the

CVO's evaluation and recommendation. Liability generally lies with recommendations for decisions and decision-making.

Consulting Services

Some CVOs employ competent, experienced and credentialed staff who can offer expert consulting services on designing systems and programs for credentialing activities.

TO OUTSOURCE OR NOT TO OUTSOURCE TO A CVO

To outsource a service traditionally performed in-house frequently involves both raw economics and more ephemeral philosophical, focus, and risk considerations. There are numerous cost benefits to outsourcing and also the potential for some loss of control over processes.

Cost Benefits

The cost benefit of outsourcing a labor intensive clerical function is easy to justify. A larger CVO has already expended the capital outlay for access to numerous electronic databases, which are, in some cases, expensive to install and keep current. In addition, these electronic connections require critical access to competent information systems technologists who are not always available in-house for smaller organizations. The obvious benefit is that the overhead for these installations can be shared among numerous clients rather than individual organizations duplicating these expenses.

Efficiencies of Scale

When access is shared to certain databases that charge access fees, the charges can be spread out among numerous participating organizations rather than just one, resulting in savings for all participants.

Turn-Around Time

Turn-around time is generally improved in a CVO as individual employees are assigned certain tasks as full-time jobs. It is typical in a hospital medical staff services department for one individual to do multiple tasks and be subject to chronic distractions. Credentialing staff that are organized functionally assures that no other tasks are being performed and more personal attention can be given to the completion of the file verification process.

NCQA CVO CERTIFICATION

Standards

In 1996, NCQA introduced CVO standards for certification. The intent of the CVO certification process is to identify CVOs that perform credentialing activities in a manner that meets NCQA credentialing standards. Managed care organizations such as health plans, physician groups, and so on can then contract for services with a certified CVO and be relieved of the obligation to conduct audits of the CVOs' compliance with NCQA standards. The NCQA "Certified" CVO places a stamp of approval on the operations of the CVO which ensures that the standards for quality and choice of sources of information are consistent with the NCQA credentialing and recredentialing standards.

CVOs are initially surveyed by NCQA and may receive certification for one year. At the end of the first survey cycle, they are resurveyed and may receive certification for up to a three year period of time. The CVO is "certified" for the various elements of the credentials process. The individual elements cannot be certified if the overall survey of the CVO shows non-compliance with good business practices and an appropriate quality program. The oversight activity of the contracting entity is obviated only for those portions for which the CVO is certified. For example, if a CVO is not certified for the element of current, valid licensure to practice, then a contracting organization would have to provide oversight for the licensure verification portion of the process outsourced to the CVO.

There are six standards on which the CVO is reviewed.[4] Standard 1 relates to the CVO's written policies and procedures for verification, frequency of reporting, and data management of credentials. It is under this standard that the operational activities, methods, sources and processes are reviewed. NCQA has approved certain sources for the verification of various elements of the verification process. The certified CVO must adhere to those approved sources in its processes of verification. There is also a time frame which is acceptable for all verifications to be performed in order to be certified. The CVO has no more than 120 days to perform all required verifications so that the client has an additional 60 days to complete the evaluation, decision making and acceptance of a practitioner into its network.

Standard 2 reviews the internal quality program and processes based on accuracy, completeness, and meeting clients' needs. To survey this standard, the survey team pulls a random sample of completed files from the CVO's previous six months of work and reviews them in detail against the elements that the contract requires and the time frames within which the files are completed. While NCQA MCO standards require all elements of verification to be in the files, allowances are made for individualized contracts so that the CVO can perform only the scope of services under contract and not be held accountable for those pieces of verification that the contracting client might prefer to perform by means of an alternative method.

Standard 3 requires that aggregate data sources used be inspected so it is clear that the most recent source documents are being checked, that a tape or CD-ROM library of all previously utilized information is in a chronological file, and that logs are kept to indicate replacement dates and dates of use. This standard also addresses NCQA approval of the data sources for both individual as well as aggregate queries. Individual queries are database queries based on a per practitioner request. Aggregate database queries are arrangements in which CVOs purchase an entire database on a periodic basis and use that data for some period of time before "refreshing" the database with an entirely new set of replacement information.

Standard 4 requires organizational protection of confidentiality and integrity of practitioner files. This area of review includes physical security of computer systems, data security of computer systems and building security, physical access issues, as well as back up systems for data, personnel confidentiality, appropriate disposal of confidential materials, personnel orientation on confidentiality, disaster retrieval systems and a host of other implications of storing and handling confidential information.

Standard 5 reviews the CVO-developed application format for specified elements of information to be collected from applicants and includes areas of concern such as illegal drug usage, Americans with Disabilities Act legislation concerning accommodation for disabilities (see Chapter 17), loss of licensure, felony convictions, disciplinary activity, licensure limitations, and an attestation statement of accuracy and completeness.

Standard 6 discusses the process and procedures for reporting ongoing adverse actions to managed care clients who are under contract for this monitoring and where such notification conflicts with state or federal law. Some CVOs contract to monitor on an on-going basis new information being received through some methodology on previously processed practitioners. Those contracts include advising all clients under contract for this service of the receipt of new negative information on any of their previously processed practitioners. This is not a required component of a CVO service, but if it is offered as a service, the standards are applicable. The statement concerning conflict with state or federal law is merely a generic nudge for local CVOs to know their own local peer review statutes and not be in violation of them for passing on peer review information without following proper procedures.

Now also included in the certification process is recognition of the scope of service of the CVO. The CVO can be certified for processing for managed care organizations (MCOs), managed behavioral health organizations (MBHOs) and physician organizations (POs). As the MBHO standards and the PO standards have been more recently introduced than the original CVO standards, there are some certified CVOs that have not yet had the opportunity to be surveyed for all sets of standards.

ELEMENTS FOR CERTIFICATION

The ten elements for which a CVO may receive certification are as follows:

License to Practice
Drug Enforcement Agency Registration
Hospital Privileges
Board Certification/Residency Completion/Graduation from Medical or
     Professional School
Malpractice Claims History
National Practitioner Data Bank (NPDB) Query
Medical Board Sanctions
Medicare/Medicaid Sanctions
Practitioner Application Processing
Malpractice Insurance

A CVO may request certification on any or all of the above elements. Therefore, when a health care organization contemplates using a CVO, the organization must match the elements for which they want to outsource with the elements for which the CVO is certified.

THE NCQA SURVEY

The survey is typically scheduled after an application is received and a pre-survey assessment is completed, which includes a description of the business, standard contract forms, lists of practitioners credentialed during the previous six months, employee job descriptions, policies and procedures, and a host of other material. A CVO must have been in business with policies and procedures in place at least six months before it is eligible for survey.

The survey team is composed of two members. One member is an NCQA staff representative and usually performs the administrative review of the CVO. The second member of the team is a Certified Medical Staff Coordinator and generally limits his or her portion of the survey to the actual review of the credentials files for the elements of the contract, the timeliness of the turn-around time, and the accuracy of the material provided for clients.

The survey is scheduled for one day and begins with a pre-survey conference. The survey includes a total review of administrative and operational functions of the CVO. A minimum of 75 credentials files are reviewed against the time frame allowed for the CVO to provide the verifications to the client (120 days). The accuracy and completeness of the credentials file is compared to the contract with the client.

The survey concludes with the equivalent to an exit conference during which the surveyors summarize findings. No indication of the outcome of the survey is discussed at the exit conference as the written findings are forwarded to the NCQA review committee and final determination on certification is made by that body.

A survey draft report is forwarded to the CVO after a few weeks and the CVO may comment on the reported findings. This presents an opportunity to correct any findings prior to the issuance of the final report. After the reply is received by NCQA, a final determination is made and results are forwarded to the CVO approximately 90 days post survey dates.

Successful initial surveys result in certification for a maximum period of one year. After a second survey, the CVO may be certified for up to three years for a maximum of the ten elements specified. If the CVO does not meet the general thresholds of the survey, it cannot be certified in any of the elements. However, having met the baseline criteria, the CVO can be certified for the number of elements it qualifies for within the certification process, based on survey findings in the review of each element.

The survey process is voluntary on the part of the CVO applicant and, as the surveys are costly, is undertaken with serious intent of success. The survey process has become virtually vital to any commercial CVO with plans to contract with any type of managed care organization. Due to the significance of certification within the managed care industry, it is virtually impossible to obtain a managed care CVO contract without maintaining CVO certification. The NCQA is clearly the leader in the industry in terms of general acceptability among managed care clients.

AAHCC CVO CERTIFICATION

In April of 1998, the American Accreditation HealthCare Commission (AAHCC), formerly the Utilization Review Accreditation Commission (URAC), approved standards for the accreditation of CVOs.[5] Actually the program offers two types of accreditation, one for CVOs that just handle verification of information and one for those that also conduct practitioner office site reviews. A significant additional component of the standards includes guidelines for site visits of practitioner offices. All other standards tend to closely resemble NCQA's certification standards and are designed to assess the same areas. They include the organizational structure, employee training, practitioner information collected, methods of verification, time frames for completion, security and confidentiality of information as well as the physician office site review.

One additional feature of this accreditation program is that AAHCC specifically addresses Preferred Provider Organizations (PPOs). The CVO standards, therefore, tend to have a slant toward the PPO industry.

AAHCC accreditation is much less prevalent than that of NCQA because, at the time of the writing, the program is new. It remains to be seen how well accepted this certification program will become and if CVOs will be forced to seek dual certification because of client demand (which will probably be driven by payer relationships). There does not seem to be any substantial difference between NCQA and AAHCC in terms of performance expectations of the CVO and duplication of this accreditation program with no acknowledgment of AAHCC's certification program by NCQA adds to the cost of doing business for CVOs.

JCAHO CVO GUIDELINES

JCAHO does not have an accreditation program for CVOs, but acknowledges that hospitals and other health care organizations may choose to use the services of a CVO. Therefore, JCAHO offers guidelines that it expects hospitals to use when outsourcing credentials verification to a CVO. Since 1996, the JCAHO *Comprehensive Accreditation Manual for Hospitals* has included a set of guidelines to be used by hospitals in determining qualifications of CVOs to perform credentialing verification services. In the 1997 standards, this issue is addressed in MS.5.4.3.2[6] and is described as "Eight Principles" for evaluating agencies that provide CVO services. The eight principles were published in an article by JCAHO in the *Federation Bulletin*[7] in 1996. The principles include:

1. The agency makes known to the user what data and information can be provided by it.

2. The agency provides documentation to the user describing how its data collection, information development, and verification process(es) are performed.

3. The user and agency agree on format for transmission from the agency of credentials information about an individual.

4. The user can easily discern what information transmitted by the agency is from a primary source and what information is not.

5. For information that can become out of date (for example licensure, board certification), the agency will provide the date that the information was last updated from the primary source.

6. The agency certifies that the information transmitted to the user accurately presents the information obtained by it.

7. The user can discern whether the information transmitted by the agency from a primary source is *all* the primary source information in the agency's possession pertinent to a given item or, if not, where additional information can be obtained.

8. The user can engage the quality control processes of the agency when necessary to resolve concerns about transmission error, inconsistencies or other data issues that may be identified from time to time.

There was no indication from JCAHO that these guidelines will be incorporated into the medical staff standards but rather are given as an example of standard MS 5.4.3.2, which discusses the hospital's process for initial granting of clinical privileges.

A comment about the foregoing guidelines is that items three to eight all tend to refer to methodologies of doing business in which not all CVOs are engaged. As mentioned elsewhere in this chapter, some CVOs choose to abstract data and send summary reports to clients rather than original documentation. This practice has been generally accepted in the managed care arena as opposed to the acute care client setting, which has traditionally demanded originals, or at the very least, copies of all documentation. CVOs that provide summary information, rather than originals or copies of all documentation, must recognize the potential liability associated with failure to disclose complete information. For example, if a CVO provides a summary report to a client that erroneously states that a practitioner has no Medicare sanctions but the practitioner does have sanctions, the CVO could be held liable for this error.

CVO OPERATING MODELS

There are many operating models for CVOs and the models reflect issues of client base, technological sophistication, size, capitalization, profit status, commercial status, public status, and captive status.

With over 250 CVOs in the marketplace at last approximation, it would be an exhaustive exercise to try to review the wide range of variations and permutations that characterize these varying businesses.

However, a few general comments follow related to some significant variations.

1. Certain CVOs were initiated in the managed care industry and are built for big business, high volume, streamlined services with no ability to customize the deliverables based upon individual client requests.

2. Other CVOs grew up in the physician professional organization environment and were primarily intended to service hospitals. These are sponsored by medical societies as non-profit, value added adjuncts to professional organizations.

3. CVOs have been created in some integrated delivery systems and are proprietary to entities within the health care systems.

4. Still other CVOs are sponsored by hospital trade organizations, again as value added services in a non-profit environment to member organizations.

5. In-house service departments have been built by several large insurance companies offering health care network insurance. Some have undergone CVO certification status but only service their internal organizations and in some cases, perhaps offer the service to physician groups with whom they have contracts.

6. Yet another variety are commercial organizations with private or public financial backing offering services as a for-profit business unit or organization to various categories of clients.

7. The final CVO model that comes to mind is the small independent operator, contracting with a small number of clients in a low overhead environment (cottage industry) which might be of service in a limited way to a much smaller client base with less sophisticated needs.

CVO COMPUTER OPERATIONS

Use of information systems technology within the various models of CVOs are as variable as is the technology and financing to support them. All CVOs need automation. The decision, then, that all CVOs have to make is whether to design and build a system in-house, or whether to purchase a software program that is available on the open market.

A good working system generically, at a minimum, should include a solid database design with a well-thought-out number of fields for pertinent information that needs to be captured. This will allow for the end result of report writing and processing that can be performed on a timely and convenient basis. The system also needs a good registration system that captures a full complement of information from applications that might be needed in reporting, tracking, prompting, expirations and exception reporting, time frames and tickler systems. It also should produce information fill for form letters of query and tracking on the number of attempts to verify information. Open memo fields are also desirable for notes to files from telephone contacts and other non-computerized functions of the process. If extremely high volume is anticipated, a scanning and indexing operation might also be in order for document management and retrieval.

Canned systems can have the drawback of canned reporting with little ad hoc reporting capabilities. Some use report writing software but the average credentialing technician is not generally sufficiently experienced in computer technology to be able to produce ad hoc reports. Therefore, in a small CVO using a canned reporting system, the obvious drawback could be the inability to produce reports for clients in formats desired or with the information needed or wanted. A well-designed system with open-ended architecture and a strong information system support staff can overcome this obstacle and produce ad hoc reports for clients as needed and in formats desired on a wide variety of information segments. These systems should be able to produce exception reports on a periodic basis to track and update time sensitive documentation as well as automatic prompts for recredentialing activities. Tracking various processes such as general mailings of applications or reapplications and their responses should be a computerized function of a well-designed system.

Attention also should be devoted to assessing various levels of reports from the database to include processing and tracking reports, management reports, volume reports, productivity reports by operator, and, of course, reports to assess turn-around time for processing, client specific practitioner lists, and any configuration of that data.

Some of the more sophisticated systems include application gathering via Internet data fills directly from applicants' offices. Previously completed applications can be re-sent electronically for updates at reappointment cycles and the paper exchange can be eliminated.

The scanning capabilities of some canned systems or stand-alone scanning systems can provide additional CD-ROM exchange of scanned documents. Some of the more advanced systems offer OCR (optical character reading) technology which implies the ability to digitize the scanned documents such that retrieval in actual text can be performed.

The long and the short of all of this readily available technology is that a prospective client should assess all needs of the operation and compare the available technology with the receptive technology of the CVO to determine if this is an easily accessible technology to the application from the end-user vantage point.

Electronic Transfer Capabilities

A wide variety of systems are available for transferring information, visual files, and application forms in an electronic format. Various methods available include diskettes of captured data from a credentialing software system, Internet transportation of documents as files through modem transfers, graphics transfers on either modem lines or CD-ROMs, and dial-up systems for direct extraction from a database with a limited access based on security levels. Much of the technology available is not particularly new to the world of technical industries, however, it is quite new in the arena of acute health care facilities. The only real issues to be assessed are not so much related to whether or not a particular methodology is available within the world of technology, but rather, is it practical given the constraints of the client base and the primary sources.

With such a wide variety of sophistication among both users and providers of information, it becomes awkward to be too out in front of the technology parade. If a user organization has excellent information systems support staff and a state-of-the-art system (rare in acute care health care facilities), the high technology operations of a CVO become something of a moot point.

Also, of course, main stream primary source operations such as the Education Council for Foreign Medical Graduates and the American Medical Association are anything but technically advanced in their provision of data. So having a state-of-the-art system at the CVO level is almost overkill and, of course, costly to operations in an already tight market. Few things are impossible to accomplish technically in this age of information. The more salient questions to address are feasibility, cost effectiveness, and ability to access the level of technology explored.

Dial-up Systems into CVO Database

Some CVOs make available a dial-up system technology, generally through a Citrix Server arrangement which allows clients to dial into the CVO's database to search on status of various elements of information that pertains to their practitioner base. The important information to query regarding these dial-up systems would be: how often is the database information refreshed; how is the database updated; what is the periodicity of the renewal of the information; what are the sources of the updated information, and other such information. This type of information-seeking allows the prospective client to understand fully the quality and timeliness of the information being provided by this type of "resalable" information.

Many CVOs operate on the assumption that the only way to break even on a verification service is the resale of information that is gathered for one client and used for additional clients. Other CVO operators do not believe that older information should be resold when it may not, in fact, be totally current and, therefore, currently valid information for the decision-making process.

SECURITY OF PRACTITIONER DATA

The security of practitioner data covers several areas of concern for a prospective client. There is, of course, the security of the practitioner data in the database applications. This type of security is implicit in the nature of access security to the actual database in which the information is housed.

There is also the issue of protection of paper information that passes through hands from the primary source that verifies the information to the housing of the information at the CVO. This process involves a number of policies of storage protection of the paper, copies of the completed files, and access to the physical storage as well as building security, disaster recovery plans, and appropriate disposal of paper and information.

There are CVOs developed by business-minded individuals who are totally unaware of the legal implications, case law, or legislative climates regarding traditional medical staff protections of peer review information. Procedures to take advantage of the protections to safeguard confidential and sensitive peer review information are usually well understood and followed in the hospital environment. Caution should be exercised in dealing with CVOs where it is apparent that there is inadequate knowledge and expertise in this area.

HOW TO SELECT A CVO THAT MATCHES YOUR BUSINESS OBJECTIVES

From all of the foregoing discussion, how then does one assess a prospective CVO for use in conjunction with a particular type of health care organization. It would seem clear that a search for philosophical and business matches should occur prior to making a decision to contract with any CVO.

Many categories of organizations are required to perform some level of credentialing activity in this age of managed care and mergers and acquisitions. The CVO of choice should not be selected only with an eye to economics but also from the perspective of understanding the nature of the entity with whom it seeks to contract.

Turn-around times, cost factors, integrity of data, compatibility of philosophy, service standards, industry knowledge, and a host of other considerations should be thoroughly demonstrated by an organization outsourced to perform this important function for a health care entity.

A recommended course of selection would be to first identify what the organization's needs are and communicate its priorities. It is difficult to address such intangibles if they are not stated by the contracting health care entity. If speed and cost are the most important requirements, then a CVO should be selected that can demonstrate the ability to dependably perform in that area. If depth of knowledge of the industry, consulting and integrity of data are at issue, then those areas should be plumbed prior to contracting. If electronic access is important, then it is important to bring technical personnel into the decision-making process to assess the capabilities of the proposed contractor.

There is also an issue of whether an organization is interstate in its business abilities. If, for instance, a health plan prefers to outsource primary source verifications and it operates on a national basis, it would be important to query a potential CVO to ascertain whether the CVO has experience and ability to perform outside of the state in which it is located, as there are some state-related differences in performing the duties of the contract.

NOTES

1. National Committee for Quality Assurance, *1998 Surveyor Guidelines for the Accreditation of Managed Care Organizations* (Washington, DC: National Committee for Quality Assurance, 1998).

2. Ibid., 1997.

3. National Committee for Quality Assurance, *1997 Standards for Certification of Credentials Verification Organizations* (Washington, DC: National Committee for Quality Assurance, 1997).

4. The American Accreditation HealthCare Commission/URAC, "About URAC" (Washington, DC: The American Accreditation HealthCare Commission/URAC Web site). Available at http:\\www.urac.org. Accessed April 30, 1998.

5. Joint Commission on Accreditation of Healthcare Organizations, *1998 Comprehensive Accreditation Manual for Hospitals*, August 1997 (Chicago: Joint Commission on Accreditation of Healthcare Organizations) MS-36

6. A. S. Buck, R. J. Corteau, P. Van Ostenberg, and P. M. Schyve, "Evaluating Agencies That Verify Practitioner Credentials - The Joint Commission Perspective," *Federation Bulletin* 83, (1996) 1.

Chapter 10

The Role of the Medical Staff in the Assessment and Improvement of Patient Care

Opal Reinbold

INTRODUCTION

The role of the medical staff in the measurement, assessment and improvement of patient care has been in the evolutionary process for a number of years. The medical staff has traditionally been delegated the responsibility for ensuring that the same level of appropriate, high-quality care is provided throughout the health care organization with which they are affiliated. In past years, most of the focus for the medical staff review process has been only on the care rendered by the physicians in the organization. Starting in the late 1980s, the focus of quality review programs has broadened to encompass not only physician care and credentialing, but review of the entire care process for patients and families. This broader process is commonly referred to as "quality improvement." Figure 10-1 illustrates the evolution of approaches to quality assessment in health care organizations from the 1960s to the present.

Advent of Quality Improvement

"Although individual competence and performance remain important, good patient care and acceptable (or better) outcomes are viewed as the product of all individual actions *and interactions* that relate directly or indirectly to the care received by the patient. Performance is thus a reflection of a variety of internal organization systems and subsystems that underlie essential day to day functions. Human error may occur within these often complex systems, but remedial actions are usually most appropriately directed to the system, not the human."[1] "Although identifying and solving isolated problems will always be a concern, quality improvement recognizes that the more significant advances will result from focusing on important functions and processes in order to improve the norm of performance."[2]

183

Figure 10-1. Evolution of Approaches to Quality Assessment.

IMPLICIT REVIEW
(Morbidity and Mortality Review)

TIME LIMITED STUDIES
(Retrospective Audits)

ONGOING MONITORING AND EVALUATION
(Quality Assurance)

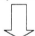

INTEGRATED PROGRAM OF CONTINUAL IMPROVEMENT
(Quality Improvement/Agenda for Change)

The role of medical staff leaders has changed with the advent of quality improvement. Organizations, whether they be acute care hospitals, physician groups, for profit or not for profit, have been called upon by regulators, consumer groups and the general public to provide ongoing data validating the quality of care given and, when possible, providing comparative data with other, similar facilities.

As noted by J. Castro in a *Time* magazine cover story, "There are two kinds of prices in America today; regular prices and health care prices.... America's medical bills are something else. They flow from a surreal world where science has lost connection with reality, where bureaucracy and paperwork have no limit, where a half-hour tonsillectomy costs what an average worker earns in three weeks."[3] This closer public focus has created a need for more systematic, integrated review of the care process which is characterized in the quality improvement process.

In the traditional "quality assurance" (QA) programs, regulatory and accrediting agencies placed the majority of the responsibility for the review of care on the medical staff. Most QA programs consisted of inspection systems, which differed somewhat by facility, and focused on "negative incidents of care" in order to attempt to identify low quality events, practitioners, or individual providers whose care or practices may have been unacceptable compared to their peers. This list of negative incidents of care, bad results or deviations from what might be considered "the standard of care," when compared to a provider's peers, initiated a review of the provider's care, most often by a retrospective review of the patient's medical record. This review was usually done by a peer, with the intent of identifying the "bad apples" and taking action to address the care provided by the physician. Most of the individual cases reviewed were deemed to be appropriate, given the circumstances at the time of the care given. Over a period of years, this system yielded few actions that improved the overall care for patients nor did it address the complex systems issues that most often contribute to the negative incidents of care.

As Donald Berwick stated, systems are frequently the root-cause of quality problems in health care facilities. "A test result lost, a specialist who cannot be reached, a missing requisition, a misinterpreted order, duplicate paperwork, a vanished record, a long wait for a CT scan, an unreliable on-call system—these are all-too-familiar examples of waste, rework complexity, and error in the doctor's daily life…For the average doctor, quality fails when systems fail.[4]

The past focus of QA on individual case review, subjective results (which may differ by facility), and a segregation of the review process by physician, nursing, or other disciplines, did not provide the overall data needed to present ongoing patient care outcome results or the quality improvement process to a public that was demanding more information to assist them in their care choices.

The following chapter presents summary information, examples, and suggestions for a structure to address this broader focus. The opportunities for the medical staff services department in this more broadened focus are many.

COMPONENTS OF THE MEDICAL STAFF QUALITY IMPROVEMENT PROCESS

Definition

Whether an organization chooses to call their process quality assurance, quality assessment, or quality improvement, the process as defined should include, but not be limited to, the following:

1. a process that is integrated with all care providers, led by the medical staff, for ongoing, systematic review of all care and service;

2. a process that involves an identification of the key processes of care and services (i.e., assessment of patients, the use of medications, operative and other invasive procedures, the education of patients and families);

3. a process that provides for an identification of indicators that determine the effectiveness of the care process, which are observable, measurable and consistent whenever possible;

4. a process for documented assessment of the results of the data collected from the indicators; and

5. a consistent reporting process for conclusions, actions and follow-up designed to identify opportunities to improve care and service, through improvement of systems, and by addressing individual performance issues, when they occur.

Structure

The structure of the quality improvement process will vary by organization. The board of trustees has the ultimate responsibility for the quality of care. The board delegates the review of clinical care to the medical staff leaders, and the review of hospital and support systems to the administrative team members. Most traditional QA structures have provided for medical staff and clinically-related information to flow through the medical staff structure, to the medical executive committee (MEC), then to the board. The hospital-re-

Figure 10-2. Quality Assurance Information Flow.

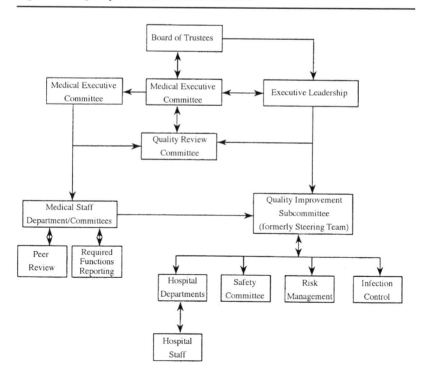

lated information, then, flowed through the hospital departments, to the management group, through executive leadership, and then to the board (see Figure 10-2).

In this structure, nature of the reporting, which was based on individual case review, dictated that the information was specific to medical staff performance and was not appropriate for information sharing outside of the medical staff.

The traditional process encouraged the segregation of information and activity in response to the review process. In the early 1980s, with the introduction of the concepts of "continuous quality improvement," the focus for the review process was recognized to be inadequate.

If 80 to 90 percent of the issues identified were related to systems problems as the quality improvement process indicated, then the focus of the review process on individual performance, departmental activities, and discipline-specific review did not encourage collaborative review and improvement activities. The new, continuous improvement processes review has created a change in the structure for the quality process, for the reporting of information, and for the follow-up activities that are generated out of the review.

(It is essential to note here that the individual case review, assessment and follow-up process remains in the medical staff structure. If the review of over-all data, through more intense assessment, reveals that there may be an individual performance issue, this process remains inside the medical staff peer review process for follow-up and in rare cases, disciplinary procedures.)

The changes, as reflected in Figure 10-3, provide for an integration of systems-related information through the introduction of a "quality council." A quality council is made up of medical staff leaders and hospital leaders, and in that way, provides a means for the review of the overview data sets and a collaborative approach to the prioritization and follow-up of any improvement opportunities.

The structure for the process includes:

1. Board of Trustees (Figure 10-3, 1);

2. Medical Executive Committee (Figure 10-3, 2);

3. The Quality Council (Figure 10-3, 3);

4. The Quality Review Committee (Figure 10-3, 4);

5. The Medical Staff Departments and Committees (Figure 10-3, 5);

6. Quality Improvement Subcommittee (Figure-3, 6);

7. Multidisciplinary teams (Figure 10-3, 7).

Figure 10-3. Performance Improvement Information Flow.

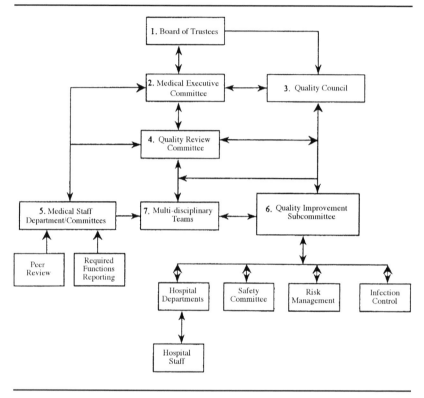

The functions of the various committees in the structure follows.

Board of Trustees

As indicated, the board of trustees has the ultimate accountability for the quality of care in the organization. Most boards choose to create a sub-committee to review this information in-depth, which includes overview data for the organization's process, and the credentialing information for the medical staff. The subcommittee may be identified as the quality sub-committee of the board or the joint conference committee of the board, and is made up of representatives from the board, medical staff leadership, and hospital leaders. The subcommittee's major function is to review information provided on the data collection, assessment, and improvement activities of the organization; to assure that appropriate mechanisms for follow-up are in place; and to ensure that the information is being used to improve care and provide for competent care by credentialing the medical staff and through the competency process for the organization.

At least annually, this group should review the quality plan and the evaluation by the leaders in the organization of their own effectiveness in the quality process. The board should also perform a self-assessment to identify any areas for improvement in order to ensure that appropriate oversight for the process is provided.

Medical Executive Committee (MEC)

The role of the MEC is similar in the new process to that of the traditional role. The overall data, in the aggregate, trended format, is presented to the MEC for review and comment, with recommendations from the medical staff quality oversight committee represented here by the quality review committee (QRC) for any approvals or actions by the MEC. Information in a summary format is also provided to the MEC for information sharing at a department or committee level, which includes any multidisciplinary activity in place to address systems issues, new policies and procedures recommended to address issues, and recommendations sought to move forward on team- or systems-related activities from the quality council or QRC of the medical staff.

On a scheduled basis, each of the medical staff departments or divisions should report a summary of their improvement activities and overall data from the peer review process. This information may include the multidisciplinary activities, the departmental activities (including any appropriate policies and procedures for approval), and an overview of the peer review activities. The overview of peer review activities may include a listing of the top three types of cases that fell out of criteria for review and any special studies generated out of peer review activity. A separate section of this report may include any disciplinary or educational actions taken to address individual case review with recommendations for approval by the MEC.

Quality Council

As indicated on the information flow diagram in Figure 10-3, the quality council provides information and feedback to the MEC. The overview data sets addressing the quality improvement process are presented to the quality council for review and input (with the exception of the peer review summary information) prior to submission for approval to the MEC. This committee is made up of medical staff leaders assigned by the MEC, executive leadership, board members when assigned by the board, and three or four managers. This group reviews the summary reports from the hospital departments, updates from the performance improvement teams that have been assigned, and rec-

ommendations from the scheduled reports from the safety committee, hospital departments and any multidisciplinary improvement teams (i.e., formed
for improvement activities) in the organization. The quality council's function is to assure (1) that the overall process is integrated and coordinated, and
(2) that there is a prioritization of improvement activities based on the available resources and the organization's strategic goals and recommendations
from the medical staff as to the most important issues to address to improve
patient care. The inclusion of the quality council in the process allows for
ongoing communication and review of the systems issues that most often underlie the performance issues in organizations.

Quality Review Committee

This is a medical staff committee made up of representatives of the key
departments or divisions of the medical staff, and the chairman of the required
review functions sub-committees that might include infection control, pharmacy and therapeutics (P&T), procedure review, and so on, depending on the
size of the organization.

Because the MEC has broad responsibilities for the business aspects of the
medical staff, even in smaller facilities and organizations it is recommended that
a separate committee review and address the quality-related activities in organizations. Even if this committee chooses to meet only on a quarterly basis, it is
important that the information and recommendations be carefully considered at
this level and then summarized for review and presentation to the MEC. This
committee reviews summarized information from medical staff departmental
review, required functions review, and pertinent information from hospital departments and safety activities, addresses any follow-up for the individual case
or peer review process by the medical staff, and addresses the review and follow-
up of any sentinel events in the organization that relate to clinical care.

It is helpful to expand the membership of this group to include key individuals responsible for hospital-related processes such as nursing, pharmacy,
infection control, quality, and others, to insure good multidisciplinary input
for the review of the information presented.

The specific data as related to individual case review may be addressed in
an executive session at the end of each meeting in which the majority of the
non-physician representatives are excused.

Medical Staff Departments and Committees

Although many medical staff organizations continue to require meeting
attendance as one of the obligations of medical staff membership, most regu-

latory organizations have removed set requirements for meeting attendance. Although the Joint Commission on Accreditation of Healthcare Organizations (JCAHO) no longer has set meeting requirements, the organization is still required to show evidence that information is being collected, assessed, reviewed, and acted upon in a timely manner. Therefore, in last few years, most medical staff organizations made an effort to consolidate their meeting processes and reduce the number of departments and committees, and therefore meetings, in the medical staff process. To demonstrate compliance with accrediting bodies and regulators, the health care facility must present information to the medical staff that is organized, aggregated, trended, and summarized for the medical staff's review and input prior to their meetings. This function, with examples and formats, will be addressed more completely in the section on the role of the medical staff services department in this chapter.

Many medical staff organizations have expanded the membership of the clinical departments or divisions to include key representatives from the hospital departments that interface with the medical staff on an ongoing basis. This has allowed for a more multidisciplinary approach to the data presented and the activities involved in addressing systems issues and multidisciplinary follow-up. The data sets presented to the medical staff departments or divisions on at least a quarterly basis (see Table 10-2) represent a performance data set for all of the disciplines involved in the care of patients in that department or division. Based on the data and the assessment performed on an ongoing basis, the group can work together to identify opportunities to improve care and service and assure that the process in place is coordinated and integrated.

Many medical staff organizations have this multidisciplinary forum, which meets on a quarterly basis, and have identified an "executive committee" of the department or division to address business and peer review issues on one of the off-months that these meetings are not held. When there is a need for review of these issues by a broader forum, an executive level session held can be held at the end of the regularly scheduled quarterly departmental meeting to ensure broader representation by the medical staff. This multidisciplinary participation better represents the need for all of the care givers to work closely together in the review and improvement of care in order to make a significant difference in the care process.

Quality Improvement Sub-committee

In the past, the quality structure in most health care facilities has created either a void of information or a glut of information for the medical staff. Either the hospital quality system provided little, if any, information to the medical staff concerning the hospital-based activities in place to address the improvement of care and service, or pages and pages of information were provided that gave little concrete information that was meaningful to the medical staff. Regulatory and accrediting bodies have required organizations to provide training to their managers and support staff on data presentation and assessment for the past seven to ten years. In most facilities, this has resulted in more meaningful information sharing by the hospital staff to the medical staff in relation to the quality activities that affect their patients.

It is essential that the information presented to the medical staff from the support areas be well-assessed, summarized, and meaningful in order for the medical staff to meet the facility's expectation to assist the organization in addressing concerns. The role of this sub-committee of the medical staff QRC is to review reported information from all of the required hospital review functions, summarize it, and present information that is pertinent to the medical staff in their review process. A report from this group should be shared quarterly with the QRC in a summarized fashion and then the information for further sharing can be recommended by the QRC. As Figure 10-3 reflects, this is pertinent information from the safety, risk, hospital infection control functions, and any relevant information from hospital quality review activities.

Multidisciplinary Teams

When issues are identified through the review of data at any level that include multiple departments or disciplines, recommendations for team activity may be made. These recommendations are forwarded to the quality council for review and prioritization, and a structured team process is then approved to address the issues.

Not all issues identified in the review process are appropriate for team activity. Often, activities must be prioritized to assure adequate resources and staffing for the activities that the teams may address. Organizations should have specific criteria for prioritization that has been reviewed and approved by the QRC, MEC, and board.

QUALITY PROCESS—LEVELS OF REVIEW AND REPORTING

In order to provide the data and information necessary to identify and address performance issues in organizations, several levels of review are necessary, all of which require involvement from the medical staff. The following section addresses each of the levels of review, with examples of data sets that may be used.

Introduction

A description of each level of review will follow. It is important to note that each level of review is supported by data from the next. The premise of the review process as outlined is that each level of review contains more specific detail than the one preceding it. For example, the first level of review, which is an overview of key functions that support the care of patients, is based on the results of the review process at lower levels in the organization. The first level of review, then, represents indicator review that addressees the outcomes of the key patient care processes at a high level. The results of the first level of review are reported to the board and MEC, as will be demonstrated. If there are any variances from the norm at this level, the expectation is that the departments and staff at lower levels will perform a more complete review of the data and provide conclusions, actions, and follow-up to the data at a later time. Examples will be given for each level of review.

Review of Key Processes

As identified earlier in the chapter, the quality improvement process, as it has evolved in health care from the concepts of Dr. W. Edwards Deming and others, is based on the premise that 80 to 90 percent of the problems identified in health care are systems-related problems instead of problems related to individual performance or human error. The first level of review is focused on key processes in the organization that affect the care and service of patients and families. Depending on the organization and its focus, inpatient care, outpatient care, provider clinic sites, and others, these key processes will vary. A good way to identify the processes that the organization considers most important is to identify the processes that most contribute to the success of the organization in meeting the needs of its customers. For example, in a clinic site, the organization may chose to focus on the registration process or the process in place to provide information to other physicians involved in the care of the patient. In an outpatient surgical center, the organization may choose to focus on the pre-admissions process for patient, the pre-anesthesia assessment process, and the post-procedure, education process.

In order to assist organizations in this area, the JCAHO has identified what they determined to be the most important processes in providing care to patients. These processes are outlined in the various accreditation manuals for health care organizations, but the JCAHO has standardized these processes across settings to be included under the patient-focused functions or processes: patient rights and organizational ethics; assessment of patients; care of the patients, which includes a number of key patient care related processes; education of patients and families; and the continuum of care. Under the functions or processes that support patient care, the JCAHO has included: improvement of organizational performance; leadership; the environment of care; human resources; infection control; and the management of information.

The first level of review, a review of general indicators of success for the key functions or processes as identified above, should be reported to the board and MEC levels of the organization.

The reporting calendar in Exhibit 10-1 presents the reports that are generally required for presentation to the board and other levels of the organization in order to meet regulatory and accreditation requirements as required at this writing. Table 10-1 illustrates a sample report format and includes information that should be forwarded to the board.

A few key indicators (see Exhibit 10-3 for examples of indicators) are selected from those available for reporting at this level. Additional indicators may be reviewed at a lower level. For example, there will probably be a more extensive list of indicators for procedures review at a lower level of the organization, but a few representative indicators will be reviewed and reported at this level to ensure that all key processes are being addressed. This information reviewed at the board and MEC level gives the recipients an overview of key processes performance that may lead to further review.

The overview set of indicators should be reviewed and revised on an annual basis with input from the board, MEC, quality council and QRC of the medical staff.

The indicator sets may vary with a focus in a given year or the requirements of a regulatory body or accreditation or certification organization. For example, the National Committee for Quality Assurance, another key accreditation organization for managed care organizations, has a set indicator list that is required for review by their accredited organizations. The indicator set may vary due to the development of a new clinical service, or because of careful review of performance of an area due to some quality issues from the previous year, or from a serious sentinel event that may need to be followed-up. The example presented is abbreviated but it is important to keep this report as brief as possible in order not to lose the value of its easy-to-review format and concise information about actions taken.

Level Two—Required Functions Review

The next level of review addresses the review of the functions in the organization that are required by regulators or accreditation agencies. These required review functions are listed on the Calendar of Reporting in Table 10-1.

As identified earlier in the chapter, the quality improvement process has an expanded review process. In the traditional quality assurance process, it was required that *the physician's performance* in reference to the areas of required review be addressed. In the expanded review process, the overall processes involved in these required functions must be addressed, with the realization that individual physician performance is affected by the over-all integrity of the processes in these key areas.

For example, the physician's use of medications and the results of medication use as it affects the care of the patient has long been required by JCAHO

Exhibit 10-1. Reporting Calendar for the Quality Improvement Process.

Reporting Matrix Calendar

	Board	MEC	Quality Review Committee	Quality Council	Medical Staff Department	Managers Hospital Department
1. Board Quality Report	Quarterly	Contribute	Contribute	Contribute	Contribute	Contribute
2. Safety Report	Quarterly	Quarterly		Quarterly	If Relevant	
3. Conpetency Report	Required Annually					
4. Required Reprots—Operative/Other Use of Medication Use of Blood Medical Records UR Pt. Satisfaction RM/Safety Quality Control Use of Restraints	Summary Part of #1 —	Quarterly QRC Report to MEC —	Required Functions Report Quarterly/On Rotation —	If Relevant —	If Relevant to the Dept. —	Contribute Quarterly Quarterly—as Relevant Quarterly
5. PI Team Results	Summary Part of #1	Summary from Quality Council Quarterly Report	Summary from Quality Council Quarterly	Monthly On Rotation	As Relevant	Monthly On Rotation
6. Departmental Improvements (MS or Hospital Departments)	Summary Part of #1	Summary from ORC for Medical Staff Dept.	Summary On Rotation	Summary of Hospital On Rotation	As Relevant and MEC	Monthly Hospital On Rotation—Summary
7. Quality Control	Part of #1 As Relevant	Summary As Part of ORC Report	Summary On Rotation	Summary On Rotation	As Relevant	As Relevant
8. Peer Review Case Review	As Relevant	Summary Part of ORC and Dept. Reports	Oversight As Needed Review and Reporting			
9. Sentinel Events	As Relevant	As Relevant to the Medical Staff	As Relevant to the Medical Staff	As Relevant to the Overall Organization	As Relevant	As Relevant

for review by the medical staff. In the new quality improvement process, the overall processes that address the use of medications must be included. The quality assurance process would have provided special studies by the P&T committee concerning the physicians' ordering practices and outcomes of high-risk medications. In the new process, the medical staff receives aggregate, trended data concerning not only the medical staff's role in the process, but also receives indicators addressing such things as: the effectiveness of the preparation process; the administration of medications, the wait times associated with each, and the wait times for out-patient medications for patients; the effectiveness of the teaching process by pharmacy, nursing, and dietary in reference to drug-food interactions; and a variety of other possible indicators, depending on the results of overview data and the request of the medical staff.

Each of the required functions reviews have been expanded to address the key processes that may affect the success of the medical staff in their coordination of the care process for patients. The results of this review process provides value for patients and families and also addresses what may have been system-related issues in which the medical staff had little or no ability to effect change in the past.

Table 10-1. Sample Quality Improvement Board Report.*

QUALITY IMPROVEMENT
QUARTERLY REPORT CARD

"REPORT CARD"	A concise snapshot of key indicators for the quality of clinical, service and financial performance.
PURPOSE	To identify key indicators of success for the issues that directly affect the success of the strategic objectives and the mission of the organization.
INDICATORS	Key measures of success for high volume, high risk patient populations, customer satisfaction, and business performance.
BENCHMARKS/ Goals	Whenever possible, national benchmarks and/or comparative data from external sources are listed. Data from the organization's performance of the same indicators from 1997 are listed when available.
DEFINITIONS	Each indicator has a definition listed to ensure data integrity.

---

*Source: Opal Reinbold, © BDO Seidman. Reprinted with permission.

Table 10-1. Sample Quality Improvement Board Report. *(continued)*

QUALITY IMPROVEMENT REPORT CARD 1998 Performance Measure	Bench-mark or Goal	1998 FY	Q1 Jul-Sep '99	Q2 Oct-Dec '99	Q3 Jan-Mar '99	Q4 Apr-Jun '99	1999 YTD
I. Service Quality							
1. Patient Satisfaction (overall%)							
2. Physician Satisfaction							
Significant Findings Identified							
Conclusions: (for any positive or negative variances) Actions: Follow-up:							
II. Human Resources							
1. Past Due Performance Evaluations %							
Conclusions: Actions: Follow-up:							
III. Clinical Measurements							
A. Operative/Invasive Procedures							
1a. PTCA as Second Procedure after							
B. Case and Care Management							
1a. Target CPG Cases as % of Total							
C. Utilization Review							
1a. Lost Income for Denied Days							
D. Skilled Nursing							
E. Psych							
IV. Medical Staff							
A. Blood/Tissue							
B. Medication Usage							
C. Medical Records							
D. Mortality Review							
E. Medical Management							
F. Restraints use							
1. Unscheduled re-admissions							
2. Unplanned returns to OR							
Conclusions: Actions: Follow-up:							
V. Safety/Risk Management							
Conclusions: Actions: Follow-up:							
VI. Market Share							
Conclusions: Actions: Follow-up:							
VII. Financial/Strategic							
Conclusions: Actions: Follow-up:							
VIII. Outpatient							

QUALITY IMPROVEMENT REPORT 1999	
JCAHO PREPARATION UPDATE	
CLINICAL PRACTICE GUIDELINE UPDATE	
MULTIDISCIPLINARY TEAM UPDATE	
OTHER KEY ISSUES	

Source: Opal Reinbold,© BDO Seidman. Reprinted with permission.

A good rule of thumb for what will be required for review, no matter what type of facility is involved, would be

1. processes that are high risk or high volume (those processes which if done poorly, represent the highest risk of poor outcomes for the most patients, or perhaps more importantly, those processes if done well, will provide the most benefit for patients and families);

2. problem prone processes;

3. those key quality control processes (for example, the accuracy of lab results or the safe levels of radiation in imaging processes).

The required functions review usually includes at least the following:

1. Operative and other invasive procedures that place a patient at risk. Whether the environment is an inpatient setting, a clinic site, or an outpatient setting, these types of procedures pose considerable risk to patients. The processes in place to identify the appropriateness of a procedure, the effectiveness of the preparation processes, the outcomes of the procedure, the post-procedure care, and education provided to patients and families should be considered for identification of measures to be reviewed and assessed on an ongoing basis.

2. Medication usage—the processes in place to ensure the safe and effective use of medications. Because research has shown that the majority of negative patient outcomes on a national basis result from the inappropriate use of medications, this is a very high risk area. The key processes to be measured for medication usage include appropriate prescribing and ordering of medications, preparation and dispensing of medications, administration of medications, and monitoring the effects of the medications on the patient.

3. The use of blood and blood products. Because the use of blood is not only potentially beneficial but also carries a substantial risk for patients, the processes in place to address blood ordering, the distribution, handling, and dispensing of blood, the administration of blood and blood products, and monitoring the effects of blood and blood components on patients should be reviewed and addressed.

4. Other areas that are often considered for required review include the timeliness and appropriateness of patient care documentation, the appropriate use of resources in providing care, information concerning risk and claims management in an organization (to include any unusual events that deviate from regular care that result in serious injury or loss of function for

patients (sentinel events), the results of quality control activities, and the results of feedback on the satisfaction of all key customer groups, with a focus on patients and families.

Organizations, depending on their size, have several options concerning how they wish to address the review of required functions. This review has traditionally been addressed by having medical staff committees review this information in detail and provide conclusions, actions, recommendations, and follow-up directly to the MEC or to a committee similar to the QRC described in this chapter. Many organizations choose to continue addressing the required functions review process in this way. However, organizations now can choose to combine committee functions (for example, P&T and infection control) and meet quarterly to address the data and issues raised (if not critical) or address the functions by custom reports for each medical staff department or division.

However organizations choose to address the detailed review of these key required functions, the following should be kept in mind:

1. A review of current regulations and standards should be done at least annually, to assure that all required data is addressed.

2. The indicators for review for the required functions should be reviewed and revised at least annually by the MEC or the oversight committee similar to the QRC addressed in this chapter.

3. The trended data format as evidenced in Tables 10-1 and 10-2 should be utilized for presentation of the required review quarterly reports.

4. Documentation must be present for the follow-up and resolution of any issues identified in the required functions review activities. These review processes will always be part of any review by state, federal, or accrediting agencies.

5. Opportunities for multidisciplinary improvement activities, based on this review, should be sought to ensure an integrated approach to the improvement of care and improvement activities supported by all constituents.

6. The results of the review process should be reported to the MEC and in summary to the board, at least on a quarterly basis, with clear evidence of appropriate actions taken when warranted.

Level Four Review—Medical Staff Departments and Committees

As indicated earlier in this chapter, each of the medical staff departments may identify a multidisciplinary data set to review the performance of its de-

Table 10-2. Sample—Departmental Quarterly Report Format.

Indicator	Comparison Data		1999					
	Comparative	1998	1Q	2Q	3Q	4Q	Total	
REQUIRED								
OPERATIVE & OTHER INVASIVE PROCEDURES								
C-Section Rate								
VBAC Rate								
TISSUE REVIEW								
Pre/Post								
Pre/Path								
MEDICATION USE								
Adverse Drug Reactions								
BLOOD UTILIZATION								
C/T Ratio								
Units not meeting criteria (Gyn only)								
Transfusion Reaction Rate								
RESOURCE UTILIZATION								
ALOS – Maternal								
Maternal Transport								
INFECTION CONTROL								
Group B Strep								
CLINICAL OUTCOMES/QUALITY OF CARE								
Neonatal Mortality Rate								
Low Birth Wt. Infant Rate (<2,500 gm)								
Neonatal Readmission								
Maternal Readmission within 30 days								
Fetal Demise Rate								
PATHWAYS								
(Indicator/if in place)								
TEAM PROJECTS UPDATE (SEE ATTACHED)								
MEDICAL RECORDS								
Delinquency Rate								
H&P								
Operative Reports								
PATIENT BASED OUTCOMES-SATISFACTION SURVEYS								
What is your overall opinion of the quality of care received (OB)								
Did the hospital staff prepare you to manage your care at home? (OB)								
What is oyour overall opinion of the quality of care received (PED)								
1. Conclusions								
2. Actions								
3. Follow-up								

partment, service or product line as related to key patient populations. The data set may include indicators of performance for all of the disciplines involved in the care of the patients, as well as indicators related to the required functions, if appropriate, and any outcomes information that may be the result of clinical path data review or special studies of certain patient populations.

(Each of the clinical departments will also have a list of case review criteria that will be used to identify cases for the medical staff review process, which will be addressed in the peer review portion of this section.)

A review of the overall data will be completed with an identification of any or recommendations made or actions that need to be taken. If the data indicates that additional review of an area is needed, the committee will assign the follow-up review and a goal date for completion. This information will then appear on the medical staff follow-up sheet (see Exhibit 10-2) which

---

Exhibit 10-2. Sample—Medical Staff Follow-up Format.

MEDICAL EXECUTIVE COMMITTEE ACTION LIST

MEETING: (date) _____

COMMITTEE MEMBER: _____

FOLLOW-UP ACTION ASSIGNED	PERSON/DEPT	REQUESTED COMPLETION BY
CARRIED OVER FROM (date) MEETING:		
CARRIED OVER FROM (date) MEETING:		
(date), 1999 ACTION ITEMS:		
NEXT MEETING: (date)—(time)—(place)		

---

accompanies each set of the departmental minutes. This information remains on the follow-up sheet until it is resolved, which acts as a reminder of outstanding issues and assists the medical staff in their follow-up process.

If the committee identifies an opportunity to address an improvement issue by using a multidisciplinary team, a recommendation is made to the quality council for review and approval.

Any hospital-related activities are reported in summary fashion in the quarterly departmental meeting. Additionally, any policies and procedures that may be appropriate for review and approval can be presented at this time.

When the scheduled quarterly report of the summary of activities for this clinical department is presented to the medical staff oversight committee (as represented in this chapter by the QRC), the chair of the department or committee should attend to present the information or the department liaison for that area can make the presentation. A summary of this information is then sent to the MEC.

It is important to note that each time information moves to the next level of reporting, it is summarized and the key issues for resolution or recommendations are highlighted.

Level Five—Medical Staff Peer Review/Individual Case Review

The quality assurance programs for the medical staff have previously been based on the individual case review by the physician's peers. This was a process based on a retrospective review of charts identified using general sets of indicators to identify variances in care that might need to be addressed in the peer review process. Most often, the first level of review was provided by

Figure 10-4. Sample—Medical Staff Peer Review Flow Diagram.

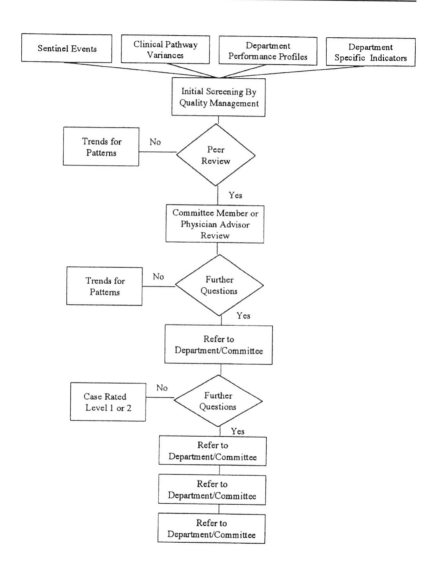

nurses in the quality or utilization department and based on 100 percent review of patient records. This very labor-intensive work usually created a process that was tedious for the medical staff and most often resulted in a validation of the care provided. This process almost never addressed the systems problems that may have contributed to the variation in care in the first place. Berwick characterized this process as follows: "We spend altogether too much time throwing out burned toast....Let's fix the toaster."[5]

Although the peer review process is identified as the fifth level of review, it is important to note that this level by no means reflects the importance of the individual peer review process in the review of care. The quality improvement process is data driven by design. Figure 10-4 illustrates the peer review process.

Just as the overall process of review has been broadened, the peer review process now encompasses *the review of data identified in conjunction with the medical staff to identify trends in the variances of care and outcomes of patient care as well as a more limited review of individual cases identified by serious events that deviate from the care process.* The process (as outlined here) begins with a review of general data sets, which if well designed, will highlight any areas of concern that may need to be addressed in-depth. See Exhibit 10-3 for example. The individual review of care stemming from serious variation in the care process, by unexpected negative outcomes of care, or by the identification of trends that leads to questions concerning the individual performance of physicians is, and always will be, a very important part of the process. However, cases that are identified for review will be fewer by the nature of the data collected concerning overall care, and the review process is thus much more meaningful for the physicians involved and should result in actions taken in a more timely fashion.

Each medical staff organization will have an individualized approach to the process of identifying data for overall review and the key set of indicators for individual case review. This process will depend on the size of the organization, the make-up of the patient population, the resources available to support the review process, and the historical process the organization has gone through to reach this level of review. For example, if the first level of review has traditionally been provided by the utilization review nurses, it may be important that they continue to be involved in the process to foster the trust level of the medical staff in any new approach to be taken.

Whichever process the medical staff may choose, the following issues should be addressed:

1. The medical staff should take the lead in identification of the overall indicators for departmental and committee review to insure that they will pick up relevant trends in the care process.

2. The process should be consistent across departments.

Exhibit 10-3. Sample—Individual Case Review Indicator Set.

SAMPLE
SERIOUS EVENTS
(Requiring Individual Case Review)

1. Any unexpected deaths.
2. Any discrepancies between procedures consented for and those performed.
3. Any surgical/invasive procedure complications such as:
   a. Any retained foreign body.
   b. Unresolved incorrect surgical counts.
   c. Injuries obtained during procedure (burns, perforations).
4. Any neurologic impairment post admission.
5. Any suicides or attempts.
6. Any conscious sedation complications.
7. Any unplanned returns to operating room/delivery room.
8. Any unplanned transfers to special care.
9. Any transfusion reactions.
10. Discrepancies between pre & post procedure diagnosis, post & pathological diagnosis.
11. Referrals from Pharmacy and Therapeutics review such as:
    a. Adverse drug reactions.
    b. Incorrect drug usage.
12. Referrals from Infection Control.
13. Referrals from case management/utilization review which may include physician identified trends such as:
    a. Over Utilization
    b. Under Utilization.
    c. Readmissions within 30 days for same or related condition.

3. Each department should identify and approve the set of criteria for the identification of the cases for individual review at least annually to be sure of the relevance of the criteria.

4. An identification of any case that qualifies as a "sentinel event" in the JCAHO review process should have a complete root-cause analysis and be addressed in a formal and timely fashion through the medical staff peer review process.

5. Each department or division should identify how it will determine which physician will provide the individual case review when it is needed.

6. It is essential that any issues identified have appropriate, timely, documented resolution.

7. A summary listing of the top three to five cases that do not meet criteria for review should be presented to the medical staff departments on an ongoing basis to help focus any continued review activities.

8. The process should focus on educational activities and address disciplinary actions after educational efforts have not achieved results.

9. The information should be used in the reappointment process.

10. The information should be kept confidential at all times.

Level Six—Quality Control

All licensed organizations are required to address the quality review functions in an organization. State licensure requirements, federal requirements, and all accrediting organizations require quality review activities that relate to the ongoing review of quality control activities in the radiology department, the laboratory functions, and the security and storage of medications, for example.

It is important that the calendar of reporting include the required reports related to these quality control activities and that the organization has documentation available concerning any issues that have arisen as well as the reporting of the resolution of the issues.

Most often, a summary report of any key issues of concern reported to the appropriate committee on a scheduled basis will suffice with the appropriate back-up documentation in the department. If, however, there are any serious issues identified, the issues must be addressed in a timely manner and their resolution reported up through the process.

Level Seven—Review of Reappointment Data

As was indicated earlier in the chapter, the quality improvement process serves to provide information to identify opportunities for improvement in the over-all care and service of the organization and to assist the medical staff and the hospital leaders in assuring that the providers of care are competent to deliver care to patients and families.

The final level of review, which much of the preceding information references, addresses how the information from the quality improvement process is used in the review of the competence of medical staff care providers at the time of reappointment.

In the past, reappointment was based on a summary listing of case review that was done for each medical staff member. An example is shown in Exhibit 10-4.

The sample presented in Exhibit 10-4 was usually accompanied by a listing of the cases that did not meet criteria for review for the physician with any comments, and in those organizations that utilized a rating system, the number of cases that rated in the lowest two review categories. This information did not provide comparative data that would give the physician making the reappointment decision any kind of objective data on which to base his decision, and therefore, make appropriate recommendations for any changes in privileges, if warranted.

The quality improvement data-driven process allows the medical staff to work toward a more objective review process.

As evidenced in the sample provided in Exhibit 10-5, this profile provides activity data; performance data with internal and external comparative data (when available); data concerning the provider's performance in reference to the required review functions; and the results of cases reviewed as compared to the practitioner's peers. The profile may also include comparative resource utilization data, and other information as deemed appropriate by the medical staff clinical departments.

This level of data review and assessment assures that the process in place for reappointment staff is based on data and a complete review of care with comparative data whenever it is available.

KEY MEDICAL STAFF SUPPORT FUNCTIONS

The role of the medical staff services department in the quality improvement process is vital. The best performance improvement program will fail in an organization that does not include the medical staff services department as a vital partner in the process. Following are some key reminders to enhance the success of any organization's improvement efforts as well as the ability of the medical staff services department to act as a liaison between the medical staff and the key organizational constituents.

Medical Staff Leader Education

"Physician leadership is the scarcest asset available to health care organizations today."

—*Robert Rowland,* Former Administrator, Sutter Medical Group

The success of the quality improvement process begins with a well-informed, educated leadership and support function. From the time incoming medical staff leaders are identified, it is essential that they be involved in some kind of education process to familiarize them with the over-all concepts of quality improvement and of the organization's process to address it. This education process can be addressed in a number of ways:

Exhibit 10-4. Sample—1993 Quality Assurance Reappointment Profile.

PHYSICIAN PROFILE

RUN DATE:
RUN TIME:

Physician Number:
Physician Name:
Specialty: PEDIATRICS

PROFESSIONAL PERFORMANCE

21 # of Admissions
0 # of Discharges
2 # of Consultations
0 # of Delinquent Medical Records
0 # of Procedures With Complications

0 # of Readmission within 14 days
   (28 for newborns)
0 # of mortalities
   Average Length of Stay
0 # of Surgical Procedures Performed

CLINICAL REVIEW

0 # of Cases reviewed by PMC
0 # of Cases reviewed by Department PEDIATRICS
0 # of cases with major post procedure tissue discrepancies
0.00 Crossmatch to transfusion ratio
0 # of units ordered   0 # of Units Given

Cross Match to Transfusion Ratio
   # of Units Ordered   # of Units Given
   # of Units not meeting Appropriateness Criteria

Physician Number:
Physician Name:
Specialty: PEDIATRICS

PROFESSIONAL PERFORMANCE

# of Admissions
0 # of Discharges
0 # of Consultations
0 # of Delinquent Medical Records
0 # of Procedures With Complications

0 # of Readmission within 14 days
   (28 for newborns)
0 # of mortalities
0.00 Average Length of Stay
0 # of Surgical Procedures Performed

CLINICAL REVIEW

0 # of Cases reviewed by PMC
0 # of Cases reviewed by Department PEDIATRICS
2 # of cases with major post procedure tissue discrepancies
0.00 Crossmatch to transfusion ratio

1. Many health care facilities plan for the progression of their medical staff leaders by involving the incoming chief of staff in the quality improvement process right away. Organizations accomplish this by requiring that the chief of staff-elect serve as the chair of the QRC in the period prior to his or her appointment as the chief of staff. This has been very successful

Exhibit 10-5. Sample—Current Reappointment Profile.

PRACTITIONER PROFILE

Department: _____   Section: _____

Practitioner Name: _____   Practitioner #: _____   Status: _____   Time Period: _____

This confidential reappointment profile has been produced to assist in assessing members of departments/sections who have applied for reappointment. Department and Section chairs may request details with regard to any information on this report from the Quality and Medical Staff Services Department.

Activity Data (#/%)	Practitioner Specific Data	Peer Comparison Data	Top 3 DRGs/ Diagnosis/ Procedure	Practitioner Specific (Rate)	Peer Comparison (Rate)	Benchmark (i.e., Maryland QI Project)
Attending physician: Inpatient Discharges			Primary C/S			
Attending physician: Average LOS			VBAC			
Attending physician: Total Deliveries			Top 3 DRGs/ Diagnosis/ Procedure	Practitioner Specific (Avg. LOS)	Peer Comparison (Avg. LOS)	Benchmark (i.e., Maryland QI Project)
Observation Visits			Normal Vaginal Deliveries (ICD 9)			
Consultations Rendered			Dept. Specific Performance Measures	Practitioner Specific	Peer Comparison	Benchmark (i.e., Maryland QI Project)
Inpatient Surgical/Invasive Procedures Performed			Stillborns			
Outpatient Surgical/ Invasive Procedures Performed			Birth Traumas			
Mortalities			RN Deliveries			
Denials			Eclampsia			

Exhibit 10-5. Sample—Current Reappointment Profile. *(continued)*

OB Practitioner Profile

Practitioner: _____   Time Period: _____

Quality/Performance	Practitioner Specific Data			Peer Comparison Data			Actions Taken/ Comments:
	Cases Reviewed	Met Criteria	Peer Reviewed	Cases Reviewed	Met Criteria	Peer Reviewed	
Operative and Procedures: Tissue Discrepancies Screening for Appropriateness Returns to O.R.							
Documentation Review							
Medication Usage Review (1) (2)							
Blood Usage Review Screening for Appropriateness							
Conscious Sedation Review Compliance with Documentation Requirements							
Mortality Review Unexpected Unexpected, but not surprising							
Nosocomial Infections Post procedure							

for organizations and for ensuring that the chief of staff is familiar with the process and has been actively involved at the time of his or her progression to role of the chief of staff.

2. Following the chief of staff's one to two year stint as chief, organizations have invited the chief of staff to sit on the quality council to provide continuity in the process.

3. The orientation of the new officers in each term of office should include training on quality improvement tools and an introduction to the organization's process and tools.

4. On at least an annual basis, many organizations have chosen to either send their officers to a quality improvement course off-site, or have provided some kind of on-site training for the medical staff leaders to help them in their roles in the quality improvement process.

Exhibit 10-5. Sample—Current Reappointment Profile. *(continued)*

Practitioner Profile

Practitioner: _____   Time Period: _____

Verification of Credentials

| Malpractice Claims ( )Yes ( )No # of claims: _____ | National Practitioner Bank Clear ( )Yes ( )No | ( ) Current Medical License | ( ) Current DEA | ( ) Liability Insurance | ( ) CME | # Days Suspended ( ) Reason: _____ |

TO BE COMPLETED BY THE DEPARTMENT CHAIR

	Yes	No	Comments:
1. Has the physician complied with Department Rules and Regulations, applicable Hospital policies and Medical Staff Bylaws?			
2. Does the physician appear to be in sound physical and mental health?			
3. Has the physician been the subject of any disciplinary action?			
4. Has the physician been the subject of repeated complaints by patients, hospital staff, or members of the Medical Staff?			
5. Are there any indications of impairment which might affect his or her ability to perform professional duties?			

The following category is recommended: [ ] Provisional [ ] Active [ ] Courtesy [ ] Consulting [ ] Physician Administrator [ ] A.H.P. [ ] Not recommended for reappointment (Explain)

Remarks/Comments: _____

I have reviewed the information in this physician's clinical profile including diagnoses attended and procedures performed, results of medical staff quality assessment/case review, risk management profiles, and medical staff citizenship. Based on this review, this practitioner has displayed clinical competence, professional performance and sound judgement, and is qualified for the privileges requested.

Section Chair's Signature: _____   Date: _____

Section Chair's Comments: _____
_____
_____

Department Chair's Signature: _____   Date: _____

Department Chair's Comments: _____
_____
_____

Partnership with the Quality Improvement Staff

The quality improvement process is successful only if the medical staff services department staff and the quality review staff are partners in the process. The over-all process will vary by facility but whether there is representation by the quality improvement staff at all medical staff meetings, which is the ideal, or just a reporting function on a quarterly basis, the information shared must be well-communicated by the quality review staff to medical staff services staff.

The information reported and the conclusions, actions, and follow-up taken by the medical staff must be clearly documented and presented in the minutes of the medical staff process.

Often, it is the attentive medical staff services professional who alerts the quality improvement staff to a request from the medical staff for follow-up or more information on an issue.

Many medical staff clinical departments now meet only on a quarterly basis. If there is not good coordination of information and follow-up, this can mean that it may sometimes be six to nine months before important issues are brought to resolution. If not addressed, these delays can have an impact on the licensure or accreditation status of health care facilities.

The calendar of reporting, as identified in Exhibit 10-1, should be a collaborative tool between the medical staff services and quality improvement staff members.

The partnership with the medical staff services department also ensures that all issues are brought to resolution and are well documented in the minutes. The preparation and review of the minutes should be a shared responsibility with medical staff services and quality staff to ensure that quality and peer review information is addressed and presented in the best manner possible.

Communication and Information Sharing

As medical staff organizations are re-organizing and having fewer meetings and structured information-sharing opportunities, the medical staff services department serves as a liaison for essential information sharing between the executive hospital leaders and medical staff leaders and between the medical staff leadership group and the rank and file in the medical staff organization. To facilitate this exchange of information, it is highly recommended that the medical staff services professional be an ongoing member of the executive leadership group of the hospital. The role of the individual in providing assurance to the medical staff, and current, appropriate information, is essential to the success of the organizational improvement efforts. Additionally, if at all possible, even small hospitals should provide some kind of newsletter to the general medical staff. Because of the lack of requirements for structured meetings, without some kind of standardized information sharing mechanism, many of the medical staff members will not be well informed and may feel isolated and uninvolved.

A well-informed, involved medical staff services department is the first step in involving and informing the medical staff on an ongoing basis.

CONCLUSION

As Henry Ford once said, "Coming together is a beginning; Keeping together is progress; Working together is success."

The continued success of organizations in a highly competitive market is reliant upon every organization's ability to accurately and cooperatively present information about its success in providing excellent, cost-effective care to ensure their patient populations are in the best health possible. The quality improvement function, and the necessity for medical staff leadership in that function, are important factors in the long term success of medical staffs and organizations that support them. A clear, simple process that is integrated, coordinated, and data-based provides the foundation for appropriate review and information-sharing. The success of those efforts is greatly enhanced by the strong support and involvement of the leaders of medical staff services departments.

NOTES

1. J. S. Robert and P.S. Schyue, "The View and Role of the Joint Commission," *The Quality Letter* (May 1990).
2. Joint Commission on Accreditation of Healthcare Organizations, *An Introduction to Quality Improvement in Healthcare* (Oakbrook Terrace, IL: Joint Commission on Accreditation of Healthcare Organizations, 1991):
3. J. Castro, "Condition: Critical," *Time* (November 25, 1991): 35.
4. D. M. Berwick, "Continuous Improvement as an Ideal in Health Care," *New England Journal of Medicine* 320 (1989): 53.
5. D. M. Berwick (From a presentation by William Fifer, M.D., "The Quality Phoenix," Estes Park Institute, Fall, 1992.)

Chapter 11

Program-specific Accreditation

Cindy A. Gassiot, CMSC, CPCS

The major functions of a medical staff organization and health care organization accrediting groups have been discussed in earlier chapters. This chapter will focus on other medical staff functions, specifically, the functions performed by institutional review boards, cancer and trauma committees, and continuing medical education programs, and how the latter are accredited.

INSTITUTIONAL REVIEW BOARDS

Hospital institutional review boards (IRBs) are required to oversee protection of the rights and welfare of human subjects involved in clinical investigation of drugs and medical devices regulated by the Food and Drug Administration (FDA). These boards were formed in many community hospitals for the first time in the 1970s, when intraocular lenses were invented, but not yet approved by the FDA, and ophthalmologists began implanting them in conjunction with surgery to remove cataracts. In large teaching facilities, the IRB has a much older history.

Although there is no accreditation per se, the FDA has issued regulations that hospital IRBs must follow governing the protection of human subjects involved in research on products regulated by the agency. Additionally, other federal agencies and departments, and some states, have regulations that govern human subject protection. The medical staff services professional (MSSP) should be familiar with those regulations that apply to research being done at his or her institution.

Products under investigation include drugs that are being evaluated by the FDA and medical devices not yet fully approved by the agency. (The research must be based on adequately performed laboratory and animal experimentation and on thorough knowledge of the scientific literature.) When physicians use investigational products in the hospital (and sometimes on an outpatient basis) they must do so under carefully controlled, scientific principles. The IRB's functions are to review and approve, require modification in, or disapprove research activities. Among other duties, the IRB ensures that risks to subjects are minimized, that risks are reasonable in relation to anticipated benefits and knowledge that is expected to result, that subject selection is equitable, that informed consent is obtained and documented, that appropriate data monitoring is in place, that privacy of subjects and confidentiality of data are maintained where appropriate, and that additional protections are provided for vulnerable subjects, such as those with acute or severe physical or mental illness or persons who are economically or educationally disadvantaged.[1]

Briefly, FDA regulations[2] require the IRB to

1. be established at any institution engaging in any investigation, study or research involving human subjects;

2. be composed of not less than five members with voting authority (members must be qualified by experience, expertise and diversity of background to give advice for safeguarding human subjects; the IRB may not be composed of all men or all women or entirely of members of one profession; the IRB must have one member whose only affiliation with the institution is IRB membership; there must be one member whose primary concerns are in scientific areas and at least one member whose primary activities are non-scientific, for example, a lawyer, ethicist, clergy; and no member should have conflicting interest);

3. perform two primary functions:
   - *review* and approve or disapprove of any proposed investigational study,
   - *monitor* any ongoing study (the IRB has a responsibility to ensure each study is carried out as stated in the protocol; any investigation must be followed until it is completed, discontinued or suspended);

4. follow written procedures and conduct business only if there is a quorum, which cannot be less than a majority of members of the committee;

5. maintain records sufficient to clearly describe the results of any study;

6. ensure that investigators obtain legal informed consent (the elements of which are specified by the FDA);

7. receive, investigate, and act on complaints relating to any study under review regardless of their source (e.g., subjects, the sponsor of the study, members of the medical staff, and so on);

8. make records available for inspection by authorized agents of the FDA.

To assist these committees in operating according to regulations, the FDA has developed a self-evaluation guide. The following guidelines, reproduced in part from that document,[3] should be used by the institution to determine what written policies and procedures are needed.

Policies and procedures are required describing the functions of the IRB with respect to

1. conducting initial and continuing review,

2. reporting findings and actions to the investigator and institution,

3. determining which projects require review more often than annually,

4. determining which projects need verification from sources other than the investigators that no material changes have occurred since previous IRB review,

5. ensuring prompt reporting to the IRB of changes in research activities,

6. ensuring that changes in approved research are not initiated without IRB review and approval,

7. ensuring prompt reporting to the IRB of unanticipated problems or serious or continuing noncompliance with the requirements or determinations of the IRB,

8. ensuring prompt reporting to the IRB of any suspension or termination of IRB approval.

Additional policies and procedures should describe the operations of the IRB with respect to

1. the review process:
   - All members should review the entire protocol.
   - One or more "primary reviewers" review entire protocol, report to the IRB, and lead discussion on the protocol.
   - All members should have access to the entire protocol.
   - The role of subcommittees of the IRB should be delineated.
   - Emergency studies must be reviewed.
   - Procedures for expedited review should be followed.

2. criteria for approval of investigation:
   - The risks to subjects must be minimized.
   - The risks to subjects must be reasonable in relation to anticipated benefits.
   - The selection of subjects must be equitable.
   - Informed consent must be adequate.

- Where appropriate, there should be adequate provisions to protect the privacy of subjects and maintain the confidentiality of data.
- Appropriate safeguards must be included in the study to protect the rights and welfare of vulnerable subjects.

3. voting requirements:

- A quorum is required to transact business.
- There must be quorum diversity requirements.
- Approval or disapproval of a study should require a certain percentage of the vote.
- All members must have full voting rights.
- Proxy votes should not be allowed.
- Investigators should not vote on their own studies.

IRB record requirements that the institution must maintain include

1. a list of IRB members and qualifications;
2. written procedures and guidelines;
3. minutes of meetings:

- members present,
- record of discussion of controversial issues,
- record of IRB decisions,
- record of voting;

4. protocols and consent documents as submitted and as finally approved;
5. communications to and from the IRB;
6. adverse reaction reports;
7. IRB consideration of adverse reaction reports;
8. periodic continuing reviews;
9. budget and accounting record regarding acquisition and expenditure of resources;
10. emergency use reports;
11. and statements of significant new findings provided to subjects.

Each investigator must provide information to the IRB. This information must include

1. professional qualifications to do the research (including a description of necessary support services and facilities),
2. the title of the study,
3. the purpose of the study (including the benefit to be obtained by doing the study),
4. the sponsor of the study,
5. results of previous related research,
6. subject selection criteria,
7. subject exclusion criteria,
8. the justification for use of special subject populations (e.g., the mentally retarded, children, and so on),
9. the study design (including a discussion of the appropriateness of research methods),
10. a description of procedures to be performed,
11. provisions for managing adverse reactions.

FDA Institutional Review Board Inspections[4]

In response to a Congressional mandate to expand its monitoring of biomedical research conducted under its regulations, the FDA developed the Bioresearch Monitoring Program and, as part of that effort, began an expanded review of IRBs in April 1977. The aim of the program is to ensure the protection of human subjects by ensuring the existence of well-organized and properly functioning local IRBs. The Bioresearch Monitoring Program, which encompasses IRBs, clinical investigators, sponsors, monitors, and non-clinical laboratories, is also intended to ensure the quality and integrity of data submitted to the FDA for regulatory decision making, as well as to protect human subjects of research. For this reason, the IRB regulations note that the FDA may inspect IRBs and review and copy IRB records.

Institutional Review Board Program

Under the Bioresearch Monitoring Program, the FDA conducts on-site procedural reviews of IRBs. These reviews are conducted to determine whether an IRB is operating in accordance with its own written procedures as well as current FDA regulations.

When an institution is selected for a procedural review, an investigator from one of FDA's field offices contacts a responsible individual at the institution, usually the IRB chair, and arranges a mutually acceptable time for the visit. When the field investigator arrives at the institution, he or she will show FDA credentials and present a Notice of Inspection to the chair of the IRB or another responsible official. This is done simply to let the staff at the institution know that the investigator is a duly authorized representative of FDA.

The investigator will first interview appropriate staff members and obtain information about the IRB's policies and procedures. Then the investigator will examine the IRB's performance by following one or more studies through the review process in use at the institution. IRB procedures and membership will be examined to see whether they conform to current FDA regulations. The investigator may request copies of records of IRB membership, IRB procedures and guidelines, minutes of meetings at which the studies were reviewed and discussed, materials on the studies submitted to the IRB by the clinical investigators, and any other materials pertaining to these studies. These materials become part of the field investigator's report to FDA headquarters.

After the inspection has been completed, the investigator will conduct an exit interview with the responsible institutional representative, usually the IRB chair. At this interview, the investigator will review the findings, describe any deviations from the current regulations, and suggest corrective actions. If appropriate, a List of Observations (Form 483) may be left with the institution.

After the investigator returns to the district office, a written report with recommendations for action, if necessary, will be prepared. This report will be forwarded to FDA headquarters for evaluation. When this evaluation is completed, a letter will be sent to the IRB chair or other responsible institutional officials. The letter may state that no deficiencies were found or, if the applicable regulations have not been followed, ask for correction. Where major or important corrections are needed, a written response may be required. At times, a follow-up inspection may be conducted.

A copy of the FDA's Compliance Program Guidance Manual for IRB Inspections (Program 7348.809) is available to the public by writing to Freedom of Information Staff, HFW-30, Food and Drug Administration, 5600 Fishers Lane, Rockville, Maryland 20857. This manual is also available on the Internet at the Web site http://www.nih.gov/grants/oprr/irb.

APPROVED CANCER PROGRAMS

The Commission on Cancer of the American College of Surgeons (ACS) sponsors a voluntary approval program for institutional cancer programs.[5] Although the tumor registry is the locus of a cancer program in the hospital, the MSSP may provide administrative support to the hospital cancer committee that is seeking approval for its cancer program. An understanding of the components of a hospital cancer program is helpful for performing these tasks.

In addition to approving hospital cancer programs, the ACS approves programs in small rural hospitals affiliated with larger institutions that have approved cancer programs; freestanding, nonhospital cancer centers; freestanding integrated programs, such as radiation oncology centers that have hospital partners; and managed care organization cancer programs.

The goals of the ACS cancer program are to decrease morbidity and mortality of cancer patients and to improve the quality of patient care. These goals are pursued by encouraging hospitals to improve cancer control efforts through prevention, early detection, pretreatment evaluation, staging, treatment, rehabilitation, and surveillance for recurrence of cancer, and to enhance the care of the terminally ill patient. These efforts are overseen by a cancer committee.

In order to seek ACS approval of a cancer program, the facility must be accredited by a recognized authority, such as the Joint Commission, the American Osteopathic Association, the National Committee on Quality Assurance, the Accreditation Association for Ambulatory Health Care, or the American College of Radiology, depending on the services offered by the facility. The facility must have specific resources for state-of-the-art diagnosis and treatment of cancer. Minimal cancer program resources include

1. a cancer committee,
2. cancer conferences,
3. a quality management program,
4. and data management systems.

The cancer program must have an authorized organization and management structure to ensure efficient and effective administration of the cancer program and services. A physician must be designated to provide medical direction for the cancer program and this individual may be the cancer committee chair.

The Cancer Committee

The cancer committee is a standing, multidisciplinary committee and it must be included in the medical staff bylaws. It must convene on a schedule that meets the needs of the institution and maintain documentation of its proceedings. The committee's responsibilities are to

1. develop and evaluate the annual goals and objectives for the clinical, educational, and programmatic activities related to cancer;

2. promote a coordinated, multidisciplinary approach to patient management;

3. ensure that educational and consultative cancer conferences cover all major cancer sites and related issues;

4. ensure that an active supportive care system is in place for patients, families and staff;

5. monitor quality management and improvement through completion of quality management studies that focus on quality, access to care, and outcomes;

6. promote clinical research;

7. supervise the cancer registry and ensure accurate and timely abstracting, staging, and follow-up reporting;

8. perform quality control of registry data;

9. encourage data usage and regular reporting;

10. ensure that content of the annual report meets requirements;

11. publish an annual report by November 1 of the following year;

12. uphold medical ethical standards.

The committee must publish and distribute an annual report that meets requirements outlined in the Cancer Program Standards.

Conferences

An approved cancer program includes conferences to educate the medical and ancillary staffs and provide consultative services to patients. The conferences must be patient-oriented and consultative, and didactic lectures must be limited to 25 percent of the conferences held. The cases presented must be representative of the case mix seen by the institution and the number of cases discussed must be proportional (at least 10 percent) to the annual caseload. The frequency of conferences must be appropriate to the category of approval. The majority of cases presented in the conferences must be prospective and all major cancer sites treated in the facility must be addressed. Frequency of conferences is determined by hospital category.

The standards include other requirements for oncology services, inpatient oncology units, radiation therapy services, clinical laboratory, routine diagnostic imaging services, and nursing care provided to oncology patients. Additionally, the standards address inpatient and outpatient care, requirements for supportive and continuing care services, and research.

Quality Management and Improvement

The standards require that the quality of cancer patient care be measured, evaluated and improved. Quality measures must be defined for topics considered to be high-priority opportunities for improvement, and to monitor compliance with treatment guidelines. The results of measurement activities must be evaluated by the cancer committee to determine current performance levels, assess the need for interventions aimed at reducing or eliminating undesirable performance, or to identify opportunities for refining existing processes. When undesirable levels of performance or patient outcomes are identified, or when there is an opportunity to improve already acceptable performance, actions must be taken to bring about desired changes. All quality management activities must be documented and reported to involved care givers and leadership groups.

Cancer Data Management

A system to monitor all types of cancer diagnosed or treated in an institution is a critical element in the evaluation of cancer care. The cancer registry in an accredited program must meet the standards defined in the American College of Surgeons Standards of the Commission on Cancer, Volume II: Registry Operations and Data Standards. Data must be collected and analyzed on all reportable cancer diagnoses. The registry must be staffed by knowledgeable personnel and cases must be abstracted within six months from the date of initial diagnosis. The registry must maintain patient confidentiality.

Long-term follow-up is essential to evaluate cancer care outcomes. Follow-up information must be obtained for all patients in the registry database to meet required follow-up rates. The registry must then submit data to the National Cancer Data Base, which provides benchmarking for patient care and quality improvement efforts of the individual cancer programs.

To meet the reporting requirements, the cancer committee must use the data collected for special studies and report the results to the facility medical and administrative staffs.

The approved cancer program must have public education, cancer prevention and screening programs for the community.

Members of the cancer care team in an approved cancer program are required to participate in ongoing cancer education pertinent to their specialty or field.

Cancer Program Approval

Eligible programs may initiate the approvals process by requesting consultative services. All institutions seeking initial approval of their cancer program must be evaluated by a consultant. Regionally-based field staff provide consultative services and conduct cancer program surveys. After the consultant visits the institution, a status report is prepared, including recommendations to improve the program when appropriate. Prior to approval, the institution must demonstrate one year of compliance with the standards and the registry must have accrued two years of data with one year of successful follow-up. The institution then makes a written request for a survey. At the time of the site survey, cancer program leadership is interviewed, documents are reviewed, and a summary session is held.

The surveyor's report is independently reviewed by two members of the Committee on Approvals Section of the ACS's Cancer Department. Approval recommendations are decided by a majority vote of the Committee on Approvals, followed by review and confirmation by the Executive Committee of the Commission on Cancer and the Board of Regents of the ACS.

Four year approval is awarded for programs that meet the standards. These programs are resurveyed every four years. Three year approval with contingency is awarded when a previously approved program has one or more measurable deficiencies that can be easily corrected and for which documentation of corrective action can be easily provided. One year approval is granted when a previously approved program has multiple deficiencies, and the potential and motivation of the institution's staff indicate that the deficiencies will be corrected within a reasonable time. Nonapproval is used when broad and multiple deficiencies exist in a previously approved program. Deferred status is designated when unclear or insufficient information about a cancer program is submitted, and an approval decision cannot be made.

APPROVED TRAUMA CENTERS[6]

The American College of Surgeons (ACS) Committee on Trauma has been committed to reducing trauma morbidity and mortality and published guidelines for care of the injured patient in 1976. A natural result of the establishment of trauma guidelines was the development of a verification process whereby a hospital can be surveyed by ACS trauma surgeons to determine whether the facility meets ACS criteria. The approvals (verification) program was initiated in 1987, and by mid-1993, ACS completed more than 200 surveys and consultation site visits. The goal of a trauma system "is to match a health care facility's resources with a patient's medical needs so that optimal and cost effective care is achieved."[7] The program continues to grow with more and more hospitals seeking ACS verification of their trauma services. The MSSP may assist with supporting this effort. The MSSP should be familiar with the designations made by ACS for trauma centers and have some knowledge of the respective requirements for his or her own facility's trauma level.

Trauma Center Levels

Because hospitals have varying resources and capabilities, depending upon size and location, the ACS has designated four levels for trauma services.

Level I Centers

The Level I facility is a regional resource trauma center that is a tertiary care facility. Because of the large personnel and facility resources required for patient care, most Level I facilities are university-based teaching hospitals.

Level II Centers

The Level II center is a hospital that is expected to provide initial definitive trauma care regardless of the severity of the injury. The Level II center can be an academic institution or a public or private community facility located in either an urban, suburban, or rural area.

Level III Centers

The Level III center serves communities that do not have immediate access to a Level I or II institution. Level III trauma centers can provide prompt assessment, resuscitation, emergency operations, and patient stabilization and can also arrange for possible transfer to a facility that can provide definitive trauma care.

Level IV Centers

The Level IV facility provides advanced trauma life support in remote areas where no higher level of care is available prior to patient transfer.

Hospital Criteria

In order to be an ACS approved trauma facility, each hospital must meet criteria. Criteria are designated as "essential" or "desired" for the respective levels. In other words, all criteria are essential for a Level I trauma center, most criteria are essential for a Level II center, and some are desirable for Levels III and IV.

Hospital Organization

The trauma service must be established by the medical staff, which is responsible for coordinating the care of injured patients, the training of personnel, and trauma quality improvement. Privileges for physicians participating in trauma care are determined through the medical staff credentialing process. A trauma service director, who is a board certified surgeon, must be designated. A multidisciplinary trauma committee is required for Levels I and II. Hospital departments or sections of general, neurologic, and orthopedic surgery; emergency services, and anesthesiology are required for Levels I and II. Neurosurgery and orthopedic surgery departments are not required for Levels III and IV. An emergency service is not required for Level IV. Criteria also spell out the various clinical capabilities of the hospital according to level.

Criteria also address the facilities, resources and capabilities that each Level must meet. These criteria address specially trained personnel, resuscitation equipment, operating room capabilities, postanesthesia recovery room capabilities, intensive care units, radiologic and laboratory capabilities, and rehabilitation service staff and equipment, with specific requirements for each Level.

All ACS approved trauma centers must have a quality improvement program. Quality improvement activities include a trauma registry, special audits for all trauma deaths, morbidity and mortality conferences, and other reviews. A criterion for Levels I, II, and III is that an on-call schedule must be published for surgical and other major medical specialties.

There are criteria for outreach programs, prevention and publication education, a trauma research program, continuing medical education, trauma support personnel, organ procurement activity, and transfer agreements.

The Approvals Process

The designation of trauma facilities is a political process performed by the local governmental emergency medical service (EMS) authorities. The ACS approvals and consultation program is designed to assist hospitals in evaluation and improvement of trauma care but does not actually designate a facility as a trauma center. At the request of an appropriate local or state authority and of the hospital, a verification review will be performed by the ACS.

The facility applies to the ACS, completes a pre-survey questionnaire and hospital resources checklist, and the survey is scheduled. A team of two surgeons from ACS perform the site visit and report their findings to the ACS trauma department. The final report is confidential and is sent to the requesting governmental agency or to the hospital by the ACS Committee on Trauma. Maximum approval for successful facilities is for three years. Reverification is accomplished through the same review process.

The Committee on Trauma of the ACS also provides consultation to hospitals, communities, and state authorities for the purpose of identifying areas for improving trauma care or preparing for a verification visit.

CONTINUING MEDICAL EDUCATION PROGRAMS

A large number of states have mandatory continuing medical education (CME) requirements for physician relicensure or for membership in the state medical association. Some malpractice insurance plans and physician specialty organizations require participation in CME.

Since there is a significant cost to practitioners, not only in tuition but in time away from practice for participation in CME, many health care facilities provide accredited CME programs for their medical staffs. Such programs are frequently supported by medical staff services departments.

CME should play a role in a practitioner's delineation of clinical privileges, and CME programs offered should be based in part on results of the medical staff's performance improvement findings, as required by the Joint Commission on Accreditation of Healthcare Organizations.

Depending upon the sophistication of the CME program, medical staff services personnel can spend a significant amount of time assisting the CME committee with curriculum development, contacting speakers for conferences, notifying medical staff members, compiling and analyzing program evaluations, and recording CME credits for reporting to medical staff members.

The Physician's Recognition Award

To provide additional motivation to pursue CME, the American Medical Association (AMA) offers the voluntary Physician's Recognition Award (PRA). Applications are based on one, two or three years of CME, and certificates issued are valid for one, two or three years from the date of application. Criteria for the awards are as follows:[8]

Educational Options for the PRA

Activities designated by accredited sponsors as category 1 or category 2 include

1. formal activities such as lectures, seminars, and workshops;
2. CME enduring materials, such as tapes and computer-assisted learning (category 1 only);
3. journal club activities;
4. self-assessment activities;
5. journal-based CME.

Physician-designated activities—category 2—includes:

1. consultation with peers and experts concerning patients,
2. use of electronic databases in patient care,
3. small group discussions,
4. self-assessment activities,
5. journal club activities not designated as category 1,
6. teaching health professionals,
7. use of enduring material not designated as category 1,
8. medical writing,
9. teleconferences,
10. preceptorships,
11. participating in formal peer review and quality assurance activities,
12. preparation of educational exhibits,
13. formal learning activities not designated as category 1 or category 2.

Other routes to obtaining PRA certificates include

1. participating in an accredited residency program,
2. passing a board recertification examination,
3. study for a medically related degree,
4. other meritorious learning experiences,
5. reciprocity with other medical education certificates,
6. international conferences approved by the AMA for category 1 credit.

The AMA offers two PRA certificates, the standard award and one with commendation. The requirements for the certificates are listed below. Reading authoritative literature an average of two hours per week is required for all certificates.

AMA PRA Certificate with Commendation for Self-directed Learning
(Reading is *not* reportable as category 2 for the certificate with commendation.)

3-year certificate: 150 hours—60 hours category 1; 60 hours category 2; 30 hours category 1 or 2

2-year certificate: 100 hours—40 hours category 1; 40 hours category 2; 10 hours category 1 or 2

1-year certificate: 50 hours—20 hours category 1; 20 hours category 2; 10 hours category 1 or 2

AMA PRA Standard Certificate
(Reading *is* reportable as category 2 for the standard certificate.)

3-year certificate: 150 hours—60 hours category 1; 90 hours category 1 or 2
2-year certificate: 100 hours—40 hours category 1; 60 hours category 1 or 2
1-year certificate: 50 hours—20 hours category 1; 30 hours category 1 or 2

Category 1 credit refers to programs accredited by the AMA. The Accreditation Council for Continuing Medical Education (ACCME) is the organization that accredits programs for national sponsors. The ACCME is composed of representatives of the AMA, the American Board of Medical Specialties, the American Hospital Association, the Association for Hospital Medical Education, the Association of American Medical Colleges, the Council of Medical Specialty Societies, and the Federation of State Medical Boards. State medical associations survey, evaluate and accredit CME programs at community facilities whose programs meet the essentials and guidelines of approved programs. Only institutions accredited as CME sponsors by the ACCME or their state medical society may designate a CME activity for AMA PRA credit.

Accredited CME

In order to be accredited, a health care facility must meet standards called the *Essentials and Guidelines for the Accreditation of CME Sponsors.* These are briefly described below.[9]

Essential 1—Institutional Commitment and Mission

The institution must demonstrate an institution-wide commitment to the overall CME program. Evidence of this commitment must be demonstrated through a written CME mission statement that has been formally approved by the institution's governing body. The mission statement must include the goals of the overall CME program, scope of the effort, characteristics of the physicians for whom activities and services will be provided, and the general types of CME activities and services to be provided.

Essential 2—Needs Assessment

The CME sponsor must have established procedures to identify and analyze the CME needs and interests of its prospective participants. In doing this, the CME sponsor must use data sources beyond the sponsor's own perception of need.

Essential 3—Educational Objectives and Audience Identification

The sponsor must have specific, clearly stated learning objectives for each CME activity. The target audience for whom the activity is designed must be defined. The objectives must be compatible with the prospective participants' knowledge levels, professional experience, and preferred learning styles.

Essential 4—Educational Design and Planning

Educational activities must be planned and designed in a manner that will most effectively accomplish the stated objectives. The CME sponsor must use competent faculty and appropriate educational facilities.

Essential 5—Evaluation

The sponsor must evaluate its overall CME program and each of its educational activities. Evaluation methods must be used to assess the extent to which objectives were met, the quality of the instructional process, and the extent to which participants feel the activity will improve their professional performance. The sponsor must demonstrate that evaluation data are used in CME planning.

Essential 6—Program Management and Resource Allocation

The sponsor must demonstrate that appropriate management procedures and adequate resources are available and used to accomplish the CME mission. There must be a CME committee, administrative support, provisions for continuity of the program, a budget and resource allocation, and CME records.

Essential 7—Joint Sponsorship

An accredited CME sponsor may be asked by non-accredited entities to jointly plan and present CME activities. This essential outlines the requirements for co-sponsoring a program with a non-accredited facility.

CME Accreditation Process

A health care facility seeking accreditation of its CME program can obtain information and application forms from the state medical association or society. The first step in the accreditation process is completion of a pre-survey questionnaire. If the pre-survey questionnaire demonstrates significant compliance with the Essentials, the state medical association then invites the facility to complete the application forms. Completion of these forms is time-consuming and provides an exhaustive look at the CME program of the facility. If the application meets with approval by the state medical association CME committee, a site survey is then scheduled. Representatives of the state's CME committee conduct the site survey, meeting with the CME committee chair and members and CME support staff, visiting educational facilities, and reviewing documentation.

Provisional Accreditation is awarded for two years to an initial applicant that successfully completes the accreditation process. Full Accreditation is awarded for up to four years to an accredited institution following completion of the provisional period and a second review and site survey. Probationary Accreditation is awarded to a fully accredited institution, following formal review and a site survey, when the CME committee determines that the institution is not in substantial compliance with the Essentials. Non-Accreditation is given to an initial applicant following a review that reveals that the institution is not in substantial compliance with the Essentials.

NOTES

1. *Federal Register* (June 18, 1991) Vol. 46.111.
2. *Federal Register* (June 18, 1991) Vol. 46.107.
3. U.S. Department of Health and Human Services, Public Health Service, National Institutes of Health, *Protecting Human Research Subjects: Institutional Review Board Guidebook* (Washington, D.C.: Government Printing Office, 1993).
4. U.S. Department of Health and Human Services, Public Health Service, Food and Drug Administration, *FDA IRB Information Sheets* (Washington, D.C.: Government Printing Office, 1989).

5. American College of Surgeons, Commission on Cancer, *Standards of the Commission on Cancer, Volume I: Cancer Program Standards* (Chicago: American College of Surgeons, 1996).

6. American College of Surgeons, Committee on Trauma, *Resources for Optimal Care of the Injured Patient:1993* (Chicago: American College of Surgeons, 1993).

7. Ibid., 8.

8. American Medical Association, *The Physician's Recognition Award Information Booklet* (Chicago: American Medical Association, 1997).

9. Texas Medical Association, *The Accreditation of Continuing Medical Education in Texas* (Austin: Texas Medical Association, 1998).

Chapter 12

Credentialing and Peer Review Issues

Vicki L. Searcy

Individuals who participate in credentialing and peer review frequently ask questions related to legal and other issues. In this chapter, questions that are often the subject of debate have been posed to a panel of experts.

Special thanks to Mark Kadzielski, Esq., an attorney with the Los Angeles office of Epstein Becker & Green; Lowell Brown, Esq., of Foley Lardner Weissburg & Aronson, Los Angeles; and Geneva Harris, CMSC, CPHQ, CPCS, Clinical Affairs Division of UC Davis Medical Center, Sacramento, California, who served as experts in answering the following questions.

CREDENTIALING QUESTIONS

Q: Do all health care organizations consider the same type of credentialing information?

A: While all organizations consider some information, such as licensure, board certification, controlled substances registration and professional liability insurance, managed care organizations (MCOs) and hospitals also have separate interests.

MCOs review office practices that have traditionally not impacted hospitals. They are more likely to be concerned with a provider's financial stability and geographic location in terms of other providers and patients. Hospitals, on the other hand, are more likely to consider location in terms of distance from the hospital.

Hospitals extend specific clinical privileges to providers, thus necessitating information related to current clinical competency to exercise specific privileges, while MCOs verify credentials to allow providers to function in the managed care setting. Hospitals most often relate to providers as independent contractors, while MCOs may employ or contract with providers for services.

Q: If several organizations require the same information, is it necessary for physicians to be credentialed by each one?

A: Yes, each provider must be credentialed by each organization. If a physician contracts with 14 health maintenance organizations, for example, he or she must submit credentialing documentation to each one, even though much of the information sought is identical for each.

Q: Is credentialing a one-time process?

A: Most hospital privileges and MCO contracts are subject to renewal at specified intervals—two years for organizations that are accredited by the National Association for Quality Assurance (NCQA) or Joint Commission on Accreditation of Healthcare Organizations (JCAHO). In hospitals, continuation of privileges is based on "demonstrated competence" or "acceptable quality of professional performance" as specified in the bylaws. In the absence of evidence to the contrary, however, most hospitals assume physicians are competent and the continuation of privileges is generally a *pro forma* action.

MCOs are required by NCQA standards to consider member complaints, quality review results, utilization management, member satisfaction surveys, medical records reviews and site visits to practitioners' offices during recredentialing. Recredentialing also must include primary source verification.

Q: Are health care organizations required to do all their own credentialing, or can the responsibility be delegated?

A: Hospitals typically do their own credentialing, but it is not unusual for MCOs to employ a third party for some or all credentialing duties.

In that case, NCQA standards require that MCOs verify their oversight of any delegated credentialing functions in writing, indicating the responsibilities of the MCO and the delegated entity, what activities have been delegated, the process the MCO uses to evaluate the delegated entity's performance and what actions will be taken if the delegated entity fails to meet its obligations. As evidence of oversight, the MCO is required to review 5 percent or 50 of the delegated entity's credentialing files, whichever is less. This auditing requirement is waived when the delegated entity is an NCQA-certified credentials verification organization.

JCAHO does not have specific standards for delegated credentialing. Instead, it addresses the delegation of any function in general and does provide some guidelines to be used in selecting a credentials verification organization (CVO).

In either case, however, the delegating body must retain the right to make key decisions regarding provider services, including revocation or restriction of privileges when required.

Q: What should hospitals do (if anything) to credential physicians in other states who are providing services to patients via telemedicine?

A: Telemedicine (long-distance medicine) started as phone consultations between practitioners at different facilities. It has blossomed to include many kinds of off-site medical consultations, such as videoconferencing between providers and patients in real time. Other telemedicine methods include radio links to emergency medicine personnel, teleradiology, interactive computing, computer-based patient records, and many other audio, video, and data transmission technologies.

There is no federal law regulating telemedicine, nor is there any uniformity among state laws impacting telemedicine. Physician licensure is the key issue when medicine is practiced across state lines through media such as videoconferencing.

Some states have statutes specifically permitting limited telemedicine physician consultations in their states by physicians licensed only in another state. Other states specifically prohibit such consultations, and still other states have no statutes on the subject. Consultants licensed in the patient's home state do not face this obstacle.

If the "practice of medicine" is taking place, a license is required. Therefore, hospitals must first examine the interaction between all the physicians and patients involved to determine whether acts have, or will, occur that constitute the practice of medicine. Then the licensure status of the consulting physician must be determined.

Before embarking on out-of-state telemedicine consultations, it is prudent that an organization do the following:

Verify that all the physicians involved have specific professional liability insurance coverage for telemedicine consultations.

Make sure the out-of-state physicians providing telemedicine consultations are licensed to practice in the state in which the hospital is located, unless licensure is not required in the state by statute.

Create patient consent forms specific to telemedicine. A telemedicine consent form should inform the patient that there may be problems with telemedicine transmission, so they are assuming risks in connection with signal transmission and linkups to the satellite or cable. The patient should also consent to have another person, such as a camera operator, present during a consultation to take photos or videos of the patient.

Maintain an accurate medical record.

Have one person or department in the organization handle all telemedicine transactions in order to maintain centralized records that can be quickly accessed.

After considering all of the issues, organizations using telemedicine should draft an agreement with off-site providers that addresses the above issues, as well as other matters, such as compensation. This will help to ensure that the resulting relationship is beneficial to the patient, the providers, and the organization itself.

Q: Is it possible to expedite the credentialing process?

A: Many organizations are "fast-tracking" portions of the credentialing process. Fast-tracking usually means that the evaluation and decision-making portion of the credentialing process is expedited when verified information indicates that an applicant meets all criteria for membership and privileges and no "red flag" information (malpractice cases, disciplinary actions, time gaps, and so on) has been identified.

Organizations that fast-track typically have individuals (rather than full committees) review credentials files and make recommendations outside the committee process. For example, a department chair can review a credentials file as soon as all verifications have been completed and it can then be routed straight to the medical executive committee as long as the fast-track criteria has been met. Some organizations choose to have the chief of staff act on behalf of the medical executive committee; however, the JCAHO standards for hospitals specifically state that the medical executive committee must act on all applications for membership and privileges. It may be wise to wait until this has been clarified by the JCAHO. The JCAHO has endorsed the practice of having a designee of the governing body act on behalf of the board, however. The caveat here is that the designee should be a voting member of the board.

Fast-tracking can be an efficient way to deal with non-problematic applications for membership and privileges. It is important, however, to ensure that the integrity of the credentialing process is not sacrificed for the sake of speed.

CONFIDENTIALITY ISSUES

Q: The information revealed during credentialing and the peer review process may be very sensitive. Are there laws to protect the confidentiality of the information, as well as the sources?

A: Lacking federal confidentiality legislation, states have enacted their own laws, most of which are aimed at hospitals rather than MCOs, and many of which are conflicting. Some states protect the confidentiality of information that is shared between peer review committees without differentiating between types of committees. Others protect only hospital committees, leaving MCOs to fend for themselves.

In some cases, confidentiality guarantees may even vary within a health care system. For example, in a network that includes hospitals, surgi-centers, physician practices and other facilities, professional sources may be protected in some situations but not in others.

This patchwork of state statutes may actually harm the peer review process. States passed confidentiality laws because they recognized that immunity is essential for meaningful and constructive peer review, but the very existence of so many different laws puts confidentiality at risk.

Physicians concerned that their confidentiality could be jeopardized may be reluctant to provide the candid comments that make peer review valuable, and credentialing bodies may have significant difficulty getting the information they need.

Q: Does the problem arise only between states? Do physicians whose practice is limited to one state have credentialing difficulties?

A: They may. The information needed for credentialing belongs only to one party—the one that obtained it—but several other parties may want access to it. Depending on state laws, that may not be possible to do while maintaining confidentiality.

Most existing laws date from the 1950s, and the laws did not anticipate managed care organizations. Nearly half a century later, any proposed legislative changes must be examined closely to see how they will affect other laws that have been enacted in the meantime. Some parties—such as plaintiffs' attorneys—always oppose extension of confidentiality privileges and can create significant resistance to change.

Q: How does a credentialing body determine when to release credentialing and peer review records, given the patchwork of confidentiality laws?

A: Entities such as state licensing boards are entitled to obtain certain information, while physicians are entitled to privacy regarding other information. It is possible to balance the rights of both groups, but it requires planning and expertise.

Credentialing bodies must first determine exactly who is requesting the information before they can decide whether to provide it. For example, federal regulations specify that investigators for the Health Care Financing Administration (HCFA) have virtually unrestricted access to credentialing documentation when they survey for Medicare conditions. However, when those same investigators survey on behalf of state and local governments, the same information may be off limits.

Most states allow peer review bodies to share their findings because it is in the public interest to do so, but credentialing entities aren't required to release any information. As a practical matter, however, it is often advantageous for credentialing bodies to share information, and in many cases managed care contracts require peer review files of member physicians to be available for review by the payer.

Q: Is there any information that is always confidential?

A: Attorney-client privileged information may not be divulged to anyone under any circumstances.

Other sensitive information, such as a physician's HIV status or treatment for substance abuse, may be protected by state law. Credentialing bodies must determine what is protected before deciding whether to release such documents.

In any event, credentialing and peer review files must be maintained in such a way as to protect confidential information while allowing access to data that is not confidential.

Q: What is the best way to protect confidential information?

A: For hospitals, where access to confidential information is limited to a person or department, the records may be fairly easy to control. It is more difficult to restrict access at a credentialing verification organization (CVO), where many people can obtain records.

In either case, the credentialing body should establish a segregated filing system. This could take the form of a master file which includes general information on each physician as well as a folder or envelope clearly marked confidential. The contents of both sections may vary by state; but in general, the confidential file would contain such records as quality assessment, peer review and risk management, while the non-confidential file would include such information as the physician application, DEA certification and appointment records.

Another option is to maintain separate files, with confidential and general information kept in separate rooms or cabinets. While that method is acceptable, it does increase the risk that a surveyor may inadvertently be denied access to something that should be disclosed. That, in turn, may open the credentialing body to charges of hiding information.

Regardless of the filing system, credentialing entities should institute a clearly defined protocol for responding to requests for information. This protocol should include fail-safe measures to guard against improper disclosure, such as a decision tree that indicates how questions are to be referred upward in the organization.

Q: When information is released, what guarantee is there that it will remain confidential?

A: The reality is that the releasing organization has no control over what the recipient does with information. However, a written agreement can define expectations and provide some peace of mind. The document need not be complex, but it should establish the terms for sharing information that provide some assurance that the recipient will respect confidentiality.

PEER REVIEW ISSUES

Q: In addition to concerns that their comments on a colleague may be released inappropriately, members of peer review committees may fear retaliatory legal actions by physicians who are subject to disciplinary action. Are these fears justified?

A: The question that is paramount in any physician review is whether the physician's performance puts patients at risk. That determination should be the overriding factor in any peer review process, but fear of a lawsuit may impede effective action.

If a physician's activities warrant disciplinary action, extensive documentation of a pattern of poor performance is critical. In such in-depth assessments, patient records, incident reports, malpractice claims, and other documents may be reviewed.

What may be equally disturbing to peer reviewers are the moral and emotional burdens discipline may entail. Privilege revocation can be tantamount to ending a physician's right to practice in a community, and can have consequences including loss of livelihood and public disgrace.

However, both the courts and public opinion condemn failure to address a known performance problem, and the price for inaction is almost certain to be higher than the emotional cost for reviewers.

When the evidence indicates a problem exists, the law is clear on what steps can and should be taken. To withstand a later review, the legal requirements for due process must be met. These include the physician's right to a hearing, an impartial determination of privilege revocation, discretionary right to counsel, written statements of specific charges and of the final decision and a decision that is based on substantive evidence.

Q: Are there ways to minimize the likelihood of successful retaliatory legal action after an adverse peer review?

A: The key to defending against such lawsuits, which angry and frightened physicians are prone to file, is proof that the process was fair, objective and unbiased.

Common flaws a plaintiff's attorney will look for include conflict of interest, poor documentation, unfair determination and uneven standards.

To avoid charges of conflict of interest, physicians who participate in peer review should not be able to benefit in any way if the reviewed physician loses privileges. Direct competitors, partners of competitors and physicians with a long history of animosity toward the physician, for example, should not be included on that physician's peer review panel.

In smaller communities, where interests are more closely related, it may be necessary for the medical staff to seek reviewers from outside the community. Ideally, the medical staff and the physician being reviewed should agree on the outside reviewers selected.

When an adverse peer review result follows a gradual loss of confidence in a physician, the hospital must have a clearly documented history to avoid charges of unreasonable or arbitrary action. While a specific incident may precipitate the negative review, it may be minor when viewed out of context. Without adequate documentation, the physician may successfully claim the adverse decision was unreasonable.

A claim of bias may also be leveled at a medical staff that loses confidence in a physician and then seeks support from other physicians to revoke that physician's privileges. If the physician can prove a decision to terminate privileges was reached before the peer review hearings, the claim of bias may be upheld. Physicians who are concerned about a colleague should provide information to the peer review committee and then let the committee fulfill its function.

Finally, peer review committees must guard against a natural tendency to hold physicians with abrasive personalities to higher standards than their more affable colleagues. If the unpopular physician sues, his or her record will be compared with others to see whether peer reviewers were consistent in their application of standards.

Q: Is there any risk of liability for peer review committees in making insurance coverage decisions?

A: While most courts and legislatures have not yet taken a position on this subject, the rulings to date show a tendency to hold health plans and medical directors accountable for insurance coverage decisions.

In a number of cases, courts have ruled that in denying coverage, a medical director was actually engaged in the practice of medicine—an occupation that should properly be left to the physicians actively involved in treatment of the patient.

Peer review committees appear to have more latitude, however, when their coverage decisions are committee, rather than individual, actions.

CREDENTIALING AND DESELECTION

Q: As managed care organizations continue to expand both in size and number, they may seek to terminate physician contracts without a clear and compelling reason, such as criminal activity or gross malpractice. What standards must MCOs meet to accomplish such "without cause" deselections?

A: The most important consideration cited in court challenges is whether the deselection (or contract termination) process was fair to the practitioner. In a few states, doctors' claims that deselection unfairly impinged on their right to practice prompted "any willing provider" laws which permit any provider to offer services to MCO patients. Most states, however, have no such laws, and disgruntled providers have asked courts to uphold their contention that they are entitled to fair procedure before being terminated.

Decisions in California, New Jersey, Connecticut, and other states affirm physicians' rights to fair procedure in terminations without cause. Without fair procedure, the deselection is deemed arbitrary, and therefore illegal.

Q: What Constitutes Fair Procedure?

A: The definition of fair procedure is still evolving. A fair procedure could be a hearing that lasts 10 days and involves attorneys and witnesses. It also could be a brief meeting in which the practitioner presents his or her case to MCO administrators. Clarification as to which types of procedures are fair will emerge from the courts as more cases are decided.

Q: What other issues affect deselection?

A: Federal and state legislative thinking is strongly in favor of consumer choice when it comes to health care. Patients' bills of rights, or consumers' bills of rights, are popular legislative responses to constituent complaints.

That means MCOs that deselect physicians for business reasons risk being charged with denying patients' choice as well as with interfering with physicians' right to practice. As a result, MCOs may become less likely to deselect physicians simply because they are inefficient or inconveniently located.

More importantly, MCOs may place more significance on avoiding those practitioners in the first place. A well-planned, thorough credentialing program with carefully crafted criteria sets quantifiable standards for practitioners, making it easy for the MCO to deselect or reject a physician who doesn't meet them. For example, if a health care organization requires physicians to be board certified, achieve a certain skill level and have a certain level of advanced training, a physician who is not board certified can be rejected for failing to meet the standards – even if he or she is already under contract—provided the standards are applied fairly and equitably across the organization.

CREDENTIALING CRIMINALS

Q: How can a health care facility protect itself against physicians who may be criminals?

A: First, the facility should have clear guidelines that state in unambiguous terms exactly what behavior is acceptable. The guidelines should address whether non-medical convictions such as income tax evasion warrant the same action as medical felonies, and identify mitigating factors such as how long ago the crime was committed, whether any loss has been redressed and the overall record of the criminal. The guidelines should also state how to deal with different situations, such as a practitioner who is arrested, one who is charged with a felony and later exonerated, one who is brought to trial on felony charges and one who is convicted.

Once the policy is established, it must be set forth in language that leaves no room for misinterpretation. General statements such as "Practitioners agree to abide by the standards of their professional organizations," or "Medical staff members must be of high moral character" are too vague. The criteria must specify what characteristics constitute these goals.

Q: If a physician is arrested, what should the health care organization do?

A: After the guidelines are in place, any specific action will depend on the circumstances of the arrest. Just remember that policies do not offer blanket protection: If an organization learns of the felony arrest of a medical staff member, or an incident in an applicant's past, administrators should confer with medical, legal and credentialing staff to determine what questions are appropriate to ask the practitioner.

The practitioner must answer those questions if he or she wants privileges, regardless of an attorney's advice to the contrary. All 50 states extend privacy protections for credentialing information in this situation, so there is no reason for the practitioner not to provide full information.

Once all the facts have been established, the credentialer can decide what action is warranted, based on the facility's standards.

CREDENTIALING GROUP PRACTICES

Q: Many times, health care facilities contract with group practices to provide certain services. How can the facility be sure everyone in the group is properly credentialed?

A: The facility should require all members of the group, and all subcontractors, to obtain clinical privileges. The ultimate responsibility for proper credentialing rests with the facility, although the more sophisticated groups do their own credentialing, often having an administrator verify that the group's doctors and subcontractors have the necessary membership and privileges.

Q: What if a provider is not credentialed?

A: Problems may arise when a group provides a new physician without notifying the facility. There can be pressure on the contracting facility to look the other way in such situations, which typically arise when the group is striving to assure adequate coverage. The suggestion may be that if no harm was done, the facility could ignore poorly credentialed providers, but that is never true. The contracting facility must always ensure that its practitioners are properly credentialed.

ACADEMIC/TEACHING HOSPITALS

Q: Can credentialing be effective in an academic teaching hospital?

A: Teaching hospitals are different from community hospitals when it comes to credentialing, but they should still comply with credentialing standards.
In the teaching hospital, there are permanent department chairs and office staff, the turnover is low, and office staff can provide credentialing support. In community hospitals, by contrast, department chairs change regularly and there is typically no permanent support staff assigned to a specific department.
Physicians in a teaching hospital practice in a defined group that offers continuous support and oversight. That closeness, coupled with the constant presence of residents, serves a monitoring function as well as affords opportunities for consultations and feedback. Peer review is virtually constant.

Q: What unique credentialing opportunities arise in the academic teaching hospital setting?

A: Billing data is readily available, since the academic setting permits a professional firm to do the billing for all practices. The department chair receives a monthly report that details such facts as the number of clinic visits or types of procedures each physician has performed that month. That data offers another check on volume and usage that often isn't available in a community hospital.

The teaching structure provides more information. When residents complete monthly, quarterly or end-of-rotation evaluations of their instructors, they provide feedback for the competency summary.

In addition, teaching hospitals can track continuity of care from pre-admission through surgery and outcomes after surgery. Community hospitals don't always know what problems may arise after surgery, because patients go to their physicians' offices for follow-up care.

Q: Are there other differences between academic and community hospitals?

A: Academic hospitals regularly conduct morbidity and mortality (M&M) reviews of specific cases. JCAHO has questioned the value of M&Ms, so many community hospitals have abandoned them in favor of more general performance improvement activities.

But M&Ms have peer review value, because physicians regularly discuss individual cases in depth. This provides a close look at the attending physician's actions, and can quickly identify those practitioners who may warrant closer attention.

In addition, academic teaching hospitals must be sure research projects are not assigned to physicians who do not have the privileges to do them. Because the department chair is familiar with privileging for the staff, he or she can verify that the research is within the proper parameters for the physician seeking the protocol.

Q: What credentialing issues do academic teaching hospitals face?

A: The biggest concern is that house staff, rather than attending physicians, provide a good portion of patient care. That means that data profiles intended to assess an attending physician's performance actually reflect the work of the residents who provided the care.

The same circumstances affect patient profiles, because patient care is always provided under the name of the attending physician, rather than the name of the resident who provided the care. Discharge data is also attributed to the physician who discharged the patient, although a single patient may have been cared for by a number of residents in several disciplines before being released.

Additionally, in this setting, the dean must encourage all departments to involve credentialing staff early in the recruitment process, rather than looking at credentialing issues just before making a job offer.

Q: What steps can academic teaching hospitals take to assure the value of credentialing data?

A: One method is simply to understand the assumptions implicit in the data, acknowledge that it is flawed, and make allowances accordingly—at the same time recognizing that the attending physician is ultimately responsible for what the house staff does.

Another option is to circumvent the data by placing more emphasis on other measures. Academic teaching hospitals have unique opportunities to evaluate clinical competence, and credentialing committees can rely on areas other than data systems for information.

Q: How can academic teaching hospitals be certain that all faculty members are clinically competent at the time of reappointment?

A: Academic teaching hospitals have opportunities for evaluation that do not arise in community hospitals and that do not translate outside the academic setting. Because of the nature of the environment, assessments may be based on direct observation or assistance with care, student evaluations, or call coverage.

In academic hospitals, department chairs regularly see reports on matters such as pharmacy and therapeutics, blood usage, invasive procedures and other quality management factors for each physician. Because of the close working relationship between the department chair and the physician, the chair can provide valuable insight into the competency of the physician in question.

Beyond that, articles in faculty publications or presentations to a professional group may indicate competence.

Q: What type of privilege delineation is effective in the outpatient setting for teaching hospitals?

A: Because teaching hospitals have a long history of providing care in clinic settings, they have inadvertently delineated privileges without differentiating between inpatient and outpatient services.

Instead, they are more likely to have established permissible levels of care. For example, a category I family practitioner may be allowed to provide only basic care, while a category II board-certified doctor may do more advanced care, and a category III may provide any level of care required. The privileges apply to the doctor without regard to whether the care is provided on an inpatient or outpatient basis.

Community hospitals, which traditionally provided only inpatient care and therefore were not concerned with office practices, now are running clinics as well. That forces them to determine what physicians may do as outpatient procedures and which services must be provided only on an inpatient basis.

Teaching hospitals often employ a consultant privileging category. Consultant status is granted to those physicians who need privileges because they touch patients in the course of their teaching duties, but consultants are low-volume practitioners who may be allowed to provide only non-invasive, outpatient services.

Q: How can teaching hospitals accomplish effective proctoring when a primary care provider never admits to the inpatient setting?

A: Teaching hospitals, or indeed any hospitals that operate clinics or have a far-flung primary care network, must make some extra effort to proctor physicians who may practice an hour or two from the hospital.

If the primary care provider has privileges but turns patients over to a hospitalist when they are admitted, proctoring is of necessity limited to outpatient care.

Effective proctoring should include concurrent and retrospective observation. Proctors should be present for procedures, or review outcomes, charts, lab reports, and other records when the procedure has been completed. Patient complaints are another proctoring mechanism.

Regardless of how proctoring is done, hospitals should be certain the cases that are proctored match privilege delineation. For example, if someone has obstetrical and gynecological privileges, proctors cannot look only at obstetrical procedures.

Q: Academic institutions are often large, complex, politically charged environments. Can the structure foster communication among the administration, medical staff and board of directors?

A: Absolutely. The easiest way to open avenues of communication is to encourage cross-representation on governing bodies. The chair of the faculty executive committee, for example, can be an ad hoc member of the medical staff executive committee, and the hospital administrator should be a member of the dean's leadership council. When a representative of each branch is present at all meetings, everyone receives the same information in the same way.

In addition, the chief of staff or medical director should have equal standing in the hospital structure with the director of nursing or the director of finance. It is critical that medical directors be recognized as supervisors as well as practitioners if they are to function effectively as administrators in the academic hospital environment.

Chapter 13

The Impaired or Disruptive Physician

Cindy A. Gassiot, CMSC, CPCS

The exact numbers of physicians impaired by drug or alcohol abuse in the United States are unknown, but have been estimated to be the same as for the general population, about 8 – 10 percent.[1] Adding to the problem, aging physicians may be impaired by senile dementia or another illness that is progressively debilitating. Medical staff and credentialing services professionals will more than likely encounter this difficult problem sooner or later in their careers. Every health care delivery organization should have in place (1) guidelines and procedures to follow in motivating impaired physicians to seek treatment and (2) a monitoring program that will allow rehabilitated practitioners to return to practice. "Ignoring the value of documented recovery or correction of prior problems only causes attempts to hide disabilities, thus delaying treatment and recovery. The risk of harm to patients treated by a disabled practitioner increases unless the credentialing process recognizes rehabilitation."[2] In the case of an aging physician who no longer has the skills necessary to practice, privileges should be curtailed.

CAUSES OF PHYSICIAN IMPAIRMENT[3]

Physicians work in a state of sustained stress. Despite their medical training, or perhaps because of it, they are prone to hazards such as physical and emotional stress, long hours, irregular sleeping schedules, and constant fatigue. As a result, they often push themselves into substance addiction or other conditions that may result in illnesses or impairments in their ability to practice.

The causes of physician impairment are varied. Studies of physicians who have become impaired suggest that one potential source of impairment may be the individual's inherent personality structure. Although obsessive-compulsive traits can be a professional asset, many individuals with these attributes also demonstrate basic insecurity, dependency, depressive features, and vulnerability to stress. A physician's self-imposed demands, combined with the expectations of his or her professional role, may prove stressful. If the physi-

245

cian is unable to meet his or her needs for nurturing and intimacy, a framework for impairment may be established.

Many aspects of medical training and practice contribute to stress, including long hours with accompanying fatigue and the frustration of caring for chronically ill patients. Many physicians are never taught how to keep an appropriate emotional distance between themselves and their patients. Physicians give and give of themselves emotionally and, over a period of time, experience burnout. At-risk physicians may turn to alcohol, other drugs or

Table 13-1. A Symptom Checklist for Detecting Physician Impairment

A disturbing metamorphosis	Deteriorating job performance
Embarrassing behavior at work and social functions	Absenteeism
Emotional volatility	Complaints about physician's behavior from patients
Evasiveness	or staff
Hostility	Consistent lateness
Inappropriate euphoria	Inability to explain treatment plan
Uncharacteristic impatience or rudeness	Inappropriate chart notes
Uncooperativeness	Inappropriate orders and treatment plans
Unpredictability	Increased incidence of treatment errors
Unreliability	Rounds late at night or at other odd times
Unusually poor personal hygiene	Unreachable when on call
Withdrawal from routine activities	
Chaos at home	**Numerous trials and tribulations**
Abuse	Arrests for driving while intoxicated
Continual discord	Frequent accidents
Inappropriate spending	Frequent hospitalizations
Obsessive involvement in an outside activity -	Frequent involvement in lawsuits
gambling, for instance	Habitual self-prescribing of controlled substances
Sexual problems	Multiple physical complaints
Unexpected absences	

Source: Adapted from "What to do When a Colleague is Impaired," by Patrick H. Hughes, Martha Illige-Saucier, Eric A. Voth, *Patient Care*, vol. 29, p. 119 © by Medical Economics, July 5,1995. Reprinted with permission.

other compulsive behaviors for relief of this psychic pain. The interplay of stress, personality and genetic factors may trigger a chemical dependency.

The clues to impairment may be subtle. Table 13-1 lists the symptoms that may be displayed by a physician who suffers from impairment.

HOSPITAL BASED PROGRAMS*

A hospital has certain legal responsibilities to take action against an incompetent physician. With respect to an impaired physician, however, responsibility and liability are not as clearly defined. Administrators and colleagues often ignore or overlook signs of developing impairment in the hope that it will disappear. Only in cases of blatant impairment do they tend to intervene, and then usually in a punitive manner.

Preferable is a non-punitive approach in which the hospital works as an advocate for the physician, rather than against him, while still safeguarding patients from harm. This type of program can detect emerging impairment, offer support to the physician and his family and encourage early treatment. Helping the impaired physician is in the best interest of the hospital as well as the impaired physician himself and the hospital's patients.

Is A Hospital Program Necessary?

Whether a program at the hospital level is necessary or even feasible depends on several variables, including

1. state mandatory reporting laws,

2. geographic location,

3. size of state,

4. activities and strengths of county medical society programs,

5. activities and strengths of state medical society programs,

6. size of the hospital,

7. hospital constitution and bylaws,

8. interest and level of awareness of the medical staff and administration.

---

*The section, "Hospital-Based Programs," is reprinted from *Proceedings of the 4th AMA Conference on the Impaired Physician*, pp.27-31, with permission of the American Medical Association, ©1980.

Generally speaking, impairment is more likely to be detected at the hospital level much earlier than it is at the county or state medical society level. This is particularly true in a large state or in a densely populated area.

Small hospitals, however, may be especially resistant to initiating programs because of their size, the intimacy among staff or time constraints. This may necessitate the involvement of the county or state medical society program.

Ideally, a hospital, county and state medical society program will complement one another. For example, if a hospital working in concert with a state program is unsuccessful in encouraging an impaired physician to seek treatment, the state society may become involved and thereby assure that the physician does not evade the issue even if he changes his hospital affiliation or practice mode.

Organization

No single model is applicable to all hospitals because of the many variables in hospital bylaws, size and state laws. These differences, however, give each hospital the capability of establishing a program that is tailored to its individual needs. The local hospital association, county medical society or state medical society may be able to identify programs operating in other hospitals in the area which can be used as a model.

A formal policy on physician impairment should be incorporated into the bylaws and should include a provision for immediate suspension of privileges if a physician is a threat to himself or his patients. Legal input will assure that due process elements, informed consent, confidentiality aspects and the legal rights of both the hospital and an impaired physician are adequately addressed. Additionally, the bylaws should include a provision of immunity for those acting on behalf of the hospital program.

A program to aid impaired physicians should be organizationally separate from...credential review and peer review, although it is desirable that input from committees charged with carrying out these functions be utilized where feasible in case-finding activities.

The hospital should continually promote its advocacy program to assure visibility and use. In this regard, an ongoing education component encourages reporting from staff and other hospital personnel, and is beneficial in increasing levels of awareness, changing negative attitudes and stereotypical perceptions, and providing cognitive information on the nature and treatability of impairment. Where possible, educational programs for spouses should be initiated. The spouse is often aware, far earlier than hospital personnel, of a physician's impairment.

In addition to education and promotion, other components of a hospital-based program include case-findings, intervention, rehabilitation and re-entry. It is generally recommended that treatment be arranged on an outpatient basis or in another hospital.

Case-Finding

A hospital is responsible for implementing policies to assure that its staff members are capable of providing quality medical care, as well as procedures to assess their mental and physical health. These existing mechanisms can be the foundation for early case-finding and prevention.

Medical staff reappointments (usually made on an annual or biennial basis) offer an avenue to reviewing a physician's performance and discussing potential or existing problems.

While credentialing, peer review and medical staff [quality improvement] functions should be outside the purview of activities relating to helping impaired physicians, members of these committees can help identify physicians who are impaired or potentially impaired.

Reports about a physician who is having problems should be encouraged and accepted from nurses, colleagues, other hospital personnel and family members. For this reason, a visible contact person or contact mechanism (e.g., special "hotline") is imperative. Whether reports, in addition, are accepted from patients, and whether reports may be made on an anonymous basis, is up to the discretion of the hospital. Anonymous reports can be valuable as well as detrimental. In any event, the identity of the person who reports a physician who may possibly be impaired should be kept confidential, and provision for such confidentiality should be stressed to encourage reporting.

Several suggestions have been made with respect to the structure and composition of the specific committee to receive and act on reports of impairment and requests of help. Potential members might include

1. well-liked, respected senior staff members;
2. staff members or administrators recovering from impairment;
3. resident and student representatives;
4. hospital administrators;
5. department heads;
6. chiefs of staff;
7. president, past-president and president-elect of the medical staff (to allow for ongoing knowledge and interest).

Four basic types of committees have been identified: (a) structured, with administrative and physician members; (b) non-structured, with physician members only; (c) structured, with physician members only; and (d) non-structured, with basic members plus others added depending on the individual case. Those programs that are defined as structured have standing committee status with ongoing function, whereas non-structured committees are constituted on an ad hoc, as needed, basis.

Some people feel strongly that staff officers with disciplinary authority should not be included because their presence might deter reporting from those who fear punitive action. Others feel equally strongly that these people with "power" *should* be included because their responsibility for quality care cannot be abdicated or delegated.

The question of whether the committee should be a standing committee or be convened on an ad hoc basis is equally debatable. Both forms have merit.

Regardless of how the committee is composed, it should focus exclusively on problems relating to impairment, as opposed to incompetence or illegal activities.

A mechanism for verifying allegations of impairment should be incorporated into any program. Options include verification by a solo physician member or by a subgroup of the committee.

Intervention

Intervention at the hospital level can emphasize the human factors that have been shown to be positive elements for encouraging a physician to seek treatment. If the committee finds its efforts are hampered by loyalty, embarrassment or overprotectiveness, it may then be necessary to involve the county or state medical society in the intervention process.

If intervention is carried out within the confines of a hospital program, a special group or subcommittee should receive training in intervention techniques. The county or state medical society may be willing to provide training courses. The intervention team may also well include a colleague of the impaired physician whom the "informer" has identified as the person most likely to induce the physician to get treatment.

Basically, the intervention process should be an organized attempt to persuade the physician to get help, while conveying the hope that treatment can be effective. Sources of help should be identified, a definite treatment plan presented and a program for rehabilitation outlined. If the bylaws include a formal policy on physician impairment, this can be used as leverage to encourage the physician to seek help promptly.

If the physician refuses help, it may be necessary to refer him to the usual hospital disciplinary channels. The hospital has the "stick" of being able to restrict or suspend hospital privileges. Even then, discipline should be applied in conjunction with a plan of rehabilitation wherever possible.

Re-entry

The hospital committee should monitor the physician's treatment and recovery, and should continue its advocacy role through the re-entry phase. Once the formerly impaired physician has returned to the hospital, the committee should recommend reinstatement of his privileges based on his current ability to practice. If monitoring of his activities is thought to be necessary for hospital, patient or physician protection, the hospital committee can delineate structured re-entry points that allow for such monitoring (e.g., proctoring of surgical privileges, review of charts, supervised patient care, urine screening).

A CONTRACT WITH AN IMPAIRED PHYSICIAN

Once intervention has occurred and the practitioner has agreed to seek treatment, the hospital or medical society committee should enter into a contract with the affected practitioner. The contract (Exhibit 13-2) should specify the terms under which the hospital or medical society committee will act in an advocacy role to the state licensing board, hospital boards, medical societies, and the Drug Enforcement Agency. The purpose of the contract is to prevent any misunderstanding as to the terms and times specified. The contract should be specifically designed to meet the need of each individual and be uniquely suited to the particular circumstances.

MONITORING PHYSICIANS*

Monitoring a Physician at the Level of the Hospital Medical Staff After Treatment for Chemical Dependence

The purpose of monitoring is to assure the medical staff that a physician resuming patient care responsibilities after treatment for chemical dependence can practice medicine safely.

The medical staff must be satisfied that the physician's current health and mental health meet the medical staff's standards for appointment, reappointment or resumption of patient care.

The medical staff must acknowledge that ongoing, consistent monitoring is required for a specified period of time, (a minimum of two years) and sufficient resources of physician time and attention must be allocated for it.

*Reprinted from *Guidelines for Physician Aid Committees of Hospital Medical Staffs* by the California Medical Association, pp. 6-11, with permission of the California Medical Association, © 1988.

A monitoring plan should be drawn up and it should serve as the basis of a monitoring agreement between the designated medical staff committee and the physician. The following elements should be addressed as the plan is designed:

1. **Treatment**—The medical staff committee should satisfy itself that the physician received the kind of treatment appropriate to the problem and

---

Exhibit 13-2. Sample Contract[4]

Name _____ Date _____

1. I, _____, agree to the terms of this contract for a period of two (2) years from the date of this contract.
2. I understand that all expenses connected with my treatment are to be rendered at my own expense and are my own responsibility.
3. I agree to cease the practice of medicine until clearance is received from the Committee.
4. I agree to enter an approved treatment center for evaluation and detoxification on _____ (date).
5. I agree to Phase I of treatment, which will consist of 28 days or longer of treatment in an in-house rehabilitation center.
6. I agree to Phase II of treatment, which will consist of an outpatient program, including attendance at regular AA meetings, and attendance at the weekly Physicians' Recovery Group.
7. I agree to Phase III of treatment, which may consist of staff training, and, if necessary, gradually phasing into medical practice under the Committee's supervision.
8. I agree to completely abstain from any mood changing chemicals, (alcohol, sedatives, stimulants, narcotics, soporifics, over-the-counter drugs, and so on) except on prescription from my primary care physician, after consultation with the Committee. I will not prescribe any medication for myself.
9. I agree to provide random urine or blood samples in the presence of another physician or designee, at the discretion of the Committee.
10. I agree to identification of a primary care physician before completion of Phase I. All aspects of my case history will be made known to this physician. He will receive a copy of this contract, and agrees to meet and consult with the Committee on Physician Health and Rehabilitation.
11. I agree to the following special terms as they apply to my illness (if any are stipulated).
12. I agree that should I leave treatment, the Committee will remove itself from an advocacy position with the Board of Medical Examiners.

_____
Signature of Impaired Physician

Witness   _____
Approved: _____
Chairman, Committee Monitoring the Physician

sufficient to assure that the problem is being addressed effectively. The medical staff committee should satisfy itself that the physician's current health and mental health are sufficient to allow him/her to practice safely.

An initial course of treatment appropriate to the situation should be instituted and completed. The monitoring plan should incorporate the elements of an aftercare plan and recovery plan which have been recommended by those responsible for the initial treatment.

2. **Release of Information**—The medical staff committee should require that the physician authorize the therapist(s) to communicate information to the medical staff committee. Information should come from those responsible for primary care (initial treatment) as well as aftercare and/or on-going care.

3. **Recovery Plan**—The physician should have a specific, on-going recovery plan sufficient to the situation and to the physician's status in recovery. The monitoring plan should be designed to accumulate the information which will, over time, document the physician's participation in this recovery program.

    Regular participation in a self-help group of persons recovering from chemical dependence (where appropriate, a group of recovering physicians or health professionals) should be required.

4. **Information to be Gathered and Reviewed**—Information about the health status of the physician in recovery and about his or her performance should be gathered and reviewed. The process of gathering and evaluating such information is called monitoring. Information should come from several sources appropriate to the physician's situation, such as from:

    - the hospital work place
    - body fluid test results
    - an aftercare coordinator
    - on-going therapist
    - family
    - office colleagues

The medical staff committee should designate those who are in a position to gather and submit to the coordinator of monitoring the different kinds of information appropriate to the case. These monitors should be appointed as members of the medical staff committee for the purpose of carrying out this activity so that the peer review protections will be applicable.

5. **Regular Contact with a Knowledgeable Observer**—There should be regular, face-to-face contact between the physician and a monitor knowledgeable about chemical dependence and about what to look for in a physician with the condition being monitored. The time and place of the contact should vary. The frequency and length of contact should be determined for each case. For some, daily or even more than once-a-day contact may be indicated, especially in the first days/weeks of the monitoring process. Most usually, three times a week would be considered a minimum. The frequency would vary with the physician's status in recovery. The length of contact must be sufficient to make an observation of the physician's behavior. The record should include periodic notes based on this observation.

   The monitors should be able to create a relationship of mutual trust, support, helpfulness and respect. Monitors, however, should maintain objectivity and diligence throughout the monitoring process.

6. **Coordinator of Monitoring**—All who serve as sources of information should report to one coordinator of monitoring for the case, and that person should be a member of the medical staff committee. The function of the coordinator is to assemble all the information and to review, interpret, evaluate and respond to the comprehensive picture.

7. **Body Fluid Testing**—Body fluid testing is desirable as one element of a monitoring plan. Body fluids (most commonly urine) should be collected on a random schedule and under direct observation. NOTE: Body fluid testing alone does not comprise a sufficient monitoring plan and is not the highest priority element of the plan. Greater weight is given to regular observation of behavior by a knowledgeable monitor.

   The monitoring agreement should specify what role body fluid testing will have in the overall monitoring plan. Where body fluid testing is required, the test done must be able to detect the drug(s) which the physician might use. The agreement should describe how positive results will be interpreted and how the medical staff committee will respond to such results. The monitoring agreement should specify the costs of testing and who pays the costs. The results should be sent to the coordinator of monitoring.

8. **Regular Conferences**—There should be a mechanism for face to face conferences, at the request of any of these parties, between the monitors, the physician monitored, the coordinator of monitoring and the medical staff committee responsible for the monitoring.

9. **Re-evaluation of the Recovery and Monitoring Plans**—There should be regular re-evaluation at some interval, perhaps every six months, by the medical staff committee to assure that it is sufficient to meet the need but does not require elements no longer necessary to the situation. Changes

to the plan should be made so that it fits the current situation of the physician and his or her status in recovery.

It may or may not be appropriate to have this evaluation made by an acknowledged expert outside of the medical staff who will provide a written report. The monitoring agreement should specify the costs of this evaluation and who pays the costs.

10. **Record Keeping**—For each case where there is monitoring, there must be a record. The record should include a copy of the signed monitoring agreement between the physician and the committee. The medical staff committee must have adequate information to asses the physician's status in recovery and compliance with the elements in the agreement. This information must be accumulated in the record and must be kept in strict confidence, preferably in a locked file or other secure storage which may be accessed only by committee members. This information should be retained indefinitely, preferably as long as the physician practices in the hospital plus five years. Disclosure of this information outside of the committee should be made only at the written request of the individual involved or with the advice of legal counsel.

11. **Response to "Slips"**—The monitoring plan should take into consideration the fact that a relapse or resumption of use of alcohol or drugs (or "slip") is not an uncommon phenomenon for those recovering from chemical dependence, especially in the early phases of recovery. Statistics show that slips occur in a significant percent of cases, usually within the first year of sobriety. The response to a slip should be the same as a response to the initial diagnosis; that is, it should be evaluated by a knowledgeable, experienced evaluator and the response should be tailored to the situation. A slip alone should not be considered cause for termination of privileges or loss of employment or position. The customary response to a slip is to intensify the treatment plan, of which monitoring is a part, for a period of time appropriate to the case. It may or may not be appropriate to require that the physician take a leave from patient care for a period of time appropriate to the situation. Consideration should be given to the physician's health and to patient safety in reaching a decision about whether a leave is appropriate.

The purpose of monitoring described here is to assure the medical staff that the physician is in recovery, continues in recovery and is participating in an appropriate recovery program. Monitoring is designed to allow the medical staff to evaluate the status of the physician's recovery.

Monitoring is a service to the physician as well as to the medical staff. For the physician, a comprehensive monitoring program establishes a history of performance, with documentation, which can be invaluable in vouching for a physician's current status in recovery. For the hospital medical staff, a record is established over time, showing that the medical staff is acting in a knowledgeable, timely, thorough and responsible way to assure that the physician continues to deliver safe care.

Monitoring for Conditions Other Than Chemical Dependence

When monitoring for a situation or condition other than chemical dependence is required, all principles of monitoring described here should be adapted and applied.

Proctoring

The medical staff must also satisfy itself that the physician's clinical skills are intact. To that end, the monitoring plan should contain provisions for proctoring, appropriate to each case.

There should be concurrent peer review and regular record review for all monitored physicians, for a period of time to be determined in each case. For those with surgical privileges, or those who perform other procedures in the hospital there should be a proctor for a period of time to be determined in each case.

When the Physician Has Privileges at More Than One Hospital

The monitoring agreement should provide for notifying the appropriate medical staff committee(s) of the other hospital(s) where the physician has privileges. In an optimal situation, monitoring activities will be integrated in a way which meets the responsibilities of each medical staff without unnecessary duplication. At a minimum, each medical staff should have a monitoring agreement (or each medical staff should be a party to one monitoring agreement) and there should be regular contact with a knowledgeable observer at each hospital whose reports are submitted to one coordinator of monitoring.

Protection of the Physician's Identity

It is possible to carry out every element of monitoring described here and still protect the identity of the physician. The physician's identity and information about the situation needs to be known only to the signers of the monitoring agreement, the monitors and the medical staff committee responsible for the monitoring. Disclosure of this information may be required if it becomes relevant in a staff privilege dispute.

THE AGING PHYSICIAN

To allow or encourage a physician to work beyond his or her physical or professional capacity is a great disservice to patients. Respect for age and long-standing service to the hospital and medical community often prevent organized medical staffs from addressing the aging physician who no longer has the skills to practice. In some cases, physicians continue to practice long after they have become prone to hearing and vision losses, memory lapses, cardiorespiratory disabilities, and loss of motor skills owing to their advancing ages.[5] Age alone is not a reason for curtailment of clinical privileges, but should be a reason to take a closer look to confirm that physical ability still matches privileges granted. Medical staffs should recognize the special needs of older physicians and develop policies to direct their actions.

A policy for the older physician could contain the following provisions:[6]

1. All physicians over the age of (65 or 70) must be reappointed annually.

2. Physicians older than the agreed minimum age are required to submit with the reappointment application a letter from a private physician certifying that the physician is healthy enough to exercise the privileges requested.

3. The credentials and medical executive committees have the authority to require the applying physician to undergo a physical examination following absence or disabling illness. The examining physician shall be authorized by the applicant to report findings of the examination to the credentials or medical executive committee. The medical staff shall also have the authority to require an examination as part of the evaluation of a physician who has demonstrated a performance problem.

4. The physician health and rehabilitation committee of the medical staff will consider supportive options for a physician who needs help because of advancing age. These might include assistance in recruiting a younger associate to provide coverage for hospitalized patients or counsel in delineating clinical privileges commensurate with remaining ability.

5. The medical staff will develop honors and awards that recognize long and valuable service as part of a structured program of withdrawal from hospital practice.

THE DISRUPTIVE PHYSICIAN

For too many years, health care facilities and their workers have suffered the antics, abuse, and disruptive behavior of a small number of temperamental physicians. Examples of this behavior include instruments being thrown in the operating rooms; nurses and other health care professionals being verbally abused to the point that they cannot function in their jobs; physicians disrupting meetings; and in a few cases, actually physically assaulting other physicians, patients, or hospital staff members. These are not unusual occurrences. The behavior of a small number of physicians gives new meaning to the term "hostile work environment."

Management in health care facilities attempted in the past to deal with these bad actors by counseling and cajoling, but were powerless to take definitive action until medical staff organizations and governing bodies decided not to continue to tolerate this kind of behavior. Ten years ago, it was the rare health care facility that had an effective policy for dealing with disruptive physicians. Today, thanks in great part to The Credentialing Institute,[7] the medical staff organization that does not have an effective policy for dealing with the disruptive physician is the exception. Through education, physician leaders, senior health care managers, and medical staff services professionals have learned how to deal with disruptive physicians.

DISRUPTIVE PHYSICIANS: ENOUGH IS ENOUGH*

There are several steps hospitals and medical staff leaders can take to lay the foundation for taking action when needed [to address disruptive physician behavior].

Step 1: Board Policies on Disruptive Behavior

It must be clear to all those who work within the hospital that disruptive conduct of any kind—rude or abusive conduct toward nurses or patients, negative comments to patients about other physicians or nurses or their treatment in the hospital, threats or physical assaults, sexual harassment, refusal to accept medical staff assignments, disruption of committee or departmental affairs, or inappropriate comments written in patient medical records or other official documents—will not be tolerated. The board should adopt a policy requiring all employees, physicians and other independent practitioners to conduct themselves in a professional and cooperative manner while in the hospital.

Step 2: Medical Staff Bylaws Language

Medical staff bylaws should clearly state that the ability to work harmoniously with others is a criterion for initial appointment and reappointment,

---

*The section, "Disruptive Pysicians: Enough is Enough," is reprinted by permission of The Credentialing Institute, Pittsburgh, Pennsylvania.

and that information regarding the applicant's professional conduct will be sought from references. In addition, disruptive behavior should be included in the section of the bylaws outlining the grounds for disciplinary action.

Not surprisingly, investigations and subsequent hearings and appeals involving disruptive physicians are often themselves very disruptive to the normal operation of the hospital. The medical staff bylaws should include language that allows the medical executive committee to refer these matters to the board (without a recommendation) at any point in the investigation or hearing process. Such language not only reflects the board's ultimate responsibility to operate an efficient and effective hospital, it allows these situations to be resolved more quickly and with less trauma to medical staff leaders, potential witnesses, and other hospital employees.

Step 3: Step-By-Step Procedure to Investigate Complaints

Documentation of disruptive conduct is critical because it is usually a pattern of conduct that justifies disciplinary action. Therefore, it is important to make a written record of each instance of unacceptable behavior and the action taken. Providing a form for reporting incidents of disruptive conduct may encourage reporting, especially by hospital employees.

Follow-Up Meetings With The Physician

Whatever hope there may be of moderating disruptive behavior will best be realized by addressing it at once, before attitudes have hardened and while it is still possible to treat the matter as capable of collegial resolution. If the physician knows that his or her conduct is unacceptable and that the hospital and medical staff leaders are prepared to act, future incidents may be prevented.

However, just a surely as it is wise to address behavior problems as soon as they occur, it is also wise to do so with caution. Confronting the physician in a heavy-handed, accusatory manner is likely to invite resentment and possible retaliation. The initial approach should be undertaken as a helpful gesture. At the same time, it must be made clear that it is more than a difference of opinion; that is, if the behavior continues, more formal action will be taken to stop it.

If the medical staff president or other medical staff leaders are reluctant to meet with the physician, or, if for any other reason, the president of the medical staff or the chief executive officer determines it to be necessary, the board chairperson or another board member should meet with the physician. Having a board member meet with the physician has several advantages. It relieves the medical staff president and other medical staff leaders from a responsibility for which they usually have neither the desire, nor the experience. And, when a physician understands that he or she is accountable directly to the board for his or her conduct, it may be easier to correct the situation in an informal matter, rather than if the physician perceives that he or she would be bending to the wishes of other physicians in matters that the physician might consider none of their business.

The participants in any meeting with the physician should be as few as possible not only to minimize the doctor's feeling that he or she has been the object of widespread discussion but also to limit the targets or any attempts at retaliation.

The record should not be a catalog of ineffective oral warnings, however. Follow-up letters to the physician help to create a record that attempts were made to deal with the problem, short of terminating the physician's staff appointment and clinical privileges. It also prevents any later claims by the physician that no one had ever discussed the disruptive behavior with him or her.

Disciplinary Action Pursuant to Medical Staff Bylaws

If informal efforts to deal with a disruptive physician are unsuccessful, formal action pursuant to the bylaws should be initiated. Hospital counsel should be involved throughout the process to assure compliance with the bylaws and to eliminate from participation in the proceedings any physician or board member who might be perceived to be biased.

Determining whether a physician possesses the qualification for appointment of being able to "work harmoniously with others..." does not require medical expertise. A recommendation from the medical executive committee (or any other medical staff committee) is not necessary in these situations if there is a policy that permits the board or management to act.

If the procedure followed either through the medical executive committee or through the board is inherently fair, and complies with the bylaws, and if there is a well-documented record of the physician's conduct and the hospital's and medical staff leaders' attempts to deal with it, the disciplinary action will be upheld.

The courts have made it abundantly clear that the provision of patient care in an atmosphere of calm, order, and respect for the dignity of all need not be sacrificed to the disruptive proclivities of any appointee to the medical staff regardless of his or her clinical abilities.

NOTES

1. Richard D. Blondell, "Impaired Physicians," *Primary Care* 20 (March 1993): 209.

2. Cindy A. Orsund and Donald P. Wilcox, "Credentialing the New Applicant - Practical Advice," *Texas Medicine* 84 (April 1988): 79.

3. Texas Medical Association Committee on Physician Health and Rehabilitation, *Do you Know a Doctor Who Needs Our Help?* (Austin: Texas Medical Association, February 1996).

4. Texas Medical Association Committee on Physician Health and Rehabilitation, *Committee on Physicians Health and Rehabilitation Contract* (Austin: Texas Medical Association, 1987).

5. Daniel A. Lang with Gail B. Jara and Laurence W. Kessenick, *The Disabled Physician* (Chicago: American Hospital Publishing, Inc., 1989): 17.

6. National Health Foundation, "Fair Treatment for Senior Physicians," *The Medical Executive Committee Reporter* 5 (July/August 1990): 5.

7. The Credentialing Institute is a partnership between Hugh Greeley Associates, Ltd., and Horty, Springer, and Mattern, P.C., a Pittsburgh firm of health care attorneys.

Chapter 14

Innovations In Medical Staff Services Operations

Wendy R. Crimp, MBA

The purpose of this chapter is to discuss innovations in the approach for management of medical staff services operations. These innovations have occurred as a result of the evolving health care industry environment in the United States. Past methods for management of medical staff services will no longer adequately support the current challenges faced by most organizations. This chapter begins with a historical perspective, continues with a discussion of implications for operating design, and concludes with the identification of tools that are required to achieve successful operating outcomes.

HISTORICAL PERSPECTIVE—EMERGING MISSIONS

Historically, medical staff organizations existed to help physicians collaborate on patient care objectives and collectively participate with administration in the management of patient care delivery. Medical staff organizations were found in the hospital setting only, and provided a mechanism for formal, structured interaction of peers and colleagues who were providing care at that facility. The Joint Commission on Accreditation of Healthcare Organizations (JCAHO) provided standards, giving hospitals a framework from which to construct bylaws and procedures that guided medical staff activities and accountability.

As the mission and role of medical staff organizations expanded, more staff was required to support the various committees, educational events and other activities undertaken by the medical staff organization. The medical staff services department became the tactical arm of the medical staff organization. The department existed to staff the medical staff organization in its endeavors. Earlier support was primarily secretarial because the main support requirements were directed at meeting management. Support requirements subsequently became more complex as the scope of services being provided was expanded.

One of the emerging missions of the medical staff organization was to ensure physician competency. Hence began the process of credentialing physicians to ensure that physicians had the basic credentials, training and experience to practice in their chosen field at that facility. Later, it was determined that not only did physician competency need to be assessed as the physicians entered the organization, but also it was critical to review the physician's credentials documentation for expirations (licenses, etc.) and assess the physician's performance at periodic intervals to ensure ongoing competency. This recredentialing effort involved the verification of how current the credentials were, and the collection of quality data elements to further evaluate the performance of the practitioner.

The focus of staff efforts thus expanded from meeting management to data management. This expanded scope of services required the staff not only to record information, but also to assure that the physician leaders had been trained to appropriately use the information in accordance with legal, accrediting body, state, and federal guidelines. Therefore, the medical staff services director became responsible for ensuring that the department was proficient in the collection and management of data, and in the interpretation and application of standards. Meanwhile, other activities were gaining importance, such as proctoring and management of allied health professionals credentialing. This change and expansion in scope typifies the medical staff organization's evolution and highlights the shifting operations and information systems requirements.

CROSSROADS

At the same time that hospital-based medical staff services departments were struggling to "re-tool" their operations to meet the challenges that they faced, two additional trends evolved in the medical staff office arena that would forever change the face of medical staff services.

1. Previously, the focus on medical staff management was confined to the hospital setting. As physicians began to form larger and larger medical groups, professional staff management emerged as an area of emphasis within the medical groups. Additionally, managed care payers began to credential the practitioners in their networks; if the payers were going to restrict patients to using only their approved list of providers, it became incumbent on the payer to assure that the physicians on their approved list were competent. Initially, standards were unclear regarding the content and scope of credentialing to be performed by the managed care industry. Later, the National Commission for Quality Assurance (NCQA) emerged as the accrediting body for medical groups and payer organizations. NCQA had similar, yet varying standards for professional staff management compared to JCAHO.

2. Both horizontal integration (between like entities) and vertical integration (between disparate entities) occurred as the industry consolidated in response to changes in reimbursement and competitive incentives. This integration

has resulted in the establishment of new medical staff services organizations that are consumed with the management of physicians across the enterprise. Consequently, the professional services department has arisen. This "new" medical staff services department may be charged with monitoring the quality and competency of practitioners in payer, hospital, and private practice settings concurrently. This requires the department to deliver services while complying with both JCAHO and NCQA standards. For example, an integrated delivery system may have three hospitals, a large independent practice association (IPA) and its own health plan. If a given practitioner has relationships with two of the hospitals, the IPA and the health plan, the professional services department can be responsible for managing multiple relationships for the practitioner.

The operational challenges that many directors of medical staff services face today, compared with 10 years ago, can make the achievement of successful management outcomes seem impossible. However, there are key elements in operating and information systems design that can be helpful to directors who are trying to transition their operations to meet the new challenges. Whether you manage a single hospital medical staff services department or are involved in multiple entity professional services management, the information that follows can assist you in assuring that your operational performance meets expectations.

TOOLS AND TIPS

Step 1: Know The Organizational Intent

The most frequent mistake encountered in today's complex environment is the tendency to jump to "how" operations and systems need to operate before completely identifying "what" organizational outcomes need to be supported. The "what" component of the equation is called organizational intent.

For example, if a five-hospital health system wants to "consolidate medical staff services," the organization needs to ask itself, "What does that mean?" Is the intent to fully consolidate the various medical staff organizations into a single organization with one set of bylaws, privileging criteria, and so on? Or, is the intent just to limit consolidation to credentialing applications and source verifications via a single credentialing department and deliver files to each separate medical staff organization for them to manage internally in accordance with separate credentialing committees and governing bodies.

It is impossible to correctly identify the operating and information systems requirements in the newly consolidated department until you know what is truly being centralized and what is to remain decentralized. Skipping this critical step of analysis of organizational intent may lead to flawed operating design, the creation of duplicated efforts (as opposed to elimination of duplication), and mismatched expectations between medical staff, administration and the medical staff services department.

Many future problems can be eliminated by clearly identifying the following:

1. Is there to be any consolidation of governing bodies or committees?
2. What accreditation standards will drive the scope of services? NCQA? JCAHO? or both?
3. How will all parties participate in crafting the scope of services and methods of operation in the shared department?
4. How will the department be funded?
5. Will all participants be changing their software to enable them to utilize the same information systems platform (perhaps a wide area network)?

These types of questions begin to identify organizational intent. The answers to these (and other) questions will assist management in designing an operation that both meets expectations and has relevance to the organizational objectives.

Step 2: Identify the Scope of Services and Work Products

Surprisingly, departmental policies and procedures rarely address the most critical processing issues, such as the following issues in credentialing:

1. How are services to be accessed? Who may request or authorize an application?
2. What items are to be verified and are the approved sources specified?
3. What is the format of the final work product? An audit summary report? or a complete file copy?
4. What should happen when a verifying organization fails to respond? What is the definition of an exhausted effort?
5. Who is responsible for producing the practitioner profile and what are its specific contents?

Addressing these and other questions is critical to defining the department's scope of services and required work products. Defining these types of issues in precise terms allows the department to have measurable performance objectives, and compliance with these objectives should lead to decreased variability in services and higher, more consistent quality of services provided.

Beyond credentialing, the department needs to subject other services to the same scrutiny. Proctoring and meeting management deserve the same type of analysis. For proctoring, the following are samples of issues that should be addressed:

1. What is the organization trying to accomplish with its proctoring program (which is not required by either JCAHO or NCQA)? What are the benefits to be realized?

2. Who is subject to proctoring? What are the conditions for waiving the requirement?

3. What documentation is required? What are the time frames for completion?

4. How will progress be monitored? What will happen if a practitioner fails to meet the proctoring requirements?

The scope of services to be offered and the operating procedures utilized will impact the intensity of resources required to deliver services. A frequent question asked of consultants is, "I have 1,000 physicians and 250 allied health professionals; how much staff do I need?" Surely this is an impossible question to answer without a clearly defined scope of services and some information regarding the type of software support that the department has. The necessity of evaluating these important factors is often not recognized by senior management and physician leaders. The greater the scope of services and the intensity of practitioner surveillance, the larger the information systems and staffing resources need to be.

For example, meeting management is highly variable among organizations; some organizations support over 100 meetings per month, while others support 10 or fewer meetings per month. The resources required to support meetings are directly related to the complexity of the medical staff organization structure and frequency of meetings. Some organizations manage to create the "United Nations" of medical staff management, with virtually every contingent represented as their own department, sub-specialty department and sub-sub-specialty department. Each department has its own meetings, agendas, issue follow-up, and so on. Other organizations have managed to simplify their structure to include five or six departments with considerably fewer meetings and carefully crafted agendas.

Some organizations are beginning to question the effectiveness of the clinical department structure altogether. Helpful questions to ask oneself are "What is it we are really trying to accomplish?" and "Is there a more effective way of doing this?" The objective of these questions gives rise to another dimension to the earlier operations design questions of "how" and "what." That dimension is, "why?" It is important to ask oneself analytical questions periodically if we want to assure that the services we provide are meaningful, have a positive impact on the practice of medicine and the quality of care rendered to patients.

Step 3: How Will Work Be Organized Or "Flow" To Ensure Objectives Are Achieved?

Work flow is an important operational design feature. In the past, smaller, single-entity hospitals may have had only two or three staff members in the medical staff services department. With smaller staffs, there isn't as much opportunity to design work flow models; each staff member seems to do a "little bit of every-thing." In larger, more complex operations, work flow becomes more important as bottlenecks can quickly lead to substantial backlogs that may require a large infusion of resources to correct.

One of the most visible illustrations is in the area of credentialing. Tradition-ally, assignment of credentialing activities has been based upon alphabetical or-der (i.e. each medical staff services department member took a section of the alphabet and was responsible for all files in that section) or files might have been assigned by department. When a staff member takes complete responsibility for application management and credentials verification for all files assigned, work does not flow, rather, it cycles as shown in Figure 14-1. When the staff member is working on any given item (i.e., data entry), all other items are suspended and thus, do not progress as the attention of staff is rotated between tasks. This can lead to an operating environment that could be characterized as "management by piles." Using the "cycling" methodology may be totally appropriate in smaller (less than three full time equivalent [FTE]) entity environments. In larger (four-plus FTE) environments, a more production-oriented model may be beneficial.

The primary difference in a production-oriented model is the creation of a work flow model in which work does not cycle; nothing becomes suspended because staff are rotating their efforts between tasks. Instead, all functions are performed continuously as files are moved through a data collection process toward completion (Figure 14-2). This means that applications are continu-ously being mailed out, outbound queries are continuous, mail is continu-ously being data-entered, and completed files are continuously being evalu-ated for closure and delivery to committee. This type of work flow represents a substantial departure from the traditional approach. Its emergence is being greeted with mixed feelings from experienced medical staff services directors and coordinators who, despite knowing that their current systems aren't keep-ing pace with the organization's requirements, are reluctant to embrace an approach so completely different from anything that they have experienced in the past. Commercial credentials verification organizations (CVOs) have been

Figure 14-1. Illustration of Traditional "Cycling" Credentials Verificaiton Workflow at the Individual Staff Level.

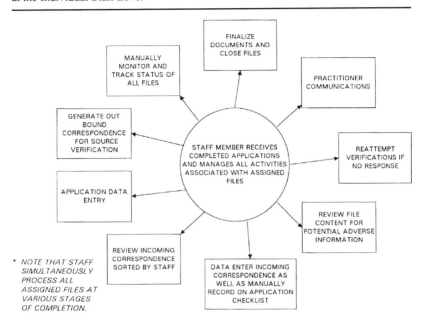

Figure 14-2. Illustration of Production-Oriented Central Credentials Verification Services Work Flow.

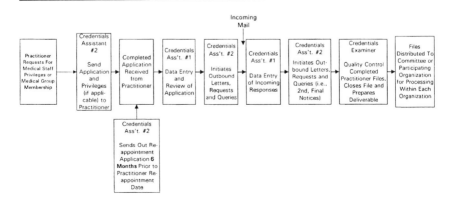

using functional work flow models for the past few years as they have had to learn how to service multiple payer, hospital, and medical group relationships for upwards of 160,000 practitioners. While the more extreme models may represent overkill when applied to smaller medical staff services departments, there are certainly elements of production-oriented or functional models that can improve the performance of any operation when properly applied.

Step 4: The Role of Software in the Emerging Operating Environment

As the complexity and scope of services has increased in medical staff services departments, the role of software as a vital tool which assists management in achieving effective operating results cannot be overemphasized. Historically, medical staff services information systems existed to print rosters and mailing labels, track meeting attendance and other such activities. More recently, the medical staff (or professional services) department has become the focal point for establishing enterprise-wide database support for the management of professional staff across entities and traditional boundaries. It is vital that the system not only be a repository for required information on each practitioner but that all transactions, affiliations and status for each practitioner be continuously tracked. This includes, but is not limited to, continuous tracking, reverification and documentation of all expirables (license, drug registration, board certification, and malpractice insurance coverage). Also, systems should be used to track work-in-process to assure that NCQA document aging requirements (verification of items is not to exceed 180 days when a decision is made regarding the practitioner) are consistently monitored and met.

Additionally, practitioner data is being linked to other organizational service interests, which increases performance pressure to assure that data is accurate, and definitions of data elements are consistent across the organization. For example, the credentialing department may become the organizational "bible" for practitioner data. Selected data collected by that department might flow to other databases and software applications within the organization; most notably, contracting, patient accounting, claims processing, physician referral services, utilization management, and others. Building interfaces that permit data to flow to other databases eliminates duplication of data entry and ensures that the entire organization is using the same set of data to manage the business by eliminating reconciliation problems. Because of the broad-reaching impact of the data collected in the credentialing department, it becomes critical that the organization of work flow ensures data integrity as data is reviewed and entered into the system. As an example, in the work flow illustrated in Figure 14-2, data entry functions are isolated. It is further recommended that data entry staff not have any phone responsibilities that might disrupt data entry and result in increased error rates. Periodic compliance audits should be performed on each staff member to assure that they adhere to acceptable levels of accuracy.

As the data is exported to other departments it will be important for everyone to utilize the same "data dictionary," which defines terminology that drives the data elements and fields across systems. The use of data dictionaries also plays a critical role within departments. For example, if the data entry of practitioner name is not standardized (i.e., with or without middle initial) the name may be entered by two individuals in different ways (Robert E. White vs. Robert White) creating duplicate records. Additionally, data security procedures need to allow for the ability to isolate which data elements can be viewed by other departments and what items are restricted only to the medical staff services department. The ability to designate specific fields as "read only" versus "read and write" will ensure that only certain individuals are allowed to update fields in accordance with specified procedures. NCQA has specific guidelines on data security, confidentiality procedures, password protection and routine back-up of databases which must be adhered to in order to meet NCQA standards.

Step 5: Assuring That Staff Is Skilled and Knowledgeable

These emerging trends in medical staff organizations has presented management and staff who currently provide support services with new career opportunities. Professional organizations are beginning to recognize changes in skills and knowledge requirements by creating special national certifications and an increase in professional seminars and publications in the field. What used to be primarily two levels of staffing (directors and coordinators) has become differentiated into multiple levels of support. Some of the emerging job descriptions include

1. the professional services director who may direct or manage medical staff services for multiple entities;

2. the compliance coordinator who may not only ensure ongoing internal compliance with JCAHO and NCQA standards, but may also be responsible for management of delegation audits for entities with whom the organization has entered into delegated credentialing authority agreements;

3. data entry coordinator whose primary focus is the entry of data and assurance of data integrity;

4. credentials examiner who is responsible for the review of files in accordance with defined criteria and the identification and flagging of potentially adverse information;

5. meeting management secretaries whose primary responsibility is staffing meetings, recording minutes and issue tracking.

These various levels of responsibility allow for differentiating experienced staff and providing potential career ladders in professional staff services that were not available in the previous flat organizations.

THE FUTURE

These are challenging times for medical staff services departments, but they are also exciting times. Changes have created a plethora of leadership and career opportunities for both management and staff.

The same changes also require expansions in technical skills and redefining the medical staff management function. The only constant in the future of medical staff services operations is the expectation for further evolution and change.

Chapter 15

Managing Medical Staff Meetings

Mimi Cruse, CMSC

As has been previously discussed, the role of the medical staff services professional (MSSP) includes providing assistance to the medical staff organization as that organization functions in a manner that complies with accrediting body regulations and fulfills responsibilities assigned to it by the governing body and the administration of the hospital. A very important part of this assistance includes coordination of medical staff committee, department, section and general meetings. Coordination involves such tasks as providing a calendar for the meetings; sending meeting notices; arranging for rooms, food, and equipment needs; preparing agendas; recording attendance and minutes; and, instituting or directing follow-up as necessary.

The number of meetings in any given time period will depend, of course, upon the size of the institution, the size of its medical staff and how that staff is organized constitutionally. For purposes of this text, imagine an institution, Central City Hospital, that has approximately 400 beds, approximately 300 physicians on staff, and numerous clinical departments, including surgery, medicine, family practice, pediatrics, obstetrics/gynecology and psychiatry. Of the departments mentioned, only surgery and medicine have organized sections. The medical staff committees include infection control, pharmacy and therapeutics, blood utilization and transfusion review, medical records, critical care, credentials, tissue and surgical practice, medical practice, and the medical executive committee (MEC), as well as other temporary ad hoc committees appointed as the need arises. (As mentioned earlier in this book, many of these committees may be unnecessary.)

MEETING PREPARATION

Scheduling

For efficient and effective scheduling, an annual calendar of medical staff meetings should be prepared and kept in the medical staff services department. The MSSP must work closely with the chief of staff and all committee and department chairs and section chiefs so that meetings are scheduled at times convenient for the chair and will facilitate the appropriate and timely flow of information between groups. One method suggested for accomplishing this is to think of the meetings as occurring on the face of a clock and then to plug that information into a calendar. For instance, if, as in Figure 15-l, the governing body meeting is at 12 o'clock, the MEC at 1, the department of surgery at 2, the credentials committee at 3, the department of medicine at 4, infection control committee at 5, and so on, there is not a smooth flow of information, since committees report to other committees, sections and departments; sections report to departments; departments (and most committees) report to the MEC; and the MEC reports to the governing body. Indeed in this scheme of things, there is considerable and unnecessary delay.

Figure 15-2 illustrates a far more reasonable schedule that allows for an expeditious flow of information. This schedule then gets transferred to a monthly calendar. It should be noted here that implementing such a meeting schedule may not always be possible for many reasons, not the least of which might be the attitude that "we've always met on the third Thursday and we see no reason to change now." The clock system is simply suggested as one method for achieving good information flow.

Figure 15-1. Clock System to Schedule Meetings: Poor Organization for Information Flow.

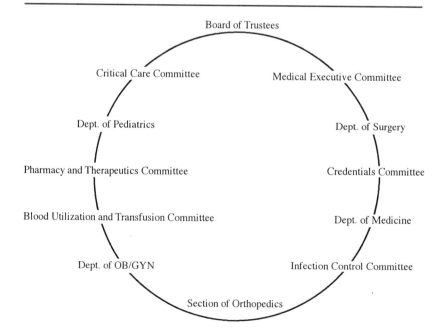

Notification

After the chief of staff or persons making appointments and assignments have completed that task, someone in the medical staff services department must notify the appointees. The notice should provide all the necessary information and permit the physicians to mark their own office calendars accordingly for the year. However, because most physicians are quite busy and patients are their first priority, most MSSPs send a reminder notification for any meeting approximately two weeks ahead of time. Computerization of committee, section and department lists can simplify this task. Along with the notice, the agenda and any materials requiring review prior to the meeting are included. (Agendas will be discussed in greater detail shortly.)

Physical Preparation

Another responsibility of the MSSP is to make arrangements for meeting rooms; order any dietary items requested by the group, such as lunch or drinks and snacks; and arrange for any special equipment the group may need, such as overhead projectors, X-ray view boxes, and the like. This should be done

Figure 15-2. Clock System to Schedule Meetings: Ideal Organization for Information Flow.

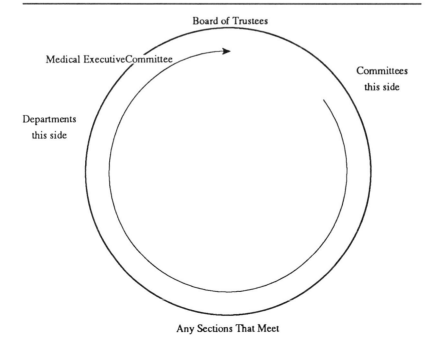

carefully, keeping in mind all of the specific needs of each different group. These arrangements must be coordinated with other departments in the hospital such as housekeeping and dietary, and preparations can be expedited through the use of forms.

In many hospitals, the various departments have their own forms. Medical staff services department personnel will simply adjust to the individual institutional policies as necessary, perhaps making suggestions for changes if the forms can be made more communicative, efficient or cost-effective. An important point to keep in mind is that with all of these preparations—the calendar, notices, and physical arrangements—the main goal is to make it as easy as possible for physicians to hold meetings required and to accomplish the assignments of the particular groups holding the meeting.

AGENDAS

When used correctly, agendas are powerful tools. By organizing an agenda before the meeting, the chair can maintain control during the meeting. The mere placement of items can influence a positive or negative outcome. For example, an item at the end of the agenda may be hurriedly discussed and voted on so the meeting can end. A negotiating principle is that 80 percent of the decisions are made in the last 20 percent of the time. Also, an item requiring lengthy discussion placed at the beginning of an agenda may mean all items after it will not be discussed.

An agenda lets other committee members prepare for items to be discussed. If a committee is to be most effective, the decisions made should reflect careful consideration. The physician who will be asked to approve a policy closing the psychiatry section to new members will need to read the policy and think about questions and concerns before coming to the meeting. Providing an agenda promotes efficiency without losing valuable input.

Another asset of a well-planned agenda is improvement in meeting minutes. Minutes that are written around the agenda allow easier retrieval of information. If a form is used for formulating minutes, the agenda item can be pretyped on the form, allowing the rough draft to be written during the meeting. Many MSSPs are now using laptop computers to expedite minute writing during the meeting.

An agenda should be clear and may state whether a given item is for information, discussion or action. In addition, the time allowed for discussion or action may also be stated. When the formulation of the agenda occurs during the preliminary planning process, the chair can tailor agenda length to length of meeting.

To ensure that items from previous meetings requiring additional time are not omitted, previous minutes must be reviewed or a reminder must be placed in an agenda item file. Committee members should be contacted or instructed to submit agenda items, allowing enough time to adequately compile the agenda.

The specific agenda format will vary, but each agenda should include some basic elements, such as approval of previous meeting minutes, committee and officer reports, old or unfinished business, new business, announcements, and the adjournment. These basic elements are explained in more detail in *Robert's Rules of Order*. When listing items under the above headings, it is important that adequate information is included for easy understanding. Use of action verbs to emphasize the expected outcome of each item is helpful.

The timing of the distribution of an agenda will normally depend upon the wishes of the chair of the group involved. However, having an agenda sent out to those who are to attend a meeting prior to the meeting is usually very beneficial. This is especially true if there are materials sent with the agenda that should be carefully reviewed before discussion occurs.

Please consider the sample agenda for a medical executive committee presented in Exhibit 15-1. The author prefers this type of agenda for MEC meetings because it not only facilitates the writing of minutes, but also ensures proper follow-up and retention of items that have not been resolved. Such items have a tendency to "fall through the cracks," especially (and understandably) when difficult issues are under discussion and members present are reluctant to take immediate action.

An effective way of keeping track of what needs to be put on the agendas of the many committees supported by the office is to establish agenda files. One file should be created for every medical staff group that meets. Everyone in the facility and the leaders of the medical staff should be made aware of the existence of these files. Any item that anyone wants considered by a specific group is sent to the medical staff services department for placement in the appropriate agenda file. The MSSP also looks over all minutes for referral items and places those in the files. The person compiling the agenda then consults the files prior to preparation, which ensures that no matter who makes up the agenda, all items of business needing consideration are there.

THE MEETING

Attendance Sheets

Because many bylaws still have attendance requirements, it is essential that an accurate record of attendance at all medical staff meetings be kept. The ideal is to have each person attending sign next to his or her name on a prepared list. The alert MSSP, however, will also note the attendees so that missing names may be filled in and initialed. Maintaining a running tabulation of attendance for each medical staff member, either on computer or manually,

---

Exhibit 15-1. A Sample Medical Executive Committee Agenda.

Central City Hospital Medical Staff
Medical Executive Committee
November 1, 1998
Agenda

_____a.m.	1. Call to order, Dr. Jones, Chair
( ) approved	2. Review of minutes of previous meeting held
( ) amended	October 4, 1998. (See attachment, pp. 1-4)
	3. CEO's report—John Smith
	4. Chief of Staff's Report—Dr. Jones
	5. Nursing Report—Mary Ward, R.N.

Unfinished Business

	6. Bylaws Committee Referral:
( ) follow-up	From Medical Staff Services: Dr. Williams is still conducting research.
	7. Blood Order Form:
( ) follow-up	From Sept. MEC minutes: "Blood order form being developed." From Oct. Blood Utilization Committee minutes: "Dr. Pontius presented draft of form for request of blood. Committee approved first draft and supports use of order form except in cases of emergency. (Draft of form distributed.)

New Business

	8. Medical Records Committee—Dr. George
( ) approved	a. Oncology On-Going Medical Form recommended by Oncology
( ) amended	Section presented for approval
( ) disapproved	
( ) deferred	
	9. Pharmacy & Therapeutics—Dr. Lock
( ) received	EPO Protocol from Nephrology Section presented for information. (See attachment, pp. 11-12.)
( ) received	10. Reports of other committees, sections and/or departments:
	Notation is made that minutes of meetings (indicated by date) are on file in the Medical Staff Services Dept., none of which contain any specific recommended actions or items needing consideration by the MEC.

Sources for agenda items are many and varied. Quite often many of the items to appear on an agenda will be dictated by what accrediting agencies such as Joint Commission on Accreditation of Healthcare Organizations (JCAHO) indicate the group should be considering at its meetings. (See Exhibit. 15-2 which indicates those items clinical departments should be considering in order to properly accomplish their monthly review of clinical practice.) There will also be unfinished pieces of business from previous meetings and referrals from other groups or persons in the facility who need to have something considered and a recommendation made or an action taken.

allows department chairs to easily access summaries to review physician citizenship at the time of reappointment. In addition to the attendance sheet itself, members present, absent, and excused may also be listed someplace in the actual minutes, above the discussion of business. It is also possible to state, "Attendance per the attached sign-in sheet" and attach a copy of the sheet to the original minutes.

Conduct of the Meeting

The MSSP does not conduct medical staff meetings; the chair does. The MSSP, however, can influence the effectiveness of the meeting by making sure the chair understands his or her responsibilities and by helping to prepare the chair. For example, it is generally useful to review the agenda and all

---

Exhibit 15-2. Sample Department of Surgery Agenda.

Central City Hospital
Agenda
Department of Surgery
November 22, 1998

I.   CALL TO ORDER—12:30 p.m.

II.   APPROVAL OF MINUTES

III.   QUALITY IMPROVEMENT REPORTS

      A.   Follow-up on Case #12345

            Response from Dr. #478

      B.   Findings from Operative & Other Procedure Review

      C.   Findings from Blood Use Review

      D.   Findings from Medication Use Review

      E.   Findings from Medical Record Review

      F.   Findings from Utilization Management

      G.   Infection Rate Report

IV.   UNFINISHED BUSINESS

      •   Revised Proctoring Protocol for department

         (See attachment)

V.   NEW BUSINESS

      A.   Revised Policy for Observing in Surgery

      B.   Need for Policy on Second Assistants in Surgery

VI.   ADJOURNMENT

materials to be considered with the chair prior to the meeting. Such a review is not always easy to accomplish, but is well worth the effort.

Many reference sources are available that define guidelines for chairs. One list of such guidelines follows:[1]

1. Start on time and work with an agenda.
2. State the reason for the meeting, briefly and clearly.
3. Ensure that members hear all sides of an issue.
4. Direct the meeting, but keep a low profile.
5. Keep the meeting moving and insist on order.
6. Speak clearly and to the group, not to individuals.
7. Summarize what has been said on an issue and aim for a decision.
8. Go for closure. Recommend additional outside work if agreement or closure cannot be reached.
9. Ask questions and clarify, but don't engage in debate with members.
10. Be sure any opinions stated are identified as such and not as directives.
11. Be sure that accurate minutes are recorded and distributed appropriately.
12. Check at the end of the meeting to assure that all subjects have been covered.

Another excellent source is *The Medical Staff Leaders' Practical Guide*.[2] Medical staff leaders who must conduct meetings may also find videotapes such as the one offered by Brighton Books: "The Hospital Medical Staff—Its Changing Form and Function."[3] Another recommended resource for overall meeting management is *How to Make Meetings Work*[4] by Doyle and Strauss. Needless to say, the better prepared a leader is to conduct a meeting, the easier is the job of the MSSP who is documenting what occurs at the meeting. Therefore, the smart coordinator helps the leader with the "homework" to the greatest extent possible.

PARLIAMENTARY PROCEDURE

The support person attending medical staff meetings should be familiar with parliamentary procedure or at least have a reference ready at hand during the meetings to help facilitate the conduct of business. Some groups will appoint their own parliamentarian, but a "hard copy" reference on hand will be very helpful if there are disputes.

Probably the most common reference work is still *Robert's Rules of Order*,[5] although some groups may prefer *Sturgis Rules Of Order*.[6] Further recommended is a very handy booklet that, because of its small size and clever design, permits quick references: E. C. Utter's *Parliamentary Law at a Glance*.[7] A brief guide to the basics of parliamentary procedure is presented in Figure 15-3, and Exhibits 15-3 and 15-4 which outline rules for handling main motions and the role of the chair.

It should be noted that the purpose of parliamentary procedure is to ensure that the majority rules while the minority is guaranteed a voice. In addition, following parliamentary procedure can assist in the orderly consideration of items and issues. Most medical staff meetings are not so formal as to require a strict adherence to proper procedure. In fact, strict adherence might be a hindrance if the procedure becomes the overriding concern, and this must be avoided. Common sense will usually dictate when the rules of order need to be invoked. The most important concerns for the support person are to use that common sense; to have a working knowledge of parliamentary procedure, and to have on hand an easy-to-use reference.

MINUTES

General Considerations

The most important purpose of preparing medical staff minutes is to document that the medical staff is in compliance with the required functions and standards of accrediting agencies. The second important purpose is to provide a means of communication between the various interacting groups of the medical staff. The person responsible for preparing the minutes needs to keep both of these purposes in mind as the minutes are prepared.

It is essential that minutes record actions taken. Surveyors for the JCAHO and other agencies will peruse minutes carefully for evidence of actions taken and resultant documentation of improvement in quality of care. This subject will be examined in greater depth shortly, but first a look at formats.

Formats

There are many formats for minutes, but the three most generally accepted are one-column, two-column or three column formats.[4] A sample of each of these formats is presented in Figure 15-4.

One-Column Format—The most traditional format. Usually a general summary of events, using either complete sentences or the briefer "fragments" style (thoughts and ideas) and one or more paragraphs for each subject. Each subject should be introduced by a title line, either underlined or entirely in upper case letters (or both). The entire width of the page is used from left to right margin.

Figure 15-3. A Guideline to the Basics of Parliamentary Procedure.*

ORDER OF BUSINESS

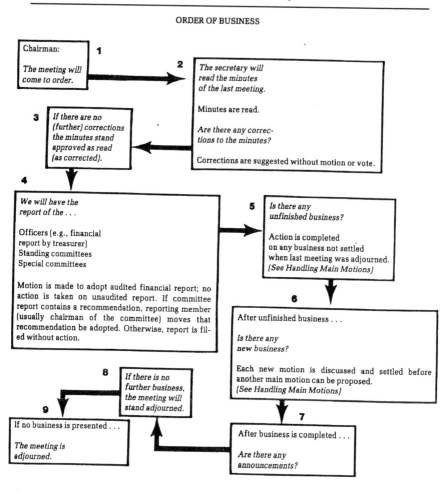

If assembly wishes to adjourn meeting before all business is completed, meeting must be adjourned by motion.

* A Quorum (the number of members necessary, according to the constitution or by-laws, to do business) must be present to hold a business meeting.

*Source: Reprinted from *Medical Staff Services Manual* by Cindy A. Orsund and Patricia J. Starr, p. 41, with permission of Cindy Orsund and Patricia Starr © 1981.

Figure 15-3. A Guideline to the Basics of Parliamentary Procedure. *(continued)*

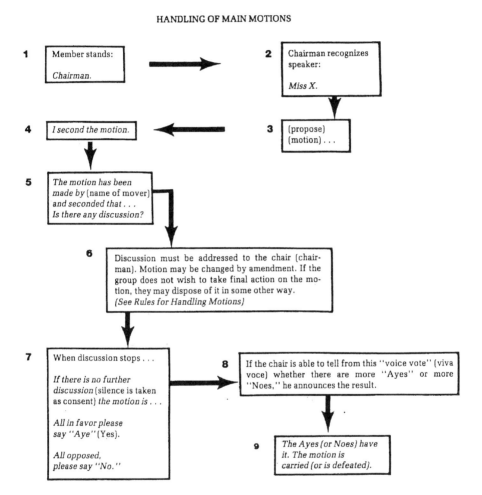

HANDLING OF MAIN MOTIONS

1 Member stands:

Chairman.

2 Chairman recognizes speaker:

Miss X.

3 (propose) (motion) . . .

4 *I second the motion.*

5 *The motion has been made by* (name of mover) *and seconded that . . . Is there any discussion?*

6 Discussion must be addressed to the chair (chairman). Motion may be changed by amendment. If the group does not wish to take final action on the motion, they may dispose of it in some other way. *(See Rules for Handling Motions)*

7 When discussion stops . . .

If there is no further discussion (silence is taken as consent) *the motion is . . .*

All in favor please say "Aye" (Yes).

All opposed, please say "No."

8 If the chair is able to tell from this "voice vote" (viva voce) whether there are more "Ayes" or more "Noes," he announces the result.

9 *The Ayes (or Noes) have it. The motion is carried (or is defeated).*

If anyone calls "Division" (questions the voice vote), the chair calls for a show of hands or a standing vote. *(All in favor raise your right hand (or stand). All opposed . . .)*

If a majority demand it, the vote may be taken by ballot.

Figure 15-3. A Guideline to the Basics of Parliamentary Procedure. *(continued)*

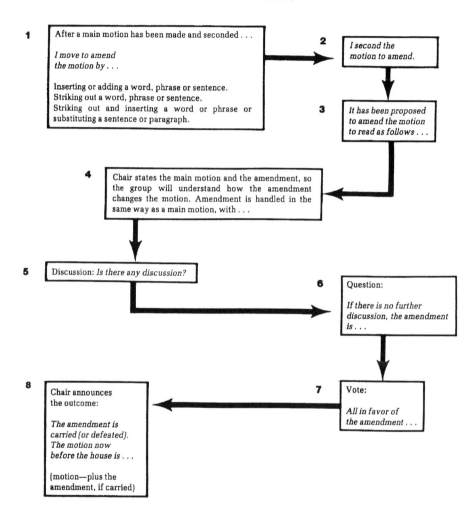

AMENDMENTS CHANGE MOTIONS

1 After a main motion has been made and seconded . . .

I move to amend the motion by . . .

Inserting or adding a word, phrase or sentence.
Striking out a word, phrase or sentence.
Striking out and inserting a word or phrase or substituting a sentence or paragraph.

2 *I second the motion to amend.*

3 *It has been proposed to amend the motion to read as follows . . .*

4 Chair states the main motion and the amendment, so the group will understand how the amendment changes the motion. Amendment is handled in the same way as a main motion, with . . .

5 Discussion: *Is there any discussion?*

6 Question:

If there is no further discussion, the amendment is . . .

7 Vote:

All in favor of the amendment . . .

8 Chair announces the outcome:

The amendment is carried (or defeated). The motion now before the house is . . .

(motion—plus the amendment, if carried)

Exhibit 15-3. Rules for Handling Main Motions.*

I. RULES ON MOTIONS
  A. MAIN MOTION
    1. It is debatable
    2. It can be amended
    3. Can be reconsidered
    4. Requires only majority vote
    5. Must be seconded

  B. MOTION TO AMEND
    • Rules same and main motion

  C. MOTION TO AMEND
     AMENDMENT
    • This motion cannot be amended

  D. MOTION TO SUBSTITUTE
    • Rules same as amend

  E. MOTION TO CLOSE OR LIMIT
     DEBATE
    1. Cannot be debated
    2. Requires 2/3 vote

  F. MOTION TO COMMIT OR REFER
    • Same as main motion except when
      already committed—2/3 vote
      discharges entire question

  G. MOTION ON PREVIOUS
     QUESTION
     (Means close debate and vote)
    1. Cannot be debated, amended or
       reconsidered
    2. Requires 2/3 vote

  H. MOTION TO LAY ON TABLE
    1. Cannot be debated
    2. Cannot be amended or reconsidered

  I. MOTION TO POSTPONE
    • Rules same as main motion

J. MOTION TO ADJOURN
    1. Is not debatable
    2. Cannot be amended
    3. Cannot be reconsidered

  K. MOTION TO TAKE FROM TABLE
    • Cannot be debated, amended, or
      reconsidered

  L. MOTION TO RECONSIDER
    1. Higher than its consideration
    2. Must be made by one voting on the
       prevailing side

  M.   MOTION TO SUSPEND RULES
    1. Is not debatable
    2. Requires 2/3 vote

  N. MOTION TO BALLOT
    1. Is not debatable
    2. Requires 2/3 vote

II. ORDER OF VOTING ON MOTIONS
  A. Fixed time to adjourn
  B. Adjourn
  C. Take a recess
  D. Question of privilege
  E. Call for order of the day
  F. Lay on Table
  G. Previous question (2/3)
  H. Limit debate (2/3)
  I. Postpone
  J. Commit or refer
  K. Substitute
  L. Amend
  M. Main motion

---

*Source: Reprinted from *Medical Staff Services Manual* by Cindy A. Orsund and Patricia J. Starr, p. 41, with permission of Cindy Orsund and Patricia Starr © 1981.

Two-Column Format—Utilizes two vertical columns, one narrow and one wide. The narrow column may be at either the left or right margin, depending on individual preference. (The right side of the page probably facilitates quick reference.) The wide column contains the "body" of minutes. Next to this, the narrow column contains either subject or action, briefly stated, often entirely in upper case letters. Either complete sentences or the briefer "fragments" style can be utilized with this format.

Three-Column Format—Newer. Utilizes three vertical columns: A wide column in the middle which contains the "body" of the minutes and one nar-

---

Exhibit 15-4. Role of the Chair.*

THE CHAIR

Calls the meeting to order.

Keeps meeting to its order of business.

Gives every member who wishes it a chance to speak.

Tactfully keeps all speakers to rules of order and to the question.

Should give pro and con speakers alternating opportunities to speak.

Does not enter into discussion.

States each motion before it is discussed and before it is voted upon.

Puts motions to vote and announces outcome.

May vote when his vote would affect the outcome or in any case when voting is by ballot.

Should be familiar enough with parliamentary law to inform assembly on proper procedure.

May appoint committees when authorized to do so or if bylaws so provide.

May assist in wording of motions if maker requests assistance.

The chair can remain seated during the meeting except at these times:

To call the meeting to order.
To put a question to vote.
To give his decision on a point of order.
May stand to recognize speakers (particularly if assembly is large).

Use of Gavel:

Rap once to call meeting to order.
Rap once to maintain order.
Rap once to declare adjournment.

In speaking to the assembly, the chair refers to himself as "The Chair."

---

*Source: Reprinted from *Medical Staff Services Manual* by Cindy A. Orsund and Patricia J. Starr, p. 41, with permission of Cindy Orsund and Patricia Starr © 1981.

Figure 15-4. Sample Formats for Minutes.*

A.   One-Column

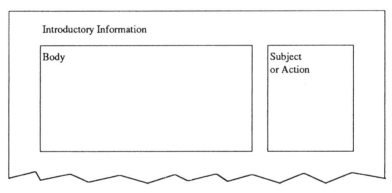

B.   Two-Column

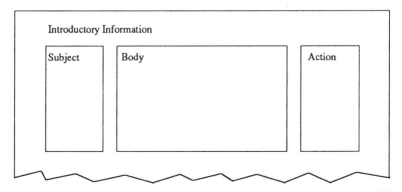

C.   Three-Column

*Description of one-column, two-column, and three-column formats is reprinted from Overview, vol. 14, no. 1, p. 8, with permission of the National Association Medical Staff Services, © 1987.

row column at each margin one of which is headed "Subject," the other "Action." Proponents of this format point out that it focuses on what was done—action taken—and contains a provision for "built-in" follow-up. Generally, the body is written in a terse, fragmentary style because of the limitations of space. This format tends to eliminate extraneous material from the minutes.

The three-column format is probably the best format for use in hospital settings today. Its advantages are fairly obvious. However, it is also possible, as the author has found, that some meetings (e.g., MEC meetings, which are longer, have many agenda items, and involve more discussion) lend themselves better to the two-column format. The recorder of the minutes, with consent of the chair, should decide on the format based on considerations of efficiency and effectiveness.

Taping

The use of a tape recorder during a meeting is often ill-advised, but occasionally can be very helpful. Such use, however, will probably require consent of the chair and even possibly the entire group. It certainly has been found that a tape can be a valuable tool when issues discussed are complicated or clouded by emotional rhetoric. There is definitely an advantage to being able to sit in the quiet of one's office and listen to the tape in order to sift out the "real meat" of such discussion. Permission given to the support person to tape a meeting implies a trust by the group. This trust, quite obviously, must be earned over time and with experience. At no time should a tape or any portion of it ever be played for anyone other than attendees who dispute the written minutes, and the tapes always should be erased for confidentiality reasons as soon as the chair has approved the minutes as prepared.

Phraseology

Great care should be taken to express the *intent* of what is expressed in minutes rather than what is actually said, especially when emotional rhetoric occurs. Most of us, being human and often speaking "off the cuff," fail to express ourselves in the most professional and diplomatic manner. The recorder of minutes can be of assistance simply by altering the phraseology while keeping true to intent.

Appropriate alterations follow:

Actual   I don't see why the bylaws committee expects us to do their work for them! Why don't they get off their royal duffs and do this themselves?"

Reported   Concern was expressed that this issue would more appropriately be resolved by the bylaws committee, and the consensus was that it should be referred to them for action.

Actual   I think this whole idea stinks! There's no way we should be involved in a project like this cockamamie idea."

Reported   One member expressed concern and suggested that the group not endorse such a project.

Actual   This is a great idea. I don't see why the committee can't be given the money and the go-ahead."

Reported   A suggestion was made that the committee be funded to investigate the project.

Actual   That's a heck of a lot of money! Let's not be stupid and spend that kind of money without really looking into it and knowing what we're doing."

Reported   One member suggested that the necessity and feasibility of the project be considered in depth prior to approval of the recommended expenditure.

Identification of Speakers

The recorder of minutes should never attempt to achieve a verbatim transcript; this is totally unnecessary and serves no useful purpose. Motions made, however, are actions taken and should be clearly stated, as accurately and as exactly as possible. If the recorder, during discussion of a motion, becomes confused as to the clear statement of the motion, clarification should be requested of the chair or the person making the motion (likewise for amendments). This can be accomplished inoffensively by addressing the chair in the following way: "Excuse me, Dr. Cureall, but I'm not totally clear on how this motion should be stated in the minutes. Could you or Dr. Doright please restate it?"

Further, there is no reason to identify by name the physicians (or members of the group) who make and second motions unless they explicitly express the desire that this be done. Indeed, some attorneys will advise against it.

As a matter of fact, there exists now a generally accepted theory that the use of names in minutes be avoided, especially when reporting items that provoked emotional outbursts. It is quite correct, however, to use names when objective reports are given ("Dr. Jones reported for the medical records committee that...."). Additionally if a member requests that his or her name be recorded, for whatever reason, then the recorder should do so. This often happens when there are dissenting votes or abstentions. In the case of clinical reviews of actual patient cases, physicians should be identified only by number. Their anonymity in these peer review situations must be protected; otherwise, the validity of the peer review process is compromised.

Content

There are certain items that minutes of any medical staff group meeting should contain. These items include the following:

1. name of institution;
2. name of group and type of meeting (regular or special);
3. date, place and time of call to order and adjournment;
4. attendance, including absences and those excused plus guests or visitors;
5. names of chair and recorder;
6. review and approval of previous minutes (with any corrections noted).

What should then follow is simply a brief description of the items discussed and the actions taken or follow-up to be done. Minutes should be simply informational and should not put anyone at risk by inclusion of gossip, hearsay, innuendo, or other potentially embarrassing statements. As Sgt. Friday used to say, "Just the facts, ma'am, just the facts."

Clinical Review Documentation

There are accreditation standards that require clinical departments to review the actual clinical practice, note problems discovered in the review, take actions to correct these problems, and track and document the results of the action taken. Whether this overall activity is called "quality improvement," "performance improvement," or some other title doesn't matter. What does matter is that the activities must be well documented in the minutes. The MSSP must be aware of current standards and keep the medical staff informed about them. The MSSP must also assist with the performance and documentation of the activities required for compliance with current standards. At the time of this writing, the JCAHO mandates that the medical staff will take a leadership role in improving the processes in the following functions:[8]

1. medical assessment and treatment of patients,
2. use of medications,
3. use of blood and blood components,

4. use of operative and other procedures,

5. efficiency of clinical practice patterns.

The performance of these functions is discussed at length in other chapters of this book. What should be noted here is that the performance or review of the performance of these functions must be reflected in minutes. There are no finite or specific rules for recording this information, at least not at the present time. Each MSSP should adopt the method or system that best suits the medical staff and the facility being served.

CONFIDENTIALITY

There exists today understandable reluctance to include peer review matters in the body of minutes—even when every attempt is made to protect the anonymity of all concerned—because it is feared they may be discoverable in a court of law. Two possible solutions are suggested:

1. Place the peer review portions of minutes on a sheet separate from the general business discussions and keep them in a separate section in the minutes book. This section is to be treated an non-releasable.

2. Keep all material dealing with clinical review and quality improvement matters in a completely separate filing cabinet and stamp them all with a stamp reading, "Privileged and Confidential. Protected by State Statute _____" (insert the appropriate number).

Each of these solutions does not absolutely guarantee that the materials will never be discovered, but each will help. The hospital legal counsel should, of course, be consulted if a subpoena is received for protected peer review documents. (See also Chapter 17.)

FOLLOW-UP

Good minutes of any medical staff group, no matter how large or small, will indicate when follow-up is required and by whom. The initiation of the follow-up will almost always fall to the person who has prepared the minutes, whether that person is doing the actual follow-up or not. There will be different responsibilities assigned in different institutions depending on the size, organization type, and other factors. For example in peer review follow-up, some MSSPs will be given the duty of preparing review forms and related letters to physicians, whereas others may only have to receive and file such items and retrieve them at reappointment time. The fact remains, however, that the minutes, if well-written, will define who is responsible and for what. The MSSP simply must keep in mind that the loop always needs to be closed— the actions taken need to have a documented result, whether favorable or unfavorable—and pending items must be pursued to that end.

CONCLUSION

The final instruction to readers seeking knowledge about the conduct of meetings and the preparation of minutes is to read as many writings as can be found on the subject. Some of these writings were noted above, but there are many others that can be of help. Mastery of the required skills depends on investigation and concentrated effort. However, the author believes that assisting a medical staff and its leaders in conducting meaningful meetings and then providing proper documentation of those meetings is not necessarily a task to be endured but can be instead an art to be enjoyed.

NOTES

1. David L. Brannon, "Making Meetings Work." (Paper presented at the annual conference of the National Association of Quality Assurance Professionals, Baltimore, October 1988).
2. Richard E. Thompson, M.D., *The Medical Staff Leaders' Practical Guide* (Marblehead, MA: Opus Communications, Inc., 1996).
3. "The Hospital Medical Staff—Its Changing Form and Function," videotape presented by William R. Fifer, M.D., (Brighton, CO: Brighton Books, 1987).
4. Michael Doyle and David Strauss, *How to Make Meetings Work* (New York: The Berkley Publishing Group, 1976) 298 pages.
5. Henry M. Robert, *Robert's Rules of Order*, edited by Darwin Patnode (New York: Berkley Books, 1993).
6. Sturgis, Alice, *Sturgis Standard Code of Parliamentary Procedure*, 3rd. ed. (New York: McGraw Hill Book Co., 1988).
7. Utter, E.C., *Parliamentary Law at a Glance: Based on Robert's Rules of Order* (Chicago: Henry Regnery Co., 1988).
8. Joint Commission on Accreditation of Healthcare Organizations, *1997 Comprehensive Accreditation Manual for Hospitals* (Oakbrook Terrace, IL: Joint Commission on Accreditation of Healthcare Organizations, 1997): MS-48.

Chapter 16

Introduction to the Law

Carla D. Thompson, Esq.

THE LEGAL SYSTEM

The legal system impacts all aspects of personal and professional life. When a check is written, a car driven, or a street crossed, laws and regulations apply. There are laws, rules, and regulations concerning the manufacture, distribution, and labeling of almost everything bought, used, or consumed. Labor laws cover most workers, most buildings must conform to building codes, and fair credit laws govern every credit card purchase made. Laws govern and regulate almost every phase of life. The legal system also provides a forum for people to use to resolve their disputes.

Criminal Law and Civil Law

Law is often defined as social control. But whereas laws prohibiting murder, arson, and theft are obviously examples of social control through government legislation, there is more to the law than the administration of criminal justice.

The law of torts, the law of contracts, and the rest of the body of law known as "civil law" is a complex system of rules that attach legal rights, responsibilities, and duties to various actions.

The criminal law segment of our legal system prohibits conduct that is contrary to the public order. Each state has its own laws defining what is a crime in that state. In the United States, there are laws dealing with the crimes of abduction, abortion, adultery, arson, bigamy, bribery, burglary, counterfeiting, disorderly conduct, dueling, embezzlement, escape, extortion, false impersonation, forgery, homicide, incest, kidnaping, larceny, malicious mischief, mayhem, murder, obscenity, obstructing justice, perjury, prostitution, rape, riot, robbery, suicide, treason and vagrancy. This, of course, is not a complete list of all crimes prohibited by law in this country.

Crimes are divided into two major categories: misdemeanors and felonies. A misdemeanor is a crime that carries a maximum penalty of less than one year in jail and/or a fine. A felony is a more serious offense that carries a term of imprisonment of more than one year. The civil actions that health care professionals may be most concerned about are tort actions and contract actions.

In a criminal case the plaintiff is always the state (sometimes called "the People.")[1]

A general understanding of the law that applies to health care administration is important so that health care personnel can protect themselves, their employers, and even their patients. Health care professionals need to be aware of the laws and regulations that define what they may or may not do.

THE COURTS

The courts are probably the most familiar part of the American legal system. Although few people have taken part in an actual trial, most people have seen a trial on television.

The court system is a complex structure of federal and state courts. In every state there is at least one federal court and an entire state court system.

Federal Courts

At the federal level the trial courts are called U.S. district courts. Each state has at least one federal district court.

The intermediate level in the federal system is called the United States court of appeals. There are 13 federal courts of appeal, and each, except for the District of Columbia Circuit, encompasses several states.

The United States Supreme Court

The final appellate court in the federal system is the U.S. Supreme Court. The U.S. Supreme Court hears appeals from the U.S. district courts and from the highest appellate court of each state. The United States Supreme Court also has jurisdiction to hear appeals involving the interpretation of a federal constitutional provision or a federal law or regulation. In very rare instances, the high court can hear appeals directly from the U.S. district courts.

In some cases, the U.S. Supreme Court also has "original jurisdiction," for example, when one state is bringing action against another state. In these rare cases the U.S. Supreme Court is a *trial court.*

There are other federal courts, such as the Court of Claims and U.S. Custom Courts. Figure 16-1 shows the federal court system structure.

State Courts

Within each state court system, there are several levels. Like the federal courts, most state court systems have three levels: the trial level, the intermediate appellate level, and the final appellate level. See Figure 16-2 for an illustration of the state court system.

In the state systems, the courts perform the same functions as their federal counterparts. Trial courts decide questions of fact, judge a defendant's guilt or innocence in criminal cases, and determine liability in civil cases. Trial courts decide if a penalty should be imposed and whether it should be a fine or a jail term. In civil cases, they determine the amount of damages to be awarded.

Appellate courts in the state system, as in the federal system, review trial court decisions to determine if the court correctly applied the law to the facts. Only rarely do appellate courts review factual determinations made at the trial level. When the facts are reviewed this is called a de novo review.

In a state system *local courts* are usually specialized and are located all around the state. Municipal courts, traffic courts, police courts, small claim courts are all examples of local courts. Their jurisdiction is very limited.

The *courts of general jurisdiction* are the basic trial courts for the community. In some states these courts are called circuit courts or district courts. In California these courts are called superior courts. In New York State the basic trial courts are oddly called the Supreme Courts.[2]

Figure 16-1. Federal Court System.

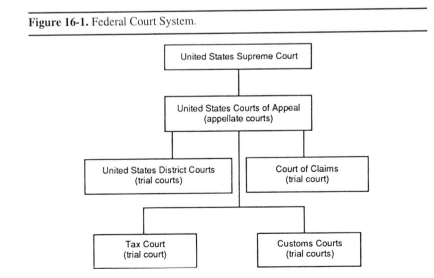

WHAT HAPPENS IN A CIVIL LAW SUIT?

How Does a Lawsuit Begin?

As previously mentioned, court actions fall into two categories: civil actions and criminal actions. *Civil cases* are those in which an individual, an organization, or a government agency sues for damages or injunctive relief from another party. *Criminal actions* are cases brought by the state or federal government against an individual who has been charged with committing a crime.

Civil actions are usually actions concerning the breach of a contract (ex contractu), or for a wrong, also known as a tort (ex delicto).

Sometimes a suit is brought for "equitable relief" rather than money damages. Equity can prohibit certain wrongful conduct with an injunction or can compel the performance of certain action with an order for specific performance. Usually money damages cannot be obtained in an equitable proceeding.

When one person has been injured by another person the injured party may consult an attorney to determine if the injury will give rise to a legal cause of action. The attorney will take the client's statement and may interview possible witnesses. The attorney will probably do some legal research to find the applicable laws and court decisions and will then determine if the client has a viable case.

If there is a cause of action, and the client wishes to proceed, the attorney will then prepare a *complaint* or a *petition* and will file it in the appropriate

---

Figure 16-2. State Court System.

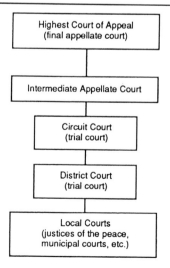

court. The attorney's client is called the *plaintiff*, and the person or organization against whom the case is filed is called the *defendant*.

The complaint states the facts of the plaintiff's action against the defendant and sets forth the judgment or money damages sought. The filing of the complaint does not prove that the plaintiff does indeed have a cause of action—that will be decided by the court.

The plaintiff's attorney also files a document called a *summons* with the court. The summons directs the county sheriff to serve a copy of the legal papers on the defendant. In some states, the summons is served as a matter of course; in others, it must be served in advance of filing the complaint; in still others, only qualified process servers may serve the summons.[3]

After the summons is served, the original document is returned to the court and it is noted whether the defendant was actually served. The serving of the summons is the defendant's official notification that a suit has been filed and that he or she has been named as a defendant. Filing the complaint and serving the summons officially commences a law suit.

The defendant is then given a certain time period in which to file an *answer* to the plaintiff's complaint.

Venue and Jurisdiction

The attorney must file the case in the proper court. A court has no authority to hear a case unless it has jurisdiction over the persons or property involved.

Some actions are called local actions, and can be brought only in the county where the subject matter of the jurisdiction is located. For example, a mortgage foreclosure can only be brought in the county where the property is located. Other actions are called *transitory actions* and can be brought in any county in any state where the defendant may be found and served with the summons. An action for personal injury is a transitory action.

Venue is the location, the county, or the district where the action will be tried. Venue may be changed (1) if there has been widespread pretrial publicity, (2) in an effort to find jurors who have not been exposed to that publicity, or (3) simply to provide a more neutral setting when there is a great deal of local sentiment about a certain case.

A *change of venue* is requested by motion and is granted or denied by the judge.

Trial Preparation

Before the trial begins, both parties can file documents with the court. Sometimes a defendant may file a pleading called a *Motion to Quash Service of Summons*, which asserts that the defendant should not have been served or was improperly served. Defendants sometimes file a *Motion to Make More Definite and Certain*, which asks the court to order the plaintiff to describe the injury more fully or to set out the facts more specifically so the defendant can answer more accurately.

Sometimes defendants ask the court to rule against the plaintiff with a *Motion to Dismiss* the case.

Before the actual trial, depositions are often taken. Depositions are out-of-court statements taken under oath, and are used for trial preparation and may be used in court. A deposition is not a public record.

Discovery is another legal term which refers to a party's attempt to get more information about the case. Sometimes parties are required to produce books or financial or medical records or submit to a physical examination.

After the pleadings have been filed, a pretrial conference is often held. Sometimes a case is settled at this conference. If not, a trial date is set.

The Trial

Sometimes the lawyers involved decide that a judge trial rather than a jury trial would be better for the case and the right to a jury trial is waived.

When a jury is requested, the lawyers and the judge engage in a process called *voir dire* to select the jury. In this process, the jurors are questioned to determine if they possess any prejudice or bias regarding the case. Each side has a certain number of challenges that can be made for any reason at all. These are called peremptory challenges. Each side also has an unlimited number of challenges that can be made for cause, that is, on the grounds that the juror cannot be termed impartial and is obviously prejudiced in some way.

Once the jury has been selected, each party makes an opening statement. Then witnesses are called to present evidence. The party calling the witness questions the witness first; this is called *direct examination*. The opposing party then questions the witness in what is called *cross examination*.

When all the witnesses have been called and examined, the parties then are allowed to make summations or *closing arguments*.

The judge then *instructs* the jury, and they begin their *deliberations*. Sometimes the jurors are *sequestered*, or isolated, from the public when they are deciding a very controversial case.

After a decision is reached, the jury returns to the courtroom and the *verdict* is read in open court.

STATUTES, LAWS, AND REGULATIONS

Hierarchy of Laws

1. United States Constitution
2. Federal Statutes and Regulations
3. State Constitution
4. State Statutes and Regulations
5. County and City Ordinances
6. The Common Law

Statutory Law

Statutory law is the body of law created by legislative acts (in contrast to the law generated by judicial opinion and administrative bodies).

Of course, the "supreme law of the land" is the United States Constitution.[4]

The structure of American government is probably familiar to all. It includes the U. S. Constitution, the national government and the individual state governments, and the three branches of government—the executive branch, the legislative branch, and the judicial branch. Administrative agencies which create administrative law are also important parts of the structure of government.

Common Law

Common law is the body of law derived from the ancient unwritten law of England. Common law consists of the principles, uses, and rules that do not rest upon any express declaration of the legislature.[5]

Courts attempt to decide cases based on principles established in prior cases. Prior cases which are similar to the case being considered are called *precedents*.

Decisions found to be unreasonable may be overturned.

Stare decisis is a legal principle that mandates adherence to decided cases. It is the policy of courts to stand by precedent and not to disturb a settled point.[6]

Lawsuits are resolved by applying decisions of previous cases. Sometimes a very slight factual difference will be used by the court to distinguish the present case from the previous cases.

Regulations

Federal Agencies

At the federal level, an administrative agency is created by a congressional act. The president, with the advice and consent of Congress, appoints the agency's director or highest official. The agency makes rules (called *regulations*), that have the force of law.

These regulations can be found in the Code of Federal Regulations (C.F.R.). The agency can interpret and enforce the regulations through administrative hearings and decisions. Federal courts can review the decisions made at an administrative hearing and can also be asked to review the regulations.

State Agencies

At the state level, some agencies are created by statute and some are created by provisions in the state constitution. The directors of these state agencies may be appointed by the governor, although the statute or the constitution might direct that the director or top agency official be elected. For example, in many states the attorney general is elected rather than appointed. In state agencies, as in federal agencies, government policies are implemented through rules and decisions. Agency rules and decisions are subject to review by the courts.

Separation of Powers

No one branch of the government is dominant over another branch. Each affects and limits the functions and powers of the others. Thus, the American government is sometimes called a "system of checks and balances." When Congress passes a bill, the president must sign it before it becomes law. And, if the president vetoes the bill, a vote of two-thirds of the Congress can override that veto. A law that has been passed by Congress and signed by the president can be declared invalid (overturned) by the U. S. Supreme Court.

The three branches of government (the executive, legislative, and judicial branches), work together to make, execute, review, and enforce the laws.

Statute of Limitations

Every civil and criminal case is subject to a specific statute of limitation, which is a time limit as to when a lawsuit may be filed. There is one exception: There is no statute of limitation for the crime of murder.

If a lawsuit is not filed within the limits of the statute, the right to sue is lost. The time to file a lawsuit will vary from state to state, and there are different times prescribed for various types of cases.

TORT LAW

A tort is a civil wrong. It is not considered a crime. The wrong-doer is called a *tort-feasor*. The purpose of tort law is to provide a method for peacefully determining liability and assessing damages to be paid to victims of wrongdoing.

There are many different torts and not all torts are recognized in all jurisdictions. In the United States, the most common torts are assault and battery, conspiracy, false imprisonment, forcible entry and detainer, fraud, libel and slander, malicious prosecution, negligence, product liability, trespass, trover and conversion, and waste.

When a person is injured or their property is damaged, the rights and responsibilities of the parties involved are determined by the law of torts. Many torts involve negligence. When a judge, or jury, or arbitrator determines one party was negligent and that the negligent conduct caused injury or property damage, the negligent party is usually required to pay for the harm done.

Simply determining that someone caused injury to someone else is not sufficient. It must be proven that a defendant was at fault. Sometimes no one was at fault as some accidents are unavoidable.

Usually a tort victim is compensated, with money, for the injury suffered. The sum most often includes medical expenses incurred or reimbursement for lost wages. If the damage was to property, the victim is usually awarded the amount of money needed to repair or replace the damaged property. Sometimes people are compensated for their pain and suffering. Although it is very difficult to assign a dollar value to the loss of a leg or an eye, in our society it has been decided that monetary compensation is the best alternative.

Categories of Torts

There are three categories of torts: intentional torts, negligence, and strict liability torts.

Most torts involve some sort of negligence, but in some cases there may be intentional wrongdoing. Intentional torts include assault, battery, false imprisonment, invasion of privacy, and the intentional infliction of emotional distress. There are also certain situations where the activity is so dangerous that it is public policy to demand absolute responsibility of the tort-feasor. These are known as strict liability torts.

Negligence

The most common tort is the tort of negligence. When a person or property is injured or damaged as a result of the actions of another person, an allegation of negligence is often made. Negligence is often divided into two degrees: ordinary negligence (which is the failure to perform as a reasonably prudent person would perform under similar circumstances) and gross negligence (which is the intentional or wanton disregard of care).

Forms of Negligence

There are several forms of negligence. *Malfeasance* is an unlawful or improper act. *Misfeasance* is the incorrect performance of a permitted act. *Nonfeasance* is the failure to act when an act is required by law or when there is a duty to act. *Malpractice* is the negligent or careless action of a person who is held to a professional standard of care. *Criminal negligence* is the willful indifference to the potential for injury or the reckless disregard for the safety of another.

Standards of Care

Professionals are held to a higher standard of care than non-professionals. A non-professional is judged by a "reasonable person" standard: What would a reasonable person do in this situation? A professional is held to a higher standard: What would a reasonably prudent person with this type of specialized training do in this type of situation?

How Is Negligence Proven in a Court of Law?

Usually, a jury will decide, based on facts presented at trial, if a person acted reasonably or negligently. Custom and common sense often determine what standard of care the jury will apply.

Sometimes the standard of care is defined by statute. If someone acted in violation of law, he or she is usually presumed to have acted negligently and is held liable for any damages that result.

Res ipsa loquitur means, "the thing speaks for itself." The doctrine of res ipsa loquitur applies when the defendant had exclusive control of the item or instrument or "thing" that caused the harm, when the plaintiff did not in any way contribute to the accident, and when the accident would not have occurred unless someone was negligent. For example, if an X-ray clearly shows that a surgical instrument was left in the chest cavity of a man who had undergone heart surgery, the plaintiff could allege that the doctrine of res ipsa loquitur applies. In this case, the mere fact that the accident happened is enough to infer that the someone (the doctor, nurse, or hospital) was negligent and will be held liable for damages.

Standards of care applicable to medical professional activities can also be found in government regulations and in accreditation manuals for hospitals and other institutions.

Sometimes the standard of care changes based on changes in statutes, rules and court cases.

In the case of *Darling v. Charleston Community Memorial Hospital*, 33 Ill. 2d 326, 211 N.E. 2d 253 (1965), the Illinois Supreme Court held that a hospital is liable for the improper review of the credentials of its staff, and that a hospital cannot limit its liability as a charitable corporation to the amount of its liability insurance, and that since the evidence supported the verdict for the plaintiff, the hospital was liable.

In the *Darling* case, a college football player was injured while playing. He was taken to the emergency room and was treated by a general practitioner who had not treated a leg fracture in recent years. X-rays were taken and the doctor set the fracture and applied a cast. The patient complained of pain. The doctor did not call in a specialist. After two weeks the plaintiff was transferred to a larger hospital under the care of an orthopedic surgeon. The surgeon found a considerable amount of dead tissue that, in his opinion, was caused by swelling of the leg against the cast. The surgeon attempted several operations to save the leg, but ultimately it was amputated eight inches below the knee.

The Illinois court held that the hospital was liable based on the evidence that the nurses at the hospital did not test the leg for circulation as often as necessary, that skilled nurses would have promptly recognized conditions that signaled impaired circulation, and that the nurses knew that the situation would become irreversible. In that situation it became the "nurse's duty to inform the attending physician and if he failed to act, to advise the hospital authorities so that appropriate action might be taken."[7]

The court also held that the hospital negligently failed to review the doctor's work and negligently failed to require a consultation with a specialist.

In the *Darling* case the court also held that the doctrine of charitable immunity did not apply and that the defendant was liable for the full judgment, even that which was in excess of its insurance coverage.

Defenses Against Negligence

A defendant may be relieved from having to pay damages, even if he or she is found to be negligent. The possible defenses are contributory negligence, comparative negligence, assumption of the risk, and release.

Contributory Negligence

The rule of contributory negligence is still the law in some states, but most states have changed to a comparative law standard. Contributory negligence was the law in all states at one time. This doctrine provided that if a person was negligent at all, he or she could not recover against another person even if that person was far more negligent.

Comparative Negligence

Since abandoning the doctrine of contributory negligence, most states have adopted a comparative negligence rule. Under this rule, one party's negligence is "compared" with the other party's negligence. Recovery of damages will be limited to an amount reduced by the percentage of fault assessed to that party. For example, if the defendant car driver was held to be 80 percent at fault but the plaintiff was held to be 20 percent at fault, the most the plaintiff could recover would be 80 percent of his or her claim.

Releases

Many times businesses will try to limit their liability by printing a release on the back of a ticket claiming they cannot be sued if there is an injury. Sometimes this will preclude a person from suing them and sometimes it will not. If the release is written in very fine print and was not noticed, the person signing will not be held to it. If it is written in a complicated way and was not understood, the person signing will not be held to it. Also, that person's right to sue will not be waived if the injuries were caused by an act of gross negligence or if the act was intentional.

Equitable Relief

In some cases involving nuisance or trespass, a plaintiff may ask the court to issue an injunction to order the defendant to stop doing something tortious.

Money Damages

As mentioned above, a tort is not considered a crime. In a tort action the plaintiff has somehow been injured. The plaintiff seeks damages (monetary compensation) for these injuries in his or her own name in a civil, not criminal, court. By contrast, in criminal law it is "the people" as a whole who seek justice. It is the state in a criminal case that brings the case, not the wronged individual. A victim of theft or rape cannot bring a criminal action against a person. The complaint is filed in the name of the state.

Tort law compensates a person with money. The person responsible for the injury is required to pay to make the harmed person whole again. Criminal law punishes the criminal who violated a law. The penalty can be a fine or imprisonment, or both.

Sometimes a Tort is Also a Crime

Some crimes are also torts. This can be confusing. Battery is both a crime and a tort. If one person strikes another person, the victim can sue to recover damages. This suit would be brought in a civil court, and if the plaintiff (the person who was hit) could prove that he or she was injured and those injuries were caused by the defendant (the person who did the hitting), the plaintiff could be compensated for the injuries. The state can also prosecute the defendant for the crime of battery, in which case the defendant might go to jail.

RESTRAINT OF TRADE

Antitrust litigation is an important legal issue for health care providers. The competition in the health care industry creates an arena for many kinds of possibly illegal actions involving the restraint of trade.

In 1890, the U.S. Congress passed the Sherman Antitrust Act, (15 U.S.C. § 1). Section 1 provides that, "every contract, combination in form of trust or otherwise, or conspiracy, in restraint of trade or commerce among the several States, or with foreign nations, is hereby declared to be illegal."

Any time there is an action to reduce market competition, or to fix prices, bar or limit members, or provide a "preferred provider" system or when there is an exclusive contract, there is the possibility of restraint of trade.

There can be a potential antitrust problem when a hospital limits its medical staff. The process a hospital uses to determine who may have staff privileges and who may not must be based on objective criteria and not on the financial advantages that may be realized by granting or denying the right to practice at the hospital.

Of course, a hospital may deny privileges to certain individuals, but the decision must be made for cause (for instance, the doctor involved has been cited for improper actions or does not possess the qualifications required for all doctors) and not merely to limit competition.

Sometimes a hospital will enter into an exclusive contract with specialty groups to provide services to the hospital. Often a hospital will contract with a pathology, radiology, emergency medicine or anesthesiology group. If these contracts are reasonable and are not made to limit competition, they are usually permitted. In several cases in which hospitals were sued, the courts held that the contracts were not against public policy.[8]

Hospitals and other health care facilities must be sure that any action or proposed action to limit access or to close its medical staff is based on objective criteria. In many states, government agencies review hospital actions regarding the granting or the denying of hospital privileges. Individual physicians and medical groups will continue to challenge hospital actions, and if objective standards are not the basis for the action, the challengers will prevail. See the following chapter for details.

NOTES

1. In any case, the title of the case is always written *Plaintiff v. Defendant.* The plaintiff (or plaintiffs), the party bringing the action, will always be listed first. Also, each case will have a citation. With the citation the case can be looked up and the complete decision read. For example, in 220 F. 2d 118, the "F. 2d" refers to the Federal Reporter, Second Series. The "220" refers to the volume, and "118" refers to the page number of that volume. The citation also can be used to learn if the case has been upheld or overturned by a higher court, and to determine if there are other cases with similar results.

2. The highest court in New York State is called the Court of Appeals.

3. In some states, a summons may only be served by a person who is over 21 years of age and who is not a party to the action.

4. United States Constitution, Art. VI.

5. *Bishop v. Unites States*, 334 F. Supp. 415 (S.D. Tx. 1971), *cert. denied* 414 U.S. 911 (1973).

6. *Neff v. George*, 364 Ill. 306, 4 N.E. 2d 388 (1986).

7. 211 N.E. 2d at 258.

8. *Jefferson Parish Hospital v. Hyde*, 446 U.S. 2 (1984). See also *Belmar v. Cipolla*, 96 N.J. 199, 475 A. 2d 533 (1984).

Chapter 17

Current Legal Issues

Joanne P. Hopkins, Esq.

INTRODUCTION

The relationship between a hospital and its medical staff, as well as the relationship between the medical staff and practitioners seeking access to the medical staff, is the subject of state and federal legislation and case law. The medical staff services professional should be familiar with the law applicable to the jurisdiction in which he or she practices. This chapter is intended to provide a general discussion of legal issues that are usually common among the states and to alert the professional to when legal counsel should be consulted.

THE MEDICAL STAFF

Relationship Between the Hospital and the Medical Staff

The hospital's medical staff is generally composed of independent practitioners who provide health care services within the hospital. The hospital's governing board groups these practitioners together as a "medical staff" to comply with legal requirements and to perform certain functions for and on behalf of the governing board. For example, accreditation and licensure requirements will compel a hospital to credential practitioners seeking to provide services in the hospital. The hospital's governing board utilizes the services of the medical staff, operating generally through medical staff officers and committees, to perform this credentialing and provide recommendations to the governing board for final decision.

Whether the medical staff is a separate legal entity has not been addressed conclusively in all jurisdictions. "Self-governance" by the medical staff may support a finding of a separate entity. Some medical staffs find it in their favor not to be construed as a separate legal entity, but to serve as an integral component of the hospital. Generally, this enables the medical staff members, when performing functions on behalf of the hospital and its governing board, to be protected under the hospital's liability insurance as an agent of the hospital. Medical staffs, however, that charge membership dues or carry other attributes of separateness may find in a particular court case that they are held to be a separate legal entity capable of being sued independently and capable of conspiring with the hospital for purposes of antitrust liability.

Medical Staff Bylaws

Again, because of accreditation and licensure requirements, the hospital must have medical staff bylaws that establish the method or manner by which the practitioners comprising the medical staff perform the functions assigned to them. There is no specific structure required of medical staff bylaws, but there are elements that must be included in the bylaws as set forth in accreditation[1] and hospital licensure standards. Additionally, for those hospitals that are Medicare providers, the Medicare Conditions of Participation[2] will address requirements for the medical staff and medical staff bylaws.

Generally, medical staff bylaws contain the following key components:

1. responsibilities of medical staff and duties of members;
2. categories of the medical staff and specialty departments/sections/services;
3. qualifications and procedures for medical staff appointment and reappointment;
4. qualifications and procedures for granting clinical privileges;
5. medical staff officers;
6. medical executive committee (and other medical staff committees if any);
7. meetings, quorum and voting;
8. corrective action and hearing/appellate review procedures;
9. peer review confidentiality and immunity;
10. amendment and adoption of bylaws and related manuals.

Medical staff bylaws also generally include, as a separate manual, a set of rules and regulations. While the bylaws contain general principles on operation of the medical staff, manuals such as the rules and regulations provide significant detail on operational requirements. Many hospitals utilize separate manuals on credentialing, corrective action, and hearing and appellate review procedures to set out the particular details for those respective areas. A separate manual may also address allied health professionals or health care practitioners who are not eligible for medical staff appointment (see Allied Health Professional Section). The process for amending a manual may differ from the process of amending the medical staff bylaws that almost always requires approval by the voting members of the medical staff and the governing board. A manual, on the other hand, may only require approval of the medical executive committee and the governing board, enabling changes to be made more easily. Therefore, the medical staff needs to be comfortable with the content of any manual since changes are not subject to approval of the entire medical staff.

Just as there are issues over whether the medical staff is a separate legal entity from the hospital, there have been court cases addressing whether the medical staff bylaws constitute a contract between the hospital or the medical staff and each member of the medical staff.[3] Some hospitals and their medical staffs prefer that the medical staff bylaws not constitute a contract with each member of the medical staff, since that may open the hospital and the medical staff to litigation based on breach of contract. Hospitals and medical staffs wishing to negate the existence of a contract may provide statements to that effect in the bylaws or, alternatively, avoid statements in the bylaws that support the allegation of the existence of a contract.

Sources of Law

State statutes or regulations may address any or all of the following issues pertinent in the medical staff setting and should be reviewed by the medical staff services professional:

1. Who can access the medical staff—are podiatrists, dentists or other independent practitioners eligible for medical staff membership or is membership limited to physicians?

2. What procedures must be afforded if medical staff appointment or reappointment is denied or if the hospital attempts to terminate or limit a practitioner's appointment or clinical privileges (e.g., "procedural due process" or notice and opportunity to be heard)?

3. Are the bylaws a contract between the practitioner and the hospital and its medical staff?

4. What may be required as a condition of medical staff appointment or what are permissible bases to deny or terminate appointment or clinical privileges (e.g., completion of a residency, board certification)?

5. What privileges of confidentiality and immunity are available for peer review actions and participants in peer review?

Case law (or court cases) in the medical staff area generally deals with either the reasons a hospital may use to exclude or terminate a practitioner from the medical staff or the procedures used to accomplish the exclusion or termination. Cases also address whether the hospital may be liable for credentialing of practitioners or for the actions of medical staff members. Depending on state law, there may be immunity for hospitals and medical staffs for credentialing and other peer review activities. Generally, this immunity will be limited to authorized actions taken in the course of peer review and will require that the actions have been taken in good faith, in the absence of malice. (See Peer Review Privilege Section.)

At the federal level, the primary law dealing with peer review is the Health Care Quality Improvement Act (HCQIA).[4] This law was intended to provide immunity for participants in peer review provided that the peer review met certain standards (see HCQIA Section). HCQIA also established the National Practitioner Data Bank (Data Bank), with required reporting by hospitals and other health care entities of professional review actions involving physicians as well as mandatory querying of the Data Bank on granting privileges or membership.

The other primary federal law that affects the medical staff is the Conditions of Participation for hospitals who are Medicare providers. The Medicare Conditions of Participation address duties and responsibilities of the medical staff, as well as operational requirements applicable to physicians and other practitioners.

MEDICAL STAFF LIABILITY ISSUES

Hospital Liability for the Practitioner

A hospital may be held liable for the actions of a practitioner who is providing services in the hospital setting. There are three primary ways this may occur.

Respondeat Superior/Vicarious Liability. This type of liability occurs when the practitioner is an employee of the hospital. Most states impose liability on the employer for the actions of the employee, even if the employer itself did not engage in any negligence. Rather, the employer is held "vicariously liable" for the actions of the employee simply by virtue of the existence of the employer-employee relationship. This liability is generally premised on the assumption that the employer is in the best position to control the employee and will do so to minimize the employer's liability.

Ostensible Agency. In this situation, a hospital may be liable for the actions of a member of the medical staff even though the practitioner is not an employee of the hospital, but is an independent contractor. Depending on the type of services provided by the practitioner, the court may find that the practitioner is an "agent" of the hospital. As an example, an emergency department physician may be an independent contractor of the hospital, but appear to the patient who presents to the emergency department for treatment as a hospital employee. In such a case, depending on the facts, the court may find that the patient had a reasonable expectation that the physician was an employee or authorized agent of the hospital and, therefore, that the patient may look to the hospital in the event the patient is injured by the emergency department physician's negligence. Ostensible agency liability is most frequently seen with hospital-based practitioners.

Independent Liability/Corporate Negligence. Separate from liability a hospital may have for the actions of the medical staff member because of its relationship to the practitioner, many states have held that the hospital has independent duties to patients which may include a duty to supervise the care provided by the medical staff and to perform proper credentialing and, therefore, liability for its own "corporate" negligence in that regard.[5] The hallmark decision in this regard is *Darling v. Charleston Community Memorial Hospital*, an Illinois Supreme Court case from 1965.[6] In the *Darling* case, there were allegations that the attending physician was not responsive to an orthopedic patient's complaints of pain and other possible complications in his treatment of the patient. Ultimately, the patient had to be transferred and undergo a leg amputation. The hospital defended against the patient's allegation of negligence by stating that only the physician could practice medicine, not the hospital. The Illinois Supreme Court, however, held that hospitals are independently responsible for monitoring, supervising and controlling care where necessary to protect the patient. The *Darling* case decision has been followed by many other states.[7]

Hospital Liability to the Practitioner

A practitioner may seek to hold a hospital liable for denying the practitioner access to the medical staff or for a hospital's decision to terminate or limit the practitioner's medical staff appointment and/or clinical privileges. The practitioner's complaints may focus on the reason for the hospital's action, the manner in which the action was taken or procedures used, or both. Lawsuits between a hospital and practitioner most commonly involve allegations of failure to afford due process, antitrust, violations of federal or state civil rights laws, breach of contract, libel, slander or defamation, and tortious interference with business or contractual relationships. Because of the importance to a practitioner of medical staff appointment to the hospital and requirements to disclose peer review or professional review actions when seeking appointment at other hospitals or managed care contracts, denied practitioners bringing suits against hospitals is not uncommon despite the state and federal law provisions on peer review immunity.

APPOINTMENT AND CLINICAL PRIVILEGES

The medical staff bylaws should contain two critical elements regarding appointment and clinical privileges: (1) the criteria or requirements, such as education, training and competence; and (2) the procedures for making the decisions. The first element deals with the basis or reason for the decision, while the second deals with the procedures used to make the decision. While a court may be inclined to defer to the hospital and the medical staff as to the reason for a decision to exclude or discipline a practitioner, it will likely scrutinize the procedures used to take the action. Key is that the procedures in the medical staff bylaws have been substantially complied with in making the decision and that the procedures are fair to the practitioner.

The bylaws should have requirements for appointment as well as requirements for clinical privileges which obviously will differ by privilege and specialty. Some hospitals group clinical privileges into categories or may have a core set of privileges generally associated with completion of a residency in the particular specialty, along with a second category of special privileges that may require additional education or training. There may be separate procedures for the appointment decision as compared to the clinical privileges decision, although many hospitals use the same process but are applying different criteria.

In challenging the basis for a credentialing or peer review action, the practitioner may allege that the action was arbitrary or capricious or being applied in a discriminatory manner. Joint Commission on Accreditation of Healthcare Organization's (JCAHO's) Medical Staff Standards require that professional criteria be specified in the bylaws and uniformly applied to all applicants.[8] The criteria are designed to ensure that patients will receive quality care. Therefore, criteria for appointment and clinical privileges should be clear and specific and applied equally to all practitioners unless otherwise provided in the bylaws.

Issues and Criteria

The following sets out some of the substantive issues that arise in credentialing and which will usually be addressed in the medical staff bylaws or related manuals.

Categories of Eligible Practitioners. The medical staff bylaws should clearly define what types of practitioners are eligible to be considered for medical staff appointment. This is most commonly done by defining the term "practitioner" or including a statement in this regard in the opening provisions of the bylaws. The hospital's governing board should be the decision-maker as to these categories, after consulting with the medical staff, so as to limit the involvement of direct economic competitors in the decision. State law should also be consulted, particularly hospital licensing statutes which may address access to the medical staff. Medical staff applications should only be provided to practitioners who are eligible to be considered. If an application is received from a practitioner who is not eligible, it should not be processed until the governing board makes a decision on whether that category of practitioners will be afforded access to the medical staff.

Residency Training. Residency training may be more logically associated with clinical privileges rather than appointment itself, however, it is frequently listed as a requirement for appointment. Some state laws specifically authorize a hospital to require that a practitioner have completed appropriate residency training to be a medical staff member.[9] In *Hay v. Scripps Memorial Hospital*, a 1986 California case, the appellate court held that it was permissible to require obstetrics residency training for obstetrical clinical privileges and, therefore, to deny those privileges to a family practitioner who lacked such training.[10] If the bylaws require residency training, it is recommended that the type of residency be specified, particularly if the requirement is tied to clinical privileges rather than appointment (e.g., a radiology residency may not be appropriate for internal medicine privileges). If tied to privileges, consideration should be given to whether there are several residencies which may be appropriate for the particular specialty or clinical privileges. Finally, state law should be checked on distinctions between residencies in medical schools and those in osteopathic schools. Distinctions or discrimination between the two in a residency requirement may be prohibited by state law or found by a court to be arbitrary.

Board Certification. Whether board certification may be a requirement of appointment or clinical privileges may also be addressed by state law. The court cases to date that have upheld exclusion of a practitioner for this reason have dealt with requirements that there be board certification or eligibility or compliance with some other alternative, not an "absolute" board certification requirement.[11] The theory generally advanced in the cases is that the requirement is arbitrary in that it assumes that a practitioner who is board certified is competent, while one who is not board certified is incompetent. Until very recently, many hospitals avoided an absolute board certification requirement because the Medicare Conditions of Participation provided that "the accordance of staff membership or privileges... [may not be] dependent solely upon certification, fellowship, or membership in a specialty society."[12] Effective April 28, 1997, the Interpretive Guidelines for the Conditions were amended to clarify that board certification may be required, but may not be the only criteria used (e.g., the practitioner may not be automatically appointed to the medical staff because of being board certified).[13] If other criteria are included and the practitioner meets all those criteria except for board certification, the

Interpretive Guidelines provide that the hospital may deny appointment based on lack of board certification. As with residency requirements, if board certification is required, consider whether any type of board certification is acceptable or whether it should be appropriate to the clinical privileges that are being sought by the practitioner. Also to be considered is whether recertification should be required if available. If board certification is an appropriate measure of competency, presumably it should be maintained.

Current Competency. JCAHO requires that the professional criteria at least pertain to evidence of "current competence," requiring that there be some process for assessing this for both new applicants and on reappointment.[14] On reappointment, the hospital should have its own internal data on the practitioner's current competence, but it may be more difficult to obtain this information at the time of initial appointment. Specific queries to other hospitals at which the practitioner has provided services may yield this information. Additionally, this is one of the primary reasons for a "provisional period," to assess the practitioner's current competence through proctoring or observation by other members of the medical staff. In order to assess current competence at the time of reappointment, the medical staff may require that certain minimum numbers of procedures be performed either at the hospital or at other hospitals, in order to maintain the specific clinical privilege.

Professional Liability Insurance. Case law has consistently upheld the hospital's authority to require that the practitioner maintain professional liability insurance for his or her actions in the hospital, because it helps ensure recovery by a patient injured by a practitioner's negligence and protects the hospital's assets.[15] Insurance requirements should be included in the medical staff bylaws with reference to minimum limits of liability which may vary by specialty if appropriate and should be consistently enforced. The bylaws may reference limits to be set by the governing board by resolution or the limits may be set out in a manual that may more easily be changed. Insurance requirements should also address the type of insurance or the type of carriers that are acceptable to ensure that the coverage will be there when needed. Additionally, there may be requirements to purchase prior acts or tail coverage if the insurance is "claims made" (or only covers claims filed during the term of the policy) to ensure coverage if the practitioner changes policies or allows the policy to terminate after he or she leaves the medical staff. Insurance that is "occurrence" based generally only covers claims dealing with incidents during the term of the policy.

Peer References. Information provided by the practitioner's peers related to current competence and other qualifications should be included in the appointment and privileging process.[16] Many hospitals obtain references from residency or fellowship supervisors and department or section chiefs at other hospitals, as well as from other peers. Inquiries to peers should be specific and request detailed information, rather than just setting out a blanket question as to whether the practitioner should be appointed to the medical staff or granted requested clinical privileges. In some states, peer references provided for purposes of peer review will be confidential under applicable peer review laws. This information, however, may need to be disclosed to the practitioner if it becomes the basis for an exclusion or termination of clinical privileges, therefore, the hospital should be very careful about "promising" the peer reference strict confidentiality. Peer references should be marked as generated for purposes of peer review and obtained in a manner that maximizes the application of state peer review privileges to the information to the extent possible.

Health Status. JCAHO requires hospitals to verify the practitioner's ability to perform the clinical privileges requested.[17] This duty may need to be balanced with the limitations on discrimination based on disability, as set forth in the federal Americans with Disabilities Act (ADA).[18] In essence, the ADA prohibits discrimination in certain settings against a "qualified individual with a disability" based on the disability. A "disability" is defined as a physical or mental impairment that substantially limits one or more of the major life activities of such individual, a record of the impairment, or being regarded as having an impairment. To be a "qualified individual with a disability," the individual must be able to perform the essential functions of the job in question with or without reasonable accommodation. If the disabled individual can perform the essential functions of the job or task with reasonable accommodation, the ADA imposes a duty to provide that reasonable accommodation.

The ADA prohibits discrimination by employers of more than 15 employees, public entities and private entities of public accommodation. Hospitals that employ practitioners will need to be cognizant of the provisions of Section I of the ADA dealing with employment. Section I's provisions relate to discrimination in the job application process, employment and termination. Where the medical staff is composed of independent contractors and not employees, hospitals will likely be subject to Section III of the ADA which addresses places of "public accommodation," but not the employment provisions in Section I. Under Section I of the ADA, employers may not ask an applicant questions eliciting information about a disability during the pre-offer stage. These questions should be reserved until a decision has been made to make an offer (or condition an offer) of employment, as must a requirement to undergo a physical examination. The ADA also prohibits discrimination based on past drug addiction or alcoholism. Questions about current illegal drug use are permissible, but otherwise the employer may only address drug or alcohol abuse as it affects the ability to perform the job functions. Some have raised concerns that the prohibition applied in the employment setting might also be applicable to providers of public accommodation under Section III. There is limited case law in this area, however, at least one case indicates that the prohibitions on discrimination would apply only to the clients and customers of the place of public accommodation (e.g., the patient), not the employees or staff.[19]

Because of some uncertainty regarding the ADA, hospitals may attempt to comply with the ADA's employment provisions even though they may be dealing with independent contractors, rather than employees. The following is a question designed to track the ADA prohibitions for purposes of assessing the health status of applicants to and members of the medical staff:

> Do you have the necessary health status or ability to perform the essential functions of medical staff appointment and exercise the clinical privileges requested, with or without reasonable accommodation, without posing a significant health or safety risk to your patients?

Some hospitals have taken an even more conservative approach and only ask about health status after a decision has been made that the applicant meets all the other criteria for appointment and clinical privileges. The offer of medical staff appointment and clinical privileges is then made conditional upon verification that the applicant possesses the necessary health status to perform the essential functions of medical staff appointment and exercise the requested clinical privileges as set forth above.

AIDS and HIV status are protected as disabilities under the ADA.[20] Using the reasoning set forth in the ADA, if a practitioner were HIV positive but could perform the essential functions of medical staff appointment and exercise the clinical privileges requested without posing a significant health or safety risk, discrimination based on HIV status alone would be problematic. With reasonable accommodation, a physician who is HIV positive may be able to meet the health status requirement. Generally, with regard to practitioners or other health care providers involved in surgery, or who come in contact with the patient's blood or bodily fluids, the courts have held that the provider cannot perform clinical privileges without presenting a significant threat to the health and safety of others and, therefore, have permitted exclusion from that practice.[21]

The medical staff bylaws should provide a mechanism to verify an applicant's or member's health status at the time of initial appointment, and reappointment as well, if concerns are raised regarding health status in the interim. Verification of health status may include documentation through a physical examination as well as drug or alcohol testing and/or testing for communicable diseases. In structuring these policies, hospitals should consult with legal counsel, since state laws may affect this analysis as well as the ADA if applicable.

Ability to Work Cooperatively with Others

The courts have generally upheld the right of a hospital or medical staff to limit a practitioner's clinical privileges or appointment because of conduct that is disruptive to hospital operations and has an adverse impact on overall patient care.[22] For this reason, most hospitals include a requirement that the practitioner document his or her ability to work cooperatively with others as a condition of medical staff appointment. Information in this regard is generally obtained through queries to other hospitals or health care entities where the practitioner has practiced, as well as peer references. In addition to addressing the ability to work cooperatively with others, the bylaws should also require that the practitioner cooperate and participate in peer review. Although not required, medical staffs usually look for evidence of a pattern of unprofessional conduct before implementing corrective action, unless a particular incident is extremely serious in nature.

Conduct or Actions at Other Hospitals

Sometimes, the medical staff is advised of an incident at another hospital involving a practitioner, either applying to or who is a member of the medical staff, that has potential implications for the practitioner's actions within the hospital. Although it is sometimes difficult to obtain sufficient information about the incident, the medical staff should be able to act on that information when indicated. The medical staff bylaws may actually provide this authority directly by requiring that practitioners maintain certain standards of conduct at other hospitals or health care entities. Regardless, the bylaws should require the practitioner to advise the hospital within a stated time period of any corrective action taken by another hospital or health care entity as to medical staff appointment or clinical privileges. If the practitioner fails to do so, corrective action may be indicated based on the failure to comply with the requirement to disclose the action (not what occurred at the other hospital). If the practitioner advises of corrective action elsewhere, the practitioner may be required to ensure that the hospital obtains detailed information about the incident so as to determine whether it has implications for the practitioner's participation at the hospital.

Distance from Hospital

JCAHO requires that each applicant to the medical staff pledge to provide for continuous care of his or her patients.[23] Many hospitals require that members of the medical staff be located within a certain distance or travel time of the hospital, so as to be available for care of hospitalized patients and when on-call for the emergency department. Proximity requirements must be carefully structured and not used as a means of limiting competition with other practitioners on the medical staff. Proximity requirements may vary by specialty based on patient care considerations. Generally, it is best to avoid general or vague requirements such as a requirement to be "close enough to the hospital," and to set specific standards that deal with mileage or travel time. If the specialty departments are involved in establishing these requirements, approval of the requirement should be required of a medical staff committee that is not composed of direct economic competitors to verify the reasonableness of the requirement.

Economic Considerations

True "economic credentialing" is generally used to refer to appointment or privileging criteria (and even contracting decisions) that deal with economic or cost issues, as compared to the competence of the practitioner or the quality of the care that he or she provides. "Cost" factors such as overutilization of hospital resources may relate to the quality of care provided by the practitioner as well, however, legal counsel should be consulted on the imposition of economic considerations or economic credentialing since this is an emerging area. (See Conract Practitioners Section.)

Hospital Utilization

Medical staffs are increasingly examining the appropriateness of minimum levels of hospital utilization as a condition for appointment to the staff. Most commonly, this is seen as a minimum utilization requirement for active staff membership. Hospital medical staffs may also consider the appropriateness of limitations on utilization for courtesy staff or other non-active staff categories. Here, the purpose may be to prevent practitioners from utilizing the full services of the hospital for their patients while escaping emergency department or on-call coverage obligations commonly imposed on active staff members. Utilization requirements that have a reasonable basis in patient care considerations or hospital operations may be justifiable, while requirements that are designed to increase use of the facility or require referrals should be questioned. As with any professional criteria, utilization requirements should be applied consistently and uniformly to all members of the medical staff.

Malpractice History

Practitioners should be required to disclose their malpractice or professional liability claims history at the time of initial appointment and to update that information at the time of reappointment. Although the fact of having malpractice claims alone may not be a basis for exclusion or termination of a practitioner, the hospital and its medical staff should examine the nature of the claims to determine if there is a basis for further inquiry and possible professional review action. In *Purcell v. Zimbelman*, the Arizona appellate court held that the hospital had failed to adequately fulfill its duty to review the qualifications of medical staff members and ensure that they were properly trained and qualified for the privileges being exercised.[24] In *Purcell*, the physician had previous malpractice lawsuits, some of which involved the procedure which had allegedly injured the plaintiff. Some hospitals query the court system to determine if the practitioner has been named as a defendant in lawsuits and/or to determine if the practitioner has properly disclosed all claims. The difficulty with these types of queries is the scope, since depending on state law, claims may have been filed in many jurisdictions making a query of the local court system inadequate.

Burden of Proof and Duty to Provide Information

The medical staff bylaws should place the duty of documenting current clinical competency and satisfaction of requirements of appointment and clinical privileges on the practitioner. Rather than making it the duty of the hospital's medical staff to show the applicant is not competent, it is the duty of the practitioner to show he or she is competent and meets the requirements for appointment and the requested clinical privileges. In some cases, the medical staff receives inadequate or incomplete information about the practitioner, making a decision as to competency or the satisfaction of other qualifications difficult. In such cases, rather than finding that the practitioner is incompetent, consideration should be given to whether the more appropriate finding is that there is not adequate information to document competency or make a decision. If the medical staff has inadequate or incomplete information, it may want to consider not processing the application, rather than denying it, since a denial implies a finding of incompetence.

The medical staff bylaws or credentialing manual should provide a clear process for identifying when additional information is needed, notifying the practitioner of the information that is needed, providing the practitioner with a specific time frame within which the information must be received, and notifying the practitioner that the application (whether it be for appointment or reappointment) will be withdrawn from processing if the information is not received within the stated time period.

Use of Institutional Criteria

Hospital medical staffs are increasingly moving toward the development of specific objective criteria for clinical privileges whenever possible. These criteria are generally classified as "minimum" or "threshold" criteria and must be met before the practitioner's application for that clinical privilege will be considered. By using objective criteria that are applied equally to all practitioners seeking the specific clinical privilege, a denial for failure to meet the criteria is not classed as a professional review action that is reportable to the Data Bank.[25] An example would be a requirement that practitioner seeking cardiac catheterization privileges document successful completion of a residency in cardiology and performance of at least 50 cardiac catheterizations within the prior two-year period. Only those practitioners who document satisfaction of the two criteria would be considered for the clinical privilege. Compliance with the criteria, however, would not be a guarantee that the privilege will be granted. As noted, the criteria are only minimum or threshold requirements and a medical staff may still examine other issues or consider other factors in determining whether to grant the clinical privilege.

The use of minimum or threshold criteria decreases the element of subjectivity that may be associated with the granting of clinical privileges. The criteria selected should have a reasonable basis and be approved by a medical staff committee that is not composed of direct economic practitioners to avoid the use of the criteria in an anti-competitive manner. Resources that may be helpful in establishing minimal or threshold criteria are state and national professional standards, board certification requirements and requirements for specialty residencies.

Provisional Period

Although the JCAHO Medical Staff Standards do not specifically require a provisional period, the provisional period is an excellent time for the medical staff to verify information it has received on new practitioners as to possession of necessary training and current competence to exercise the clinical privileges requested. If a provisional period is used, efforts should be made to make the period meaningful. There should be a formal process whereby competence can be observed and evaluated. Proctors should be required to prepare written reports, preferably using a standardized form. There should be documentation that information generated during the provisional period was considered. If a practitioner has difficulty with designated proctors, there should be provisions to appoint alternate proctors. Since the proctor must hold the clinical privilege that is being reviewed, there may be situations in which none of the medical staff members can serve as proctors. In these cases, it may be appropriate to permit proctorship at other facilities or proctoring by a practitioner who is not a member of the medical staff. In terms of reporting to the Data Bank, the imposition of proctoring or other limitations during the provisional period are not reportable to the Data Bank if those requirements are imposed on all practitioners seeking those clinical privileges during the provisional period.[26] On the other hand, limitations during the provisional period that exceed those routinely imposed on practitioners may be reportable.

"Cross" Privileging

While generally a particular clinical privilege is available in only one specialty department or service and is reviewed by that department or service, there are certain clinical privileges that may be exercised by practitioners in different specialties, therefore, several specialties may be credentialing for the same privilege. One option is to have each specialty department or service credential for the same privilege, but this may result in inconsistent criteria or judgments as to the qualifications and competence of practitioners between the different departments or services. Medical staffs that encounter this issue may find it helpful to utilize a joint or ad hoc committee to review the criteria established by the different departments or services and ensure consistency. The requirements, however, need not be exactly the same. For example, where a clinical privilege will be exercised by both gastroenterologists and general surgeons, it may be appropriate to require that the gastroenterologists provide additional documentation of specific surgical training or skill, whereas the additional requirements placed on the general surgeon may deal more with diagnosis or pathology recognition.[27] Criteria of this type acknowledge the specific skills of the different specialties, but are designed to provide for consistency regardless of the specialty. The other option is to only allow one department or service to offer the clinical privilege and require that all practitioners be reviewed by that department or service even though some will be assigned elsewhere. Unfortunately, this approach frequently is open to criticism based on the potential anti-competitive implications and the potential for "turf battles."

Contract Practitioners

In some cases, hospitals have contracted with practitioners for the delivery of professional services. Examples are emergency medical services, anesthesia, radiology and pathology. Hospitals may also contract for the services of intensivists or hospitalists or for the staffing of outpatient clinics. The courts have generally upheld the right of a hospital to contract for professional services, including on an exclusive basis.[28] Exclusive arrangements should be justified by documented patient care or hospital operational considerations, such as the need to ensure a single standard of care, facilitate scheduling of procedures or provide 24-hour coverage for the professional services. A practitioner who provides professional services pursuant to a contractual arrangement should be credentialed in the same manner as any other member of the medical staff.

A significant issue is the relationship between the contract for professional services and the practitioner's rights pursuant to the medical staff by-laws. By contract, the hospital and practitioner can agree to different rights or procedures for terminating clinical privileges or terminating a practitioner's authority to provide services in the hospital. In the absence of a contractual provision to this effect, however, the practitioner would be entitled to the rights set forth in the medical staff bylaws. Some include a provision in the medical staff bylaws providing that contract practitioners are entitled to the same rights as other members of the medical staff, in the absence of a contrary provision in the contract. In the event of a conflict between a contract and the medical staff bylaws, many professional services contracts will provide that the terms of the contract will control.

In the area of exclusive contracting for professional services, the governing board, in consultation with the medical staff, should address the following issues: (1) how are medical staff applications handled when the applicant is requesting privileges in an area which is subject to an exclusive contract; (2) what happens to the clinical privileges of the practitioners providing services pursuant to an exclusive contract when that contract terminates or, in the case of an exclusive contract with a professional association or group, when the practitioner's relationship with the association or group terminates; and (3) how does the hospital move from a situation in which there is no exclusive contract (and numerous practitioners hold clinical privileges in the particular area) to an exclusive contract (e.g., the effect on the clinical privileges of those practitioners who are not subject to the exclusive contract) and must procedural rights of review be afforded to the excluded practitioners. Although the hospital's governing board maintains final authority over decisions of contract and other business decisions, to the extent these issues can be addressed in advance in the medical staff bylaws, conflict between the hospital, the medical staff and individual practitioners may be lessened.

Allied Health Professionals

Hospitals should have a mechanism in place to verify the qualifications and competence of all individuals who provide patient care services in the hospital setting. For members of the medical staff, this is the reason for the medical staff credentialing and peer review procedures. For hospital employees, this evaluation is done pursuant to the human resources process, with the scope of each employee's practice set forth in a written job description. Allied health professionals are generally referred to as those health care professionals who are not eligible for appointment to the medical staff and who are not employed by the hospital. For these individuals, there must also be a method of credentialing or evaluating their qualifications and competence.

Particularly for allied health professionals who function independently, or without direction or supervision from another practitioner, frequently the hospital and medical staff will utilize the medical staff credentialing process for these individuals and grant them clinical privileges. For allied health professionals who are dependent, the hospital may use the medical staff credentialing process or may opt to use another process, such as a hospital multi-disciplinary committee. The hospital committee should have representation from hospital administration and the medical staff, as well as other practice areas affected by the allied's practice, such as nursing, pharmacy and surgical services. The hospital committee might issue recommendations to one or more of the medical staff committees or might issue its recommendations directly to the governing board. Whenever a system is used other than the medical staff credentialing process, there should be clear mechanisms for medical staff input into the scope of practice for allied health professionals and particularly to practitioner supervision when required either by the allied's licensing statutes or by hospital policy.

One of the most controversial areas is what types of allied health professionals should be permitted to provide services in the hospital. This decision should be one reserved for the governing board since the allieds may be direct economic competitors of the practitioners, but there should be a mechanism for medical staff input. If a request is received from an allied health professional for whom the governing board has not made a decision as to access, the request should be tabled until the governing board can decide whether that particular discipline or category of allied health professional should be permitted access. Only if the governing board has granted access should an application be considered.

Finally, in establishing procedures to credential allied health professionals, the procedures should address qualifications required, how the services provided by the allied will be monitored and incorporated into the hospital's quality improvement program, how complaints or concerns will be addressed regarding the allied's practice, how the allied's authorization to provide services may be limited or terminated, and whether the allied is entitled to any procedural rights of review. State statutes may address the procedural rights of review to which an allied may be entitled and JCAHO provides that individuals with clinical privileges must be afforded procedural rights, although these rights need not necessarily be the same as those afforded to practitioners appointed to the medical staff.[29] When using the medical staff credentialing system to credential allieds, the bylaws should be very specific as to whether the allied is entitled to the same procedural rights of review as members of the medical staff since the credentialing system usually incorporates those rights.

QUALITY IMPROVEMENT AND CORRECTIVE ACTION

As discussed earlier, a hospital's governing board has certain responsibilities for monitoring and maintaining the quality of patient care in the hospital. The governing body uses the medical staff to assist in fulfilling this responsibility through peer review and quality improvement programs. It is through the ongoing monitoring of patient care services delivered in the hospital that concerns and problems are identified. Because the hospital's governing body has overall responsibility for the quality of care, these concerns and problems involving a member of the medical staff must be addressed, if necessary, with corrective action affecting the practitioner's clinical privileges and/or medical staff appointment.

Role of Quality Improvement Data

Ideally, problems or concerns regarding the quality of services provided by a member of the medical staff are addressed through the quality improvement process, rather than by corrective action. The quality improvement process may be implemented through medical staff departments or committees or by hospital committees with medical staff representation, or some combination of the two approaches. Some mention of the quality improvement process should be included in the medical staff bylaws, particularly as to the relationship between the quality improvement process and the corrective action process. The department or committee responsible for quality improvement should have the authority to collect data regarding the practitioner and to meet with the practitioner if problems or concerns are identified. The department or committee should also have the authority to work with the practitioner to implement voluntary practice changes, if possible, to address quality improvement problems that are confirmed. The medical executive committee should be kept apprised of quality improvement activities, including the implementation of voluntary practice changes when indicated. Generally, it is only if a practitioner is unwilling or unable to address documented quality improvement concerns on a voluntary basis that the medical staff should consider the need for corrective action.

Grounds for Corrective Action

Corrective action or discipline against a member of the medical staff should be taken when actions or conduct by the practitioner have or may have a detrimental effect on the delivery of patient care services or operation of the hospital. Some common examples of situations in which corrective action is taken include

1. failure to practice in accordance with customary or accepted professional standards;

2. failure to comply with medical staff or hospital bylaws, rules and regulations, or policies (e.g., failure to cooperate in peer review or to provide required emergency services);

3. unprofessional conduct;

4. violation of professional ethics;

5. commission of crimes;

6. impairment of health status affecting the ability to exercise clinical privileges without posing a significant threat to the health and safety of others.

The authority to monitor the practitioner's hospital practice and to implement corrective action, including reasons for taking corrective action, should be specified in the medical staff bylaws, as well as the governing board bylaws (although generally in less detail).

Types of Corrective Action

The medical staff bylaws usually provide for three types of corrective action: routine, summary or emergency, and automatic. What distinguishes the different types of corrective action is whether the action is taken before the practitioner is given a right to a hearing or after or without the benefit of a hearing at all.

Routine corrective action is the most common type of action taken. With routine corrective action, the affected practitioner is given notice of the allegations and procedural rights of review prior to the corrective action being imposed, if the proposed action will adversely affect the practitioner's exercise of clinical privileges in the hospital (see Procedural Rights of Review Section).

Summary or emergency corrective action is action taken before giving the practitioner any procedural rights of review, therefore, it is usually reserved for situations that potentially pose an immediate threat to the safety of patients or staff or require immediate intervention. This form of corrective action is used in extreme situations in which it would be inappropriate to allow the practitioner to continue to practice until a full investigation has been completed and hearing held. Rather, the action is taken and the practitioner is given the right to a hearing after the fact (generally on an expedited basis). Depending on the provisions in the medical staff bylaws, summary or emergency action may involve a suspension of all of a practitioner's privileges or imposition of more limited action such as a mandatory co-admission requirement or consultation requirement. Only the action necessary to address the immediate problem should be taken.

The third type is referred to as automatic corrective action and is usually imposed in cases where there is no dispute as to the facts. For example, automatic corrective action in the form of termination of medical staff appointment would be taken if the practitioner loses his or her professional license. Since without a license one cannot practice, there would be no issues to be addressed in a hearing—either the practitioner has a license or does not. Some medical staff bylaws also provide for automatic corrective action in the case of loss of required professional liability insurance, loss of prescribing authority, and repeated or continued delinquency in completion of medical records. The key with automatic corrective action is that there is no dispute regarding whether the event or action that is the basis for automatic corrective action has occurred. Otherwise, the practitioner may be entitled to a hearing to determine whether there is a reasonable basis for the corrective action.

Corrective Action Procedures

Corrective action procedures (and related procedural rights of review) should be clearly specified in the medical staff bylaws or related manual. Generally, routine corrective action proceedings begin with the filing of a written request for corrective action. The bylaws should specify what individuals or committees may file a request and the request is usually directed to the medical executive committee. Upon receipt of a written request, the medical executive committee initiates an investigation of the events or concerns that prompted the request. Most medical staff bylaws require that the practitioner be notified of the request for corrective action and of initiation of the investigation. The investigation may be conducted by a standing medical staff committee or an ad hoc investigating committee, and will likely involve at least an interview with the affected practitioner. The results of the investigation are generally then reviewed by the medical executive committee, which issues a recommendation as to whether corrective action is indicated and, if so, what form of corrective action should be taken. The practitioner is notified of the recommended action in writing and, if the action is "adverse," given procedural rights of review or an opportunity to address the concerns through a hearing before the matter is referred to the governing board for a final decision.

When summary or emergency action is imposed, the practitioner is immediately notified and the appropriateness of the action may be reviewed by the medical executive committee or the practitioner's department as soon as possible. If the reviewing committee determines that the summary or emergency action was indicated and is adverse to the practitioner, then the practitioner is afforded a hearing while the action remains in effect. Automatic corrective action, by definition, requires no decision by the medical staff and is imposed automatically, with no right to a hearing.

The purpose of corrective action should be the furtherance of the delivery of quality patient care within the hospital and proper operation and functioning of the hospital. Corrective action should be taken after a reasonable effort to obtain information about the conduct or activities that are in question and upon the reasonable belief that corrective action is warranted by the facts. The type of corrective action taken will depend upon the severity of the problem and should be tailored to the specific circumstances. Intervention may range from an informal discussion between the department chair and the affected practitioner to formal corrective action, such as revocation of privileges, which may be appropriate in response to a more serious breach or problem.

Informal Intervention

A practitioner for whom minor deficiencies have been identified might be approached by the department chair for informal counseling and resolution, rather than resorting to corrective action. The chair should point out the deficiency(ies) and discuss alternative methods of patient care or professional conduct, depending upon the nature of the problem, and encourage the affected practitioner to take the necessary steps to improve his practice. Informal intervention is often used initially when problems are caused by a practitioner's unprofessional conduct or disruptive behavior. While this intervention may be informal in nature, a dated written record should be made by the department chair, including a general description of the problem and the essence of the intervention or counseling, and placed in the affected practitioner's confidential peer review file. It is always important to document these kinds of informal discussions, because the problem may continue or recur in a more serious manner necessitating formal corrective action. Documentation that prior attempts have been made to address the problem informally may be important to support formal corrective action. One drawback of informal intervention is that the intervention by a department chair may not be eligible for or covered by statutory immunities or protections that exist for actions by peer review committees. To the extent possible under state peer review law, informal intervention should be structured to fall within available protections, such as by having the individual act on behalf of or as agent for a peer review committee.

Additional Education or Training

In some cases, a problem with variations in patient care may best be solved by corrective action that requires the affected practitioner to obtain further education or training. For example, a practitioner might be misusing a category of drugs due to lack of knowledge about the indications and effects of the drug. The practitioner might be required to attend a continuing medical education program on the use of that category of drugs to correct the knowledge deficit. Likewise, a practitioner whose technical skill in performing a procedure is deficient might be required to attend a "hands-on" formal course to sharpen his or her skills.

Supervision and Retrospective Chart Review

A practitioner who performs a procedure with less skill than is consistent with professional standards may benefit from performing the procedure under supervision by a qualified practitioner. Supervision or observation may also be used to obtain additional information about a practitioner, such as to confirm whether the practitioner possesses the necessary technical skill to perform a requested procedure in cases where concerns have been raised. Mandatory second consultations for a limited period of time, for example, may be appropriate where a practitioner's documentation of clinical indications for admission or a surgical procedure have been questioned. A peer could also be asked to review a practitioner's medical records to determine that appropriate standards of patient care are being maintained. A record should be created of each procedure or patient whose care was observed, supervised or reviewed, with the record maintained in the affected practitioner's peer review file.

Letter of Warning

In some cases, the action needed is to formally warn the practitioner of the identified problem and advise that the problematic actions or conduct must cease. Particularly when dealing with conduct issues, it is important that the letter of warning set out exactly what is expected of the practitioner or what conduct is unacceptable and will not be tolerated.

Limitation of Privileges

A practitioner who has serious problems or complications for whom a lesser form of corrective action has been undertaken and failed (e.g., observation) or is inappropriate may require an actual limitation of clinical privileges. This may occur when it has been determined that a practitioner is performing a procedure or treating cases that go beyond his or her skill or knowledge base or has an unacceptable rate of complications from a particular procedure. For example, a cardiologist who performed permanent pacemaker implantation had several complications followed by a death while a patient was undergoing the procedure. Having noted the complications earlier, the department chair had required the affected practitioner to perform at least five procedures under supervision. The fifth patient expired while undergoing the procedure due to actions by the practitioner. The department chair then initiated corrective action, recommending that the practitioner's privilege to perform pacemaker implantation be suspended.

Revocation of Privileges and/or Appointment

A practitioner who has a documented pattern of serious problems, complications, deaths, or infractions of hospital policies or rules may be subject to a revocation of privileges, or a recommendation that all of the practitioner's privileges be removed which in effect removes the practitioner from the medical staff. This form of corrective action usually follows other unsuccessful attempts to address the practitioner's problem, but may also be the first form of corrective action if the problem is particularly serious or significant.

PROCEDURAL RIGHTS OF REVIEW

Entitlement

The medical staff and governing board recommendations or actions that will entitle a practitioner to procedural rights of review, or a hearing and appellate review, should be clearly delineated in the medical staff bylaws following review of the federal and state law requirements. Since medical staff appointment and the right to exercise clinical privileges are often essential for the practitioner to be able to engage in his profession, the law generally affords the practitioner certain procedural rights of review before the "taking" of his medical staff appointment or clinical privileges. Procedural rights of review may arise in connection with initial appointment, reappointment or corrective action. They may also arise in connection with the provisional period or a practitioner's request to increase clinical privileges during the term of appointment. Actions for which a hearing should be afforded are generally those which are "adverse" or "adversely affecting" a practitioner's clinical privileges or medical staff membership based on the practitioner's competence or conduct. HCQIA defines "adversely affecting" to include "reducing, restricting, suspending, revoking, denying, or failing to renew clinical privileges or membership."[30] The JCAHO Medical Staff Standards require a fair hearing and appeal process for "adverse decisions" regarding appointment or reappointment and the granting of initial or renewed/revised clinical privileges.[31]

If the proposed action will limit or restrict the practitioner's exercise of clinical privileges, the practitioner will usually be afforded the right to a hearing prior to imposing the adverse action (except in the case of summary or emergency action).[32] If, on the other hand, the proposed action does not interfere with the practitioner's right to practice, a right to a hearing may not be required. For example, the imposition of retrospective chart review should not limit the practitioner's right to practice or exercise clinical privileges. Requiring a practitioner to obtain the approval of another practitioner before performing surgery, however, may limit the practitioner's ability to exercise his or her surgical privileges and require affording procedural rights of review depending on the provisions in the bylaws. The bottom line is that the decision of whether to afford a hearing should *not* be addressed on a case-by-case basis, but should be specified in advance in the medical staff bylaws.

The procedural requirements for the hearing will be based on both state and federal law and should be clearly delineated in the medical staff bylaws. Many bylaws afford more procedures than are required by law. The purpose of a hearing is to provide the practitioner a fair opportunity to be heard and whatever reasonable procedures that will facilitate this process should be included in the medical staff bylaws. The reason for affording the right to a hearing or procedural rights of review is to allow the practitioner an opportunity to address the specific concerns that have been raised about his or her delivery of patient care services and or conduct, and to demonstrate that the proposed adverse action is not warranted.

Health Care Quality Improvement Act

The federal Health Care Quality Improvement Act, enacted in 1986, was intended to promote effective professional peer review for physicians. HCQIA was enacted in the aftermath of *Patrick v. Burget*, an antitrust lawsuit brought by an excluded physician in Oregon, to encourage effective and professional peer review by limiting liability for monetary damages of health care entities and participants in good faith peer review.[33] HCQIA establishes certain standards for "professional review actions" and provides that entities and individuals who comply with those standards will be entitled to certain limited immunities if sued by the affected physician.[34] (Note that HCQIA defines a "physician" as a M.D. or D.O. physician or dentist; podiatrists and other types of independent practitioners are not mentioned.[35]) HCQIA defines a "professional review action" as an action or recommendation by a professional review body in the conduct of professional review activity based on the "competence or professional conduct of an individual physician (which conduct affects or could affect adversely the health or welfare of a patient or patients) and which affects or may affect adversely the clinical privileges or membership in a professional society of the physician."[36] A "professional review action" is an "action or recommendation of a professional review body...in the conuct of professional review activity, which is based on the competence or professional conduct of an individual physician (which conduct affects or could affect adversely the health or welfare of a patient or patients), and which affects (or may affect) adversely the clinical privileges, or membership in a professional society, of the physician."[37]

The standards established for a professional review action that would qualify for limited immunity are that the action be taken

1. in the reasonable belief that the action was in the furtherance of quality health care;

2. after a reasonable effort to obtain the facts of the matter;

3. after adequate notice and hearing procedures are afforded to the physician involved or after such other procedures as are fair to the physician under the circumstances; and

4. in the reasonable belief that the action was warranted by the facts known after reasonable effort to obtain facts and after meeting the notice and hearing requirements.[38]

Compliance with the standards is not required by HCQIA; compliance is necessary, however, to invoke the immunity afforded by the statute.

With regard to the third standard providing for "adequate notice and hearing," HCQIA sets out procedures that will be deemed to meet this standard.[39] The specific procedures are set out in Appendix B and include providing notice to the practitioner of the proposed action and a list of witnesses expected to testify against the practitioner, affording the practitioner the right to representation by an attorney or other person of the practitioner's choice, and providing the practitioner with the written recommendation of the hearing panel. Immunity may be available even if a hospital or medical staff does not afford all of the specific "adequate notice and hearing" procedures set out in HCQIA, since HCQIA also allows the use of "such other procedures as are fair to the physician under the circumstances."[40] Many hospitals and medical staffs, however, have not wanted to gamble with other procedures that might be considered "fair" and have incorporated all of the HCQIA procedures in their medical staff bylaws or fair hearing plan unless they find them to be particularly burdensome. Some believe that it will be easier, in the event of litigation, for the hospital and medical staff members to assert the immunity if the HCQIA procedures have been precisely followed. Others believe that immunity will be available even if the actual procedures in the HCQIA are not complied with, if the peer review is conducted in good faith and basic hearing procedures are afforded in accordance with the medical staff bylaws. Those hospitals that have followed the HCQIA procedures should have an easier time documenting that the practitioner has been afforded procedural due process in the event of litigation. The objective, however, is to further quality patient care through the use of effective peer review, not just to avoid litigation by affected practitioners.

A hospital and medical staff may use a single "fair hearing plan" to set out the procedures to be used both for denial of appointment or reappointment and for corrective action. A hospital may vary the procedures somewhat if it is determined that different obligations should be owed an existing member of the medical staff as compared to an initial applicant. For example, the burden of proof may differ, placing a greater burden on the applicant as compared to the member. This will ultimately be a matter for the hospital and medical staff to address in consultation with legal counsel. The objective, whether there is one fair hearing plan or two, is that the plan be comprehensive, clear and fair.

LEGAL ISSUES IN CORRECTIVE ACTION AND HEARINGS

Legal challenges to medical staff privileging decisions generally fall into two categories: substantive and procedural. A substantive challenge involves the reason for the adverse action. Was there a reasonable basis for limiting or terminating the practitioner's clinical privileges or medical staff appointment? This is an area in which each case will be evaluated on its own merits and the courts generally defer to the medical staff and hospital governing board in this regard.

A procedural challenge involves the procedures followed in imposing the adverse action or affording the procedural rights of review. Were the procedures fair and did they comply with the requirements in the medical staff bylaws? As previously mentioned, the HCQIA procedures for adequate notice and hearing are an example of what would be regarded as fair. The key is to: (1) know the procedures and requirements in the medical staff bylaws (or related manuals) on adverse actions and hearings/appellate review; (2) ensure they comply with legal requirements; and (3) follow them to the fullest extent possible. Failure to follow the procedures in one's own bylaws is a common reason for litigation and yet one that can easily be avoided.

The following will highlight some of the legal considerations that may arise in connection with adverse action and affording procedural rights of review.

Documentation of the Problem

One of the most difficult aspects of adverse action, whether on appointment or reappointment, or in corrective action, is actually documenting the problem. There may be a concern regarding a practitioner, but either individuals are not willing to put the concern in writing or the time is not taken to actually examine the relevant information so as to be able to appropriately document the problem. There must be a basis for adverse action and the basis should be documented. Concerns, problems or complaints should be put in writing and there should be an objective evaluation of that information and the practitioner's practice. For example, if there is a concern that a practitioner's complication rates are particularly high with a certain surgical procedure, a retrospective review of the practitioner's cases could be performed to ascertain the actual frequency of complications and whether there are unique factors about the patient population that may explain the complication rate.

Equal Application of Requirements

Another problem area is that requirements or standards imposed on a practitioner may not be applied equally to other practitioners. Taking the surgical complication rate example above, it is entirely appropriate to intervene if a practitioner's complication rate exceeds accepted professional standards. The problem often arises, however, that there are several practitioners with similar or worse complication rates, yet action is only being taken against one practitioner. Another problem is having requirements or standards that are rarely enforced. An example is a bylaws' provision allowing termination of a practitioner's active staff membership for failure to attend medical staff meetings. If the provision is never enforced until suddenly there is a practitioner who is not liked or whose practice is "borderline," the adverse action may be subject to a challenge of arbitrariness or application in a discriminatory manner. Requirements or standards should be applied consistently.

Practitioner Involvement in Corrective Action

The medical staff bylaws should include specific procedures to be followed once a request for corrective action is filed. Frequently, the bylaws will require that the affected practitioner be advised of the filing of the complaint and may allow the practitioner to participate in the investigative process or meet with the investigating committee. These requirements are often overlooked in the corrective action process. The bylaws should be consulted immediately when there are indications of adverse action. An error in the early stages can create problems with later aspects of the action and even the hearing process. If an error is made, an attempt should be made to correct it even if a procedure or step in the process must be repeated.

Investigation

Two issues deserve mention as to investigations. First, certain professional review action reporting requirements are triggered depending on whether the affected practitioner is then under "investigation."[41] Therefore, the medical staff bylaws should clearly define when an investigation commences. The Data Bank *Guidebook* contains helpful information on what constitutes an investigation which should be reviewed in addressing this issue.[42] An investigation for purposes of imposing a professional review action (e.g., corrective action) should be distinguished from reviews that occur on a regular basis for purposes of quality improvement. Second, more often than hospitals and medical staffs like to admit, a complete investigation takes place after a hearing has been scheduled and the practitioner has retained an attorney. The proper time for the investigation is before any recommendation for adverse action is made. Once a recommendation for adverse action has been made, there should be no need for further investigation, but merely preparation for the hearing itself. The practitioner should be advised of the reasons for the adverse action at the time he is notified that adverse action is being recommended. If all information is not available when that notice letter is written or additional information identified later, the notice will need to be supplemented prior to the hearing. There may also need to be a postponement of the hearing to allow the practitioner adequate time to address the new information in advance of the hearing.

Right to a Hearing

There may be a question as to whether an action entitles the practitioner to request a hearing. This is a matter on which state law must be consulted and entitlement should be specifically addressed in the bylaws. Generally, hospitals and medical staffs opt to afford hearing rights for those actions that will be reportable to the Data Bank if subject to a final decision by the governing board. Examples of particular actions that may be overlooked in the bylaws are whether probation, consultation requirements or supervision requirements entitle the practitioner to request a hearing. Another matter that needs to be dealt with is whether termination of a practitioner's clinical privileges because of termination of a professional services contract with the hospital entitles the practitioner to a hearing. Some find it beneficial, in drafting the fair hearing plan to list those actions that are "adverse" (and entitle the practitioner to procedural rights of review) as well as those that are "not adverse."

Notice of Charges

Under HCQIA's recommended procedures, the first notice to the practitioner, advising that a professional review action has been proposed, must include the reasons for the proposed action.[43] This notice requirement is one of the most essential elements of procedural due process. The practitioner must be given adequate notice of the charges and reasons for the proposed action, so as to be able to adequately defend himself. Failure to properly advise the practitioner of the allegations or basis for the proposed adverse action may jeopardize the entire proceeding.

Notice should include a list of the hospital or patient records that support each of the allegations and will be presented in the hearing.[44] The practitioner should be given access to these records and documents upon request. Withholding information from the practitioner that is needed to prepare for the hearing raises the possibility of a procedural challenge. The practitioner, however, should not be entitled to access documents that are not related to the proposed action or allegations or to defending or refuting the allegations. Because of their importance, questions pertaining to access to documents in the pre-hearing period and during the hearing should be discussed with legal counsel and addressed in the bylaws or fair hearing plan.

Discovery and Deposition Rights

Although few cases have addressed this issue,[45] generally practitioners are not given the right to pre- trial discovery, such as depositions or interrogatories, unless otherwise provided by state law or in the medical staff bylaws. Despite appearances to the contrary, the hearing is not intended to be a mini-trial. What rights are afforded in this regard should be specifically set out in the bylaws or the fair hearing plan. This is an area where the use of a hearing officer to advise the hearing panel and handle procedural matters and objections will be helpful. Frequently the hearing officer will conduct pre-hearing conferences to address these issues prior to the hearing.

Waiver of Procedural Rights

Occasionally there are procedures, either in the medical staff bylaws or required by law, that both the practitioner and the hospital or medical staff want to modify. For example, a practitioner may be willing to waive the 30-day time period recommended by HCQIA between the notice of the date of the hearing and the hearing itself in order to start the hearing as soon as possible. If a waiver is being obtained and the practitioner is represented by counsel, both the practitioner and counsel should sign the waiver.

Hearing Panel Bias

Even before HCQIA was enacted, which limits the use of direct economic competitors of the affected practitioner on the hearing panel,[46] efforts were made to ensure that the hearing panel members could be fair and were unbiased as a key component of procedural due process. The hospital should be able to document that the individuals who will judge the practitioner in the hearing meet any requirements or qualifications set in the bylaws. Individuals who have participated in the investigation leading to or the issuance of the adverse action, or who may be witnesses, should be excluded from the panel. As mentioned, under HCQIA, direct economic competitors should also be excluded. Hospitals may find it helpful to send a preliminary questionnaire to the prospective hearing panel members requesting information necessary to determine whether the individual is qualified to serve, so that there will be adequate time to secure replacements if any problems are detected. Alternate hearing panel members may be designated in the event a member is later disqualified or cannot attend the hearing at the last minute. In addition to this process, the practitioner should be allowed to actually question the members of the hearing panel. The hearing transcript should include any questioning of the hearing panel members and other evidence as to whether they have any bias or are in direct economic competition with the affected practitioner.

Role of Attorneys

HCQIA's recommended procedures afford the practitioner the right to "representation by an attorney or other person of the physician's choice."[47] This language raises a question as to whether the use of the "or" means that the hospital and medical staff can choose between affording the right to an attorney or the right to another person of the physician's choice, or must afford both options. The other concern is whether there is any reasonable alternative to representation by an attorney that would still entitle the hospital and medical staff to the qualified immunity available under HCQIA. As mentioned earlier, HCQIA provides that, to be eligible for the qualified immunity, either the procedures detailed in the statute must be used or "such other procedures as are fair to the physician under the circumstances." But can there be any substitute for representation by an attorney—is representation by someone who is not an attorney "fair"? Some hospitals and medical staffs wishing to limit the role of attorneys allow the attorney to be present during the hearing, but do not allow the attorney to question parties or witnesses or address the hearing panel. Limiting what the attorney may do, however, may jeopardize the availability of the qualified immunity although it has been upheld under HCQIA in at least one federal circuit.[48] Public hospitals particularly should examine applicable legal requirements, since the right to representation by an attorney without limitations may be an essential element of procedural due process. If the practitioner is permitted to be represented by an attorney, the committee that issued the adverse action or recommendation is afforded the same right.

Right of Cross-Examination

The right of the practitioner to cross-examine any witnesses or evidence presented against him or her is another essential element of the hearing. The use of written statements from witnesses in the hearing may be challenged by the practitioner unless the witnesses are also available to be questioned by the practitioner at the time of the hearing. For example, use of a consulting expert's report in the hearing may be unacceptable unless the expert is available to be cross-examined by the practitioner. This also means that the use of anonymous complaints or written statements may be limited in the hearing, since to do so may be interpreted as a denial of the right to cross-examination. In some cases, if the witness cannot be available for the hearing, it may be possible to submit written questions in advance to the witness and have them answered, with the answers presented at the time of the hearing.

New or Additional Information

The reason the initial notice of charges containing reasons for the proposed corrective action is so important is that it defines for the practitioner what issues or allegations he or she must address in the hearing. If, during a hearing, additional allegations or reasons for the proposed adverse action come to light, it may be appropriate to give the practitioner the opportunity to have the hearing recessed for a reasonable amount of time to allow the practitioner to prepare to address the additional matters. HCQIA procedures may even require issuance of a new and amended notice of charges and waiting at least 30 days before resuming the hearing.

Because of the right of cross-examination, all evidence to be considered by the hearing panel should be presented to the practitioner at the time of the hearing. The hearing panel should not conduct its own "private" investigation. If the hearing panel relies on information learned other than that presented at the hearing, the practitioner may be denied the right of cross-examination. If the hearing panel decides during the hearing that it needs additional information, a request to obtain that information should be made by the panel to the parties in open session and the hearing recessed until that information can be presented.

Hearing Report

The hearing panel should issue a written report setting out its findings and recommendation according to what is required by the bylaws. The report needs to be sufficiently detailed to indicate the basis for the recommendation and may reference pertinent provisions in the hearing transcript or documents presented during the hearing. Under the HCQIA recommended procedures, the affected practitioner must be given a copy of the report and most fair hearing plans require this.[49]

Standard of Review in Appeal

An appeal is not intended to be a "second hearing." It is a limited review and the bylaws should specify those limits or the standard of review to be used. Generally, the purpose of an appeal, which should be set out in the fair hearing plan, is to determine: (1) if the recommendation is arbitrary, capricious or unreasonable or not supported by evidence in the record, and (2) if the procedures set out in the bylaws or fair hearing plan have been substantially complied with. The appeal may be before the full governing board of the hospital or a committee appointed by the board to serve as an appellate review committee. The committee reviews the hearing record, the hearing panel's report and any information considered by the medical staff since the hearing. If the practitioner is permitted to submit a written statement or make an oral presentation at the time of the appeal, this information would also be considered by the appellate review committee, and the committee who originally issued the adverse recommendation or action would be afforded these same rights. New or additional evidence should only be received and considered by the appellate review committee if the evidence was not reasonably available at the time of the hearing. In some cases, new evidence may necessitate reopening the hearing and sending the issue back to the hearing committee for a revised recommendation.

Composition of Appellate Review Committee

While there are generally limitations on who may serve as members of the hearing panel, it is not so clear whether the same restrictions apply to the individuals who conduct the appellate review. HCQIA does not address appeals or appeal procedures. Even if not legally required, it is still recommended that individuals who have been involved in the investigation or the hearing not also serve on the appellate review committee. (If nothing else, this may lessen the risk of their becoming individual defendants if litigation results.) Although there is much discretion in the composition of an appellate review committee, generally the committee is composed of the governing board or a subcommittee of the governing board. If a hospital has a joint conference committee, composed of members of both the medical staff and the governing board, frequently this committee will serve as the appellate review committee. As with the hearing, the appellate review committee should issue a written report setting out the findings required by the bylaws or fair hearing plan.

Final Decision

Unless otherwise provided in the bylaws, the governing board must issue a final decision on the adverse recommendation. Under the HCQIA recommended procedures, the decision must be in writing and include the basis or reason for the decision and a copy must be provided to the affected practitioner.[50]

PEER REVIEW PRIVILEGES OF CONFIDENTIALITY AND IMMUNITY

Privilege of Confidentiality

Many states afford some statutory privilege of confidentiality to records and proceedings generated in the course of peer review in a hospital setting, as well as in other health care settings. State statutes may be limited to those records and proceedings generated by peer review committees or may extend to individuals who engage in peer review as well. Privileges of confidentiality often extend to individuals who provide information to peer review committees for purposes of peer review. The privilege of confidentiality prevents discovery or access to the records or proceedings of peer review in a lawsuit such as a professional liability action by a patient or a lawsuit by an excluded practitioner. The purpose of this special protection is to encourage appropriate and effective peer review, and candor in the process, without fear of creating information or documents that will be used against the hospital or the affected practitioner. In some cases, the privilege applies even if there is evidence of bad faith or malice.[51]

To be protected as peer review records and proceedings, generally it must be demonstrated that the information or documents was in fact generated in the course of peer review. Hospitals and medical staffs should examine the manner in which certain information and documents are created to determine whether they would be protected under the state's peer review privilege of confidentiality. Generally, routine administrative or business records will not fall within the category of peer review records and proceedings, even if forwarded to a peer review committee. On the other hand, if generation of a particular document or report is at the specific request of a peer review committee or is generated in the peer review committee's fulfillment of its responsibilities, the document or report may be privileged.

Privileges may be waived, either by intentional act or sometimes by an unintentional act, such as unauthorized disclosure to a third party. Any provisions in the medical staff bylaws or credentialing procedures addressing the confidentiality of peer review information should also set out the procedures required to actually waive the privilege. Because of the seriousness of a waiver of the privilege, it should occur only with the approval of appropriate medical staff officers and hospital administration. Peer review privileges protect both the hospital and medical staff participants in the peer review, but also the affected practitioner who is the subject of the peer review.

As a creature of state law, most state privileges of confidentiality will apply only to lawsuits involving causes of action under state law such as professional liability. If a lawsuit is filed in federal court and involves federal causes of action, there is no obligation of the federal courts to honor the state privileges of confidentiality.[52] For this reason, it should never be assumed that particular records or proceedings will always be protected from discovery, nor should promises be made to those who participate in peer review or provide peer review information that confidentiality is absolute.

Privilege of Immunity

The same state laws that afford a privilege of confidentiality to peer review records and proceedings may also extend a privilege of immunity, or freedom from liability if sued, to those who perform peer review or participate in the process. Generally, grants of immunity are limited to actions taken in good faith or without malice, therefore, these privileges may be more limited in application than privileges of confidentiality.

HCQIA also affords immunity in the peer review process at the federal level. Under HCQIA, the following entities and individuals are not liable for monetary damages with respect to a professional review action that meets the four standards specified in HCQIA (see discussion above): (1) the professional review body; (2) any person acting as a member or staff to the body; (3) any person under a contract or other formal agreement with the body; and (4) any person who participates with or assist the body with respect to the action.[53] The limitation on liability does not apply to damages involving civil rights violations, nor to an action by the United States or any state attorney general. A "professional review body" is defined as a health care entity or a governing body or any committee of a health care entity which conducts professional review activity and includes any committee of the medical staff of the health care entity when assisting the governing body in a professional review activity.[54]"Professional review activity" is an activity to determine whether a physician may have clinical privileges or membership in the entity, to determine the scope or conditions of the privileges or membership, or to change or modify them.[55]

HCQIA also extends a second protection from immunity to those individuals who provide information to a professional review body.[56] While under the first grant of immunity, the professional review action must meet all four standards in HCQIA, the immunity afforded to those providing information is not so limited. A person providing information to a professional review body regarding the competence or professional conduct of a physician may not be liable for monetary damages unless: (1) the information provided was false; and (2) the person providing it knew that the information was false.

HCQIA Reporting Requirements

The HCQIA immunity for a professional review body may be lost for a three-year period under certain circumstances if the health care entity has failed to report professional review actions as required by HCQIA.[57] Under HCQIA, there are three levels of reporting that are required, with only the third affecting the grant of immunity to a health care entity for professional review actions. The first required reporting deals with medical malpractice payments and requires each entity (including an insurance company) which makes payment under a policy of insurance, self-insurance or otherwise in settlement or satisfaction of a judgment in a medical malpractice action or claim to report information regarding the payment as set forth in HCQIA.[58] Failure to report under this provision exposes the entity to civil monetary penalties. The second reporting requirement applies to state boards of medical examiners and requires each board which revokes or suspends (or otherwise restricts) a physician's license or censures, reprimands or places on probation a physician for reasons relating to professional competence or conduct to report the information to the Data Bank.[59] The third requirement is imposed on health care entities and requires a report from each health care entity which: (1) takes a professional review action that adversely affects the clinical privileges of a physician for a period longer than 30 days; (2) accepts the surrender of clinical privileges of a physician while the physician is under investigation by the entity relating the possible incompetence or improper professional conduct (or in return for not conducting such an investigation or proceeding); or (3) in the case of a professional society, takes a professional review action which adversely affects the membership of the physician in the society.[60] These reports of professional review actions are provided to the state board of medical examiners, which in turn forwards the information to the Data Bank. Permissive reporting of a professional review action is permitted for other licensed health care practitioners.[61] The information that must be reported on the professional review action includes the name of the physician, a description of the acts or omissions or reasons for the action or, if known, for the surrender. For significant detail and information on reporting, refer to the Data Bank *Guidebook.*

Recommendations

The following are some general recommendations to maximize the availability of applicable privileges of confidentiality and immunity in the peer review setting.

1. Mark all documents generated or received by a peer review committee as "Privileged and Confidential—for Purposes of Peer Review" or "Privileged and Confidential—Records and Proceedings of Peer Review Committee," depending upon the precise language of the applicable state statute.

2. Ensure that the medical staff bylaws authorize medical staff committees to conduct peer review and function as peer review committees, using the precise language set forth in applicable state statutes of confidentiality and immunity in peer review. If hospital or board committees conduct peer review, examine the governing board bylaws as well to ensure proper authorization.

3. Ensure that the actions of individuals in the course of peer review are taken as agents for or on behalf of peer review committees, if applicable. For example, the authority given to a chief of staff or CEO to impose summary or emergency corrective action should be taken as agent for or on behalf of the medical executive committee or the governing board. This should facilitate application of any privileges of immunity afforded to the peer review committee.

4. Limit distribution of peer review records and proceedings to those who have a need to know. When appropriate, retrieve original documents at the close of meetings. Limit copying of peer review records and proceedings to designated persons.

5. Establish policies and procedures regarding access to peer review records and proceedings, including access by the affected practitioner and other members of the medical staff. Generally, committee records and proceedings should only be available to members of the committee for purposes of carrying out committee responsibilities, medical staff committees to which that committee reports, and the governing board.

6. Identify those provisions in state statutes on confidentiality that permit disclosures to third parties. For example, the state statute on confidentiality of peer review records and proceedings may permit disclosure to licensing and accreditation agencies of the health care entity, without such disclosure resulting in a waiver of the privilege. The state statute may permit disclosure to any governmental agency which is permitted by law to access records, such as the state board of medical examiners or the licensing agency for the hospital or health care entity. These provisions should be reflected in applicable policies and procedures regarding disclosure of peer review records and proceedings.

7. In responding to requests for information from other hospitals engaged in credentialing or peer review, written authorization from the affected practitioner should be obtained (although state law may not require it). Verify

that the authorization contains appropriate language both authorizing the disclosure of information by the hospital and releasing the hospital from liability for any disclosure pursuant to the authorization.

8. Verify that a requested disclosure is permitted by applicable state law and will not result in a waiver of the privilege. If the disclosure is permitted by state law, structure the disclosure to fit within any provisions in the statute. For example, if the statute authorizes disclosure from one peer review committee to another peer review committee, require that queries from other hospitals generate from their peer review committees and that the responses be provided by your own hospital's peer review committee. Mark the response "Privileged and Confidential—Records and Proceedings of Peer Review Committee."

9. In providing information in response to a query, rely on information that is available in the credentials file, avoiding opinions and recommendations since those are more properly covered through peer references. Provide factual information that answers the questions. Avoid volunteering information except under special circumstances. Avoid general requests for information, such as "tell us anything you think might be important," and require specific questions.

10. Most applications for medical staff appointment or reappointment contain language requiring the applicant to release the hospital, the medical staff, and any individuals or committees participating in peer review from liability related to peer review actions or recommendations. Care should be taken in drafting these releases of liability to ensure that they are not more limited than the immunity afforded by state or federal law. Additionally, the medical staff bylaws should provide that operation of the release of liability is not contingent on the practitioner's signature on the document, but operates by virtue of submission of the application itself.

CREDENTIALING IN THE MANAGED CARE SETTING

Comparison to Hospital—Medical Staff Credentialing

Credentialing and peer review is no longer exclusive to the hospital-medical staff setting with the emergence of managed care organizations, provider networks and integrated health care delivery systems. As new methods develop for the delivery of health care services, these entities need to credential and frequently delegate credentialing to hospitals or other health care entities that already have significant expertise and credentialing processes already in place. While there are many parallels between credentialing in the hospital-medical staff setting and credentialing in the managed care setting, there are also several interesting differences. Credentialing in the managed care setting usually addresses the practitioner's office practice standards rather than just hospital practice. The geographic location and numbers of practitioners for a managed care organization or provider network may have different significance than the composition of a hospital's medical staff. Managed care organizations may require a different ratio of primary care practitioners to specialists than for hospitals. Economic and efficiency based criteria may be utilized by the managed care organization to a greater extent than hospitals. Finally, there may be different relationships (and consequently legal requirements) between the medical staff member and the hospital, as compared to the participating provider and a managed care organization.

Particularly in the managed care setting, factors related to economics or business may be pertinent in deciding whether to terminate a provider's participation. Examples are the provider's agreement to provide 24-hour availability and coverage to enrollees, conduct of office staff or office conditions, and compliance with utilization review appeal procedures. Often these are factors that do not relate to the clinical competence of the provider. For these reasons, there may be different processes used to deal with disciplinary action or termination of participating provider status for quality of care issues as compared to economic or business reasons.

Credentialing in both the hospital and managed care organization settings has tended to focus on independent practitioners, such as physicians, dentists, podiatrists and chiropractors. State legal requirements for managed care organizations may, however, require access and credentialing of other types of providers which will need to be incorporated by managed care organizations. State law has increased their scope of practice over the last few years in many states, and managed care organizations' financial arrangements with physicians and other practitioners may create incentives for the use of physician extenders or allied health professionals. Increasing interest in the incorporation of allied health professionals into managed care organizations will necessitate credentialing of those professionals as well.

Duty to Credential

As with hospitals, the managed care organization's duty to credential is controlled by both accreditation and licensure standards as well as case law. There are several agencies that offer accreditation or certification for managed care organizations, with the two more dominant currently being the JCAHO, through its *Accreditation Manual for Health Care Networks*, and the National Committee for Quality Assurance (NCQA) through its *Standards for Managed Care Organizations*.[62] JCAHO also accredits preferred provider organizations or PPOs, which have as their primary customer, an insurance carrier, employer, or other health care purchase that uses the PPO's panel as the source of providers for the delivery of health care services to insured individuals.[63] All these standards require that individuals permitted by law and by the entity to provide care be appointed and reappointed to provider panels through defined processes which involve an application, review of relevant documentation, verification of credentials, and office visits, if appropriate.

Just as the courts have extended various forms of liability to hospitals related to the actions of practitioners and negligent credentialing, we see the courts now applying these theories to managed care organizations. In *Harrell v. Total Health Care, Inc.*,[64] a 1989 Missouri case, a patient was injured by a health service organization urologist to whom she was referred by the organization's primary care practitioner. The appellate court found that health service organizations, like hospitals, have a common law duty to their members to conduct a reasonable investigation to ensure that practitioners are competent and capable of providing care that meets community standards. Here the health service organization had credentialed the urologist, a process which consisted of verifying licensure, admitting privileges to hospitals and authority to prescribe controlled substances. No other credentialing procedures were required or performed. In a 1992 Pennsylvania case, *McClellan v. HMO of Pennsylvania*,[65] the court ruled that the enrollee could maintain an action for negligent selection of a practitioner against the health maintenance organization (HMO). In this case, Ms. McClellan had sought treatment for a mole on her back. The HMO primary care practitioner failed to order a biopsy or histological examination of the mole tissue.

Legal Issues

Although there may be different implications in the managed care setting, many of the legal issues related to credentialing are the same. Managed care organizations must also address the issue of access to a provider network or the managed care organization. Many states have enacted legislation referred to as "any willing provider" laws which require HMOs and other types of managed care organizations to afford access to all practitioners who meet the requirements established by the managed care organization or to afford access to certain disciplines or professions. Managed care organizations must also decide what procedural rights of review must be provided if a practitioner is excluded from participation in the provider network or, if after participation is granted, a decision is made to terminate the practitioner's participation. This issue is increasingly being addressed by state laws, some of which require a minimum of written notice to the practitioner of the basis for denial or termination and in some cases an opportunity for review by a panel of peers. To some extent, the decision as to whether to afford procedural rights of review may depend on whether the managed care organization is subject to the HCQIA reporting obligations. HMOs are included in the HCQIA definition of a "health care entity" and must report professional review actions to the Data Bank, therefore, these types of managed care organizations may decide that the immunity benefits of affording adequate notice and hearing as set forth under HCQIA outweigh the burden of affording this process.[66] Managed care organizations, on the other hand, are more likely to make decisions regarding practitioner participation based on factors other than quality of care, such as costs or compliance with utilization review procedures. The only actions that must be reported under HCQIA are those relating to the practitioner's competence or professional conduct.

A final issue deals with whether managed care organizations are entitled to invoke state privileges of confidentiality or immunity for peer review. In some states, these laws may be drafted broadly enough to apply to HMOs and other types of managed care organizations, in which case credentialing and peer review by these organizations should be structured to comply with applicable privileges. In other states where the laws have been focused only on hospitals, this may be an area for future legislation as managed care organizations increasingly engage in credentialing and the litigation potential increases.

Delegated Credentialing

Frequently, the managed care organization will delegate credentialing or a portion of credentialing responsibility to a hospital or health care entity which also has established credentialing policies and procedures in place. Delegated credentialing is addressed by the JCAHO standards for health care networks as well as the NCQA standards for managed care organizations.[67] Both require that the network or managed care organization maintain authority over final decisions, such as approval of new practitioners and termination of practitioners, and that there be evidence of oversight by the network or managed care organization and evaluation of the delegate's activities. The NCQA standards actually require that the managed care organization perform a due diligence review of the delegate's credentialing activities and verify that policies and procedures of the delegate meet NCQA accreditation standards. Managed care organizations are also required to review either 5 percent or 50 of the delegate's credentialing files, whichever is less. There must be a written document describing the responsibilities of both the managed care organization and the delegate, the delegated activities, the process used to evaluate the delegate's performance, and the remedies if the delegate does not fulfill its obligations.

JCAHO does not contain specific provisions on delegated credentialing, but deals generally with delegation of any functions addressed by standards in the accreditation manual. In such cases, the network must use clear criteria and performance expectations to select contractor/delegates, must retain the right to make key decisions and actively oversee contracted or delegated activities, and periodically cooperate with the contractor/delegate to coordinate activities.

Delegation may involve delegation of the information gathering and primary source verification function and the actual evaluation of the qualifications of the practitioner, or it may involve delegation of only one portion of the function. In some cases, delegation is to a credentials verification organization (CVO), which is defined by NCQA as an organization that verifies credentials of practitioners for managed care organizations and/or health delivery organizations or practitioners.[68] CVOs generally gather information and conduct primary source verification, but do not evaluate the qualifications to the practitioner or make recommendations on whether the practitioner should be granted access to the provider network. NCQA certifies CVOs and, if delegation is to a certified CVO, the audit requirement involving review of files may be waived.[69]

There are several key legal issues in any arrangement for delegated credentialing. The first is that the arrangement should be structured to maintain the confidentiality of any peer review information generated by the delegate. If the managed care organization or network is itself eligible for privileges of confidentiality and immunity for peer review actions, state law may permit the delegate to be eligible for those same privileges when providing services on behalf of the managed care organization or network. There should be a written agreement between the two entities, clearly setting out the delegate's status as to the delegating entity. The written agreement should also set out the precise scope of duties, access to original information by the delegating entity, how information will be maintained confidentially by the delegate, and ownership and access to the delegate's information particularly on termination of the delegation arrangement. The agreement and any disclosure of information should include statements that the information generated pursuant to the delegation is privileged under applicable state law and that disclosure is not intended to waive any applicable privileges of confidentiality.

A second legal issue involves final decision-making authority. In delegated credentialing arrangements involving more than just information gathering and primary source verification, the managed care organization or network needs to ensure that it has not given so much authority to the delegate as to compromise its own responsibilities for purposes of accreditation or licensure. Generally, any form of delegated credentialing will provide for the managed care organization or network to retain final authority over decisions regarding practitioner participation.

Uniform or Centralized Credentialing

A variation from delegated credentialing is the move towards uniform or centralized credentialing. In this situation, the focus is for several organizations (which generally are related or components of an integrated health care delivery system) to conduct credentialing together, as compared to having one organization conduct credentialing on behalf of another as occurs in delegated credentialing. Uniform or centralized credentialing may be limited to use of a joint application for practitioner participation in hospitals and managed care organizations, may extend to shared or joint credentialing committees which evaluate and issue recommendations on practitioner participation, or may involve joint decision making as to a practitioner's participation in all of the components in the health care delivery system. The main benefits of uniformed or centralized credentialing are the reduced duplication and time and expense for the various components of the integrated health care delivery system as well as the practitioners. Importantly, the use of a uniform or centralized system also promotes consistent standards among related organizations, in that criteria for participation will likely be consistent among the components. As with delegated credentialing, the primary legal issues involve application of state peer review laws on confidentiality and immunity as well as assuring that each component maintains sufficient final decision-making authority so as not to jeopardize each component's individual accreditation or licensure status.

Queries for Managed Care Organizations

As credentialing moves into the managed care setting, obviously managed care organizations and networks are seeking information from hospitals and other health care entities about practitioners wanting to participate with the organizations and networks. While state peer review laws on confidentiality may permit the exchange of confidential peer review information between hospitals, these laws need to be carefully examined to determine whether peer review information may be disclosed to managed care organizations or networks without risking loss of that same privilege. In some states, managed care organizations such as HMOs are included in the statutes on privileges of confidentiality for peer review. In other states, however, this may not be the case, making it difficult to disclose privileged and confidential peer review information.

Appendix A: Significant Case Law Summary

Darling v. Charleston Community Hospital, 211 N.E.2d 253 (Ill. 1965)—Hospital's Duty To Supervise Physician

Lawsuit by patient against hospital for acts of nurses and negligence as to attending physician where patient's orthopedic injury resulted in amputation. Patient alleged that hospital was negligent in permitting physician to treat orthopedic injuries and not requiring him to update operative procedures, in failing through the medical staff to exercise adequate supervision, and in not requiring consultation especially after complications set in. Hospital defended as to physician that only physician may practice medicine, therefore hospital cannot be liable for the acts of a physician where reasonable care exercised in selecting the physician originally. The Illinois Supreme Court upheld verdict for patient, noting that hospitals do more than just provide facilities for treatment but assume certain responsibilities for the care of the patient.

Purcell v. Zimbelman, 500 P.2d 335 (Ariz. Ct. App. 1972)—Improper Review of Clinical Competence

Lawsuit by patient against hospital for failing to take action against attending surgeon when it knew or should have known that he lacked the skill to treat the condition in question. Hospital defended that could not be liable for acts of independent contractor physician where there was no reason to believe a specific act of malpractice would occur. Jury found in favor of the patient. Evidence showed that two prior cases involving similar questions as to treatment of diverticulitis had been presented to the department of surgery but no action was taken. A total of four malpractice cases had been filed against the physician and hospital prior to his treatment of Mr. Zimbelman. After describing accreditation standards and custom at hospitals as to the medical staff, the Arizona appellate court found that the hospital had assumed the duty of supervising the competence of its staff physicians. It also found that the hospital was responsible for the actions of the department of surgery since it acted on its behalf and, if the department was negligent in not intervening after the first two cases, then the hospital would also be negligent. Evidence of the filing of the four lawsuits was admissible against the hospital to show it had notice of concerns as to Dr. Purcell's competency as to the particular condition but also as to his general competency, and should have reviewed his records.

Gonzalez v. Nork, 131 Cal. Rptr. 717 (Cal. App. 1976)—Failure of Peer Review Process

Lawsuit by patient against physician and hospital for damages resulting from operation where physician did not inform patient of more conservative treatment available. Physician had history of unnecessary or negligent surgery in years prior to laminectomy on patient. Jury found for patient. Supported hospital's duty to create a mechanism by which it may discover inadequacies of its staff members.

Johnson v. Misericordia, 294 N.W.2d 501 (Ct. App. 1980), affirmed 301 N.W.2d 156 (Wisc. 1981)—Failure of Initial Credentialing Process

Lawsuit by patient against hospital for negligently granting orthopedic surgical privileges to Dr. Salinsky (physician settled prior to trial). Patient had suffered damage following physician's removal of pin fragment from hip. Despite provisions in the medical staff bylaws, no investigation was made of any of the information provided on the application form (which was incomplete). Contrary to the physician's representations on the application, he had experienced denial and restriction of privileges elsewhere (involving his orthopedic surgical privileges) and had not been granted privileges at some of the hospitals listed on the form. Expert testimony was that a hospital exercising ordinary care would not have appointed him to the medical staff. The Wisconsin Supreme Court held that a hospital has a duty to exercise due care in the selection of its medical staff: "The promotion of quality care and treatment of patients requires hospitals to perform a thorough evaluation of medical staff applicants...and further, to periodically review the qualifications of its staff through a peer review or medical audit mechanism." Delegation of the responsibility to the medical staff does not relieve the governing body of its duty to appoint only qualified practitioners and to periodically monitor and review their competency. On the initial application, at a minimum, the hospital should require that the application be complete and verify the applicant's statements especially as to education, training and experience. Additionally, it should solicit information from peers, including those not referenced in the application, determine current licensure and whether licensure has been subject to challenge, and inquire as to malpractice history.

Elam v. College Park Hospital, 183 Cal. Rptr. 156 (Cal. App. 1982)—Failure to Have Proper Supervision

Lawsuit by patient against podiatrists, coadmitting physician and hospital as a result of injuries following podiatric surgery. The podiatrists were independent contractors, not employees of the hospital. The hospital was granted summary judgment and the California appellate court reversed finding that the hospital had a duty to ensure the competency of its medical staff and to evaluate the quality of medical treatment rendered on its premises. In reaching its decision, the court examined the hospital's general duty to protect patients from harm, the statutory requirements for hospitals and accreditation standards regarding appointment, reappointment and peer review, and the public's perception that the hospital is a health care facility responsible for the quality of medical care and treatment rendered.

Mitchell County Hospital Authority v. Joiner, 189 S.E.2d 412 (Ga. 1972)—Governing Body is Ultimate Authority

Lawsuit by deceased patient's wife against physician and hospital where patient had been sent home from ER after chest pain and died later at home. Patient alleged that hospital was negligent in failing to require satisfactory proof of the professional qualifications of the physician, failing to investigate his qualifications, character or background, and failing to exercise ordinary care in determining competency and character. The hospital defended that it had delegated screening of applicants to the medical staff. The Georgia Supreme Court held that the fact that the medical staff had recommended appointment did not relieve the hospital of liability if the appointment was negligent since the medical staff acts as agent for the hospital.

Patrick v. Burget, 486 U.S. 94 (1988)—Medical Staff Peer Review

Dr. Patrick filed an antitrust lawsuit against the physicians of the Astoria Clinic alleging that they caused him to lose his hospital medical staff privileges as a result of his decision not to join the clinic and instead compete against it. While the jury found in Dr. Patrick's favor, the appellate court held that the physicians were immune from antitrust liability for even bad faith under the state action exemption. (The state action exemption applies if the action (here peer review) is articulated and affirmatively expressed as state policy and if the state actively supervises the activity.) The U.S. Supreme Court held that, although the state mandates that hospitals engage in peer review, the state is not involved in nor supervises the actual peer review decisions, therefore, the exemption did not apply and the physicians participating in the peer review could be held liable under antitrust theory.

Miller v. Eisenhower Medical Center, 614 P.2d 258 (Cal. 1980)—Disruptive Behavior

Lawsuit by a physician against the hospital for denial of medical staff membership based on inability to work with others as required by the medical staff bylaws. The physician argued that the standards for medical staff membership were so vague and uncertain as to allow for arbitrary or discriminatory application. The California Supreme Court held that even a private hospital may not permit exclusion from the medical staff on an arbitrary or irrational basis. The requirement to be able to work with others was permissible if there is a showing that the inability presents a real and substantial danger that patients might receive other than a high quality of medical care. In other words there must a link between the conduct and the potential effect on patient care. The court reversed the judgment in favor of the hospital.

Rao v. Auburn General Hospital, 573 P.2d 834 (Wash. Ct. App. 1978)—Disruptive Behavior

Lawsuit by physician against hospital for denying privileges. After a trial court held the physician was not entitled to recover, the physician appealed. The Washington appellate court held that a hospital has a discretionary right to exclude physicians whether based on lack of proficiency or a personality that will be detrimental to the working of the hospital. Additionally, the court should not substitute its evaluation of such matters for that of the hospital's governing board.

Robinson v. Magovern, 521 F.Supp. 842 (W.D. Pa. 1981), *aff'd without opinion*, 688 F.2d 824, *cert. denied*, 459 U.S. 971 (1982)—Denial of Application Not a Restraint of Trade

Lawsuit against hospital board members and certain thoracic surgeons by physician whose application for staff privileges was rejected. Allegations included violations of the antitrust law (Sherman Act) by agreements to limit thoracic surgery privileges to one group of which the department chief was a member, as well as denial of due process and breach of contract. The Court found that no hospital or surgical group had a monopoly, found a lack of evidence of specific anticompetitive intent, conspiracy or agreement to take joint action, and rejected Dr. Robinson's allegation that the hospital was an "essential facility" (denial of access creates a severe handicap for market entrants). The Court stated that (1) the hospital's policy of encouraging its medical staff to concentrate their practices at that hospital, (2) the concern regarding Dr. Robinson's contribution to the residency program, and (3) the concerns as to his alleged inability to work harmoniously with others advanced the hospital's institutional objectives of providing quality patient care and did not reasonably restrain trade. Because Dr. Robinson had open-heart privileges at other hospitals, the denial did not prevent cardiologists from referring to him or patients selecting him.

Jefferson Parish Hospital District No. 2 v. Hyde, 466 U. S. 2 (1984)—Upholding Hospital's Exclusive Contract

Lawsuit by anesthesiologist denied admission to the medical staff based on the hospital's exclusive anesthesia contract, alleging the contract violated antitrust law. The U.S. Supreme Court reversed the holding of the Fifth Circuit that the contract was illegal per se because it involved a "tying arrangement" by which the patient buying the operating room service also had to buy the anesthesia service. The Supreme Court found that the contract did not constitute an illegal tying arrangement because patients were not forced to purchase the anesthesia service, but could enter a competing hospital and use another anesthesia group. Tying arrangements are only condemned if they restrain competition by forcing purchases that would otherwise not be made. In the absence of an impermissible tying arrangement, the plaintiff must show that the challenged contract unreasonably restrained trade. There was no evidence that the price, quality or supply or demand for either the operating room service or the anesthesia service had been adversely affected by the exclusive contract or that the market as a whole had been affected by the contract.

Boyd v. Einstein Medical Center, 547 A.2d 1229 (Pa. Super. Ct. 1988)—Managed Care Organization Liable for Practitioner's Actions

Lawsuit against HMO and participating physicians following death of patient after alleged misdiagnosis. The patient's estate sought to recover against the HMO which had represented that the participating physicians were competent and evaluated for up to six months prior to being accepted into the HMO, on the theory that the physicians were ostensible agents of the HMO and therefore liable for their actions. The Pennsylvania Superior Court found that the policy reasons for holding hospitals liable for medical staff members under the ostensible agency theory applied equally to HMOs based on the limited provider list from which patients may select, the selection of the participating physicians by the HMO, the role of the gatekeeper in accessing a specialist, the fact that the patient does not contract directly with the physician but with the HMO, and the mechanics of payment for services. The court reversed the summary judgment granted for the HMO and remanded to the trial court.

Harrell v. Total Health Care, Inc., 1989 WL 153066 (Mo. App.), affirmed, 781 S.W.2d 58 (Mo. 1989)—Failure to Credential

Lawsuit by patient against health service organization for injuries as a result of malpractice during surgery based on corporate negligence and negligence in the selection of the surgeon. The appellate court examined the relationship between Total and the physician and the limited choice for the patient of physicians. The Missouri appellate court, finding an unreasonable risk of harm to subscribers if the physician is incompetent, held there was a common law duty owed to conduct a reasonable investigation to ascertain the physician's reputation for competency. The court left the extent of the investigation to be determined on a case by case basis, but said no investigation means the duty has not been met. By statute, a health service corporation was immune from liability for any negligence of a person or entity rendering health services to the corporation's members and beneficiaries, therefore, the Missouri Supreme Court affirmed the summary judgment granted for Total. The court also stated it saw no reason that a HMO might not also be a health service corporation and, therefore, eligible for the same immunity.

McClellan v. Health Maintenance Organization of Pennsylvania, 604 A.2d 1053 (Pa. Super. Ct. 1992)—Duty to Select and Monitor Providers

Lawsuit by patient against HMO based on corporate negligence and ostensible agency theory for negligence of participating physician in not submitting a mole tissue sample for testing. The Pennsylvania Superior Court held that there was sufficient evidence to submit the issue of whether the physician was an ostensible agent of the HMO based on the representations of the HMO as to the quality of the physicians and other factors. Although the court did not extend the theory of corporate negligence used with hospitals to HMOs, it held that HMOs have a nondelegable duty to select and retain only competent physicians, allowing that issue also to be submitted to a jury for decision.

Appendix B: Practitioner's Hearing Rights Under Health Care Quality Improvement Act, 42 U.S.C.A. §11112(b).

(1) Notice of proposed action

The physician has been given notice stating—

(A) (i) that a professional review action has been proposed to be taken against the physician,

(ii) reasons for the proposed action,

(B) (i) that the physician has the right to request a hearing on the proposed action,

(ii) any time limit (of not less than 30 days) within which to request such a hearing, and

(C) a summary of the rights in the hearing under paragraph (3).

(2) Notice of hearing

If a hearing is requested on a timely basis under paragraph (1)(B), the physician involved must be given notice stating—

(A) the place, time, and date, of the hearing, which date shall not be less than 30 days after the date of the notice, and

(B) a list of the witnesses (if any) expected to testify at the hearing on behalf of the professional review body.

(3) Conduct of hearing and notice

If a hearing is requested on a timely basis under paragraph (1)(B)—

(A) subject to subparagraph (B), the hearing shall be held (as determined by the healthcare entity)—

(i) before an arbitrator mutually acceptable to the physician and the healthcare entity,

(ii) before a hearing officer who is appointed by the entity and who is not in direct economic competition with the physician involved, or

(iii) before a panel of individuals who are appointed by the entity and are not in direct economic competition with the physician involved;

(B) the right to the hearing may be forfeited if the physician fails, without good cause, to appear;

(C) in the hearing the physician involved has the right—

(i) to representation by an attorney or other person of the physician's choice,

(ii) to have a record made of the proceedings, copies of which may be obtained by the physician upon payment of any reasonable charges associated with the preparation thereof,

(iii) to call, examine, and cross-examine witnesses,

(iv) to present evidence determined to be relevant by the hearing officer, regardless of its admissibility in a court of law, and

(v) to submit a written statement at the close of the hearing;

(D) upon completion of the hearing, the physician involved has the right—

(i) to receive the written recommendation of the arbitrator, officer, of panel, including a statement of the basis for the recommendations, and

(ii) to receive a written decision of the healthcare entity, including a statement of the basis for the decision.

Appendix C: Recommended References on Legal Issues

1. Health Care Quality Improvement Act, 42 U.S.C.A. §11111 et seq.

2. National Practitioner Data Bank Guide Book (NPDB Help Line 1-800-767-6732)

3. Medicare Conditions of Participation for Governing Body and Medical Staff, 42 C.F.R. §482.11-.66

4. Joint Commission on Accreditation of Healthcare Organizations, *Accreditation Manual for Hospitals*, Governing Board and Medical Staff Standards

5. State laws on

    a. health care entity licensure as applicable to medical staff

    b. peer review privileges of confidentiality and immunity, including governmental agency access to peer review information

    c. reporting of professional review actions or other issues involved physicians or other practitioners on the medical staff

NOTES

1. Joint Commission on Accreditation of Healthcare Organizations, *1998* Comprehensive *Accreditation Manual for Hospitals* (Oakbrook Terrace, IL: Joint Commission on Accreditation of Healthcare Organizations, 1998).

2. 42 C.F.R. Part 482 (1997).

3. See for example *Gonzalez v. San Jacinto Methodist Hosp.*, 880 S.W.2d 436 (Tex. App.— Texarkana 1994, writ denied) (finding bylaws are a contract); *Gianetti v. Norwalk Hosp.*, 557 A.2d 1249 (Conn. 1989) (holding are not a contract).

4. 42 U.S.C.A. § 11101 et seq. (1995).

5. But see *Agbor v. St. Luke's Episcopal Hospital*, 952 S.W.2d 503 (Tex. 1997) (holding that state peer review immunity statute applied to patient's cause of action against hospital for negligent credentialing).

6. 211 N.E.2d 253 (Ill. 1965) (See Appendix A)

7. See Appendix A for discussion of additional cases dealing with corporate negligence (e.g., *Purcell, Johnson, Elam*).

8. Joint Commission on Accreditation of Healthcare Organizations, *1998 Comprehensive Accreditation Manual for Hospitals,* MS.5.4.

9. See for example, Tex. Health & Safety Code § 241.101 (West Supp. 1998).

10. *Hay v. Scripps Memorial Hospital*, 228 Cal. Rptr. 413 (Ct. App. 1986).

11. *Kahn v. Suburban Community Hospital*, 340 N.E.2d 398 (Ohio 1976); *Hull v. Board of Commissioners of Halifax Hospital*, 453 So. 2d 519 (Fla. Dist. Ct. App. 1984); *Cameron v. New Hanover Memorial Hospital, Inc.*, 293 S.E.2d 901 (N.C. Ct. App. 1982); *Sarasota County Public Hospital Board v. Shahawy*, 408 So. 2d 644 (Fla. Dist. Ct. App. 1981); *Armstrong v. Board of Directors of Fayette County General Hospital*, 553 S.W.2d 77 (Tenn. Ct. App. 1976).

12. 42 C.F.R. § 482.12(a)(7) (1997).

13. Medicare & Medicaid Guide (CCH) ¶45,128 (1997), p. 53,189.

14. Joint Commission on Accreditation of Healthcare Organizations, *1998 Comprehensive Accreditation Manual for Hospitals*, MS.5.4.3.

15. See for example, *Stein v. Tri-City Hosp. Auth.*, 384 S.E.2d 430 (Ga. App. 1989); *Kling v. St. Paul Fire & Marine Ins. Co.*, 626 F. Supp. 1285 (C.D. Ill. 1986); *Backlund v. Board of Comm'rs*, 724 P.2d 981 (Wash 1986), appeal dism'd, 481 U.S. 1034 (1987); *Holmes v. Holmako Hosp.*, 573 P.2d 477 (Ariz. 1977).

16. Joint Commission on Accreditation of Healthcare Organizations, *1988 Comprehensive Accreditation Manual for Hospitals,* MS.5.7.

17. *Id.* at MS.5.4.3.

18. 42 U.S.C.A. Chap. 126 (1995)

19. *Menkowitz v. Pottstown Medical Center*, 1997 U.S. Dist. LEXIS 19116, *8 (E.D. Pa. 1997).

20. See for example, *Donahue v. The Melrose Hotel*, 1997 U.S. Dist. LEXIS 4877, *16 (N.D. Tex. 1997) (citing 29 C.F.R. Part 1630, App. 1996).

21. See for example, *Estate of William Mauro v. Borgess Medical Center*, 137 F.3d 393 (6th Cir. 1998).

22. See cases at Appendix A.

23. Joint Commission on Accreditation of Healthcare Organizations, *1998 Comprehensive Accreditation Manual for Hospitals*, MS.5.10.2.

24. 500 P.2d 335 (Ariz. Ct. App. 1972) (See Appendix A).

25. U.S. Department of Health and Human Services, Public Health Service, Health Resources and Services Administration, *National Practitioner Data Bank Guidebook* DHHS Pub. no. HRSA 95-255 (Washington, DC: US Government Printing Office, 1996): E-16.

26. Id. at E-20.

27. See discussion in Joint Commission on Accreditation of Healthcare Organizations, *Medical Staff Credentialing*, (Oakbrook Terrace, IL: Joint Commission on Accreditation of Healthcare Organizations, 1993): 28-29.

28. See for example *Jefferson Parish Hosp. Dist. No. 2 v. Hyde*, 466 U.S. 2 (1984); *Dutta v. St. Francis Regional Medical Center*, 867 P.2d 1057 (Kan. 1994); *Bartley v. Eastern Maine Medical Center*, 617 A.2d 1020 (Me. 1992) (See Appendix A on *Jefferson Parish* case).

29. Joint Commission on Accreditation of Healthcare Organizations, *1998 Comprehensive Accreditation Manual for Hospitals,* MS.5.2, 5.2.1.

30. 42 U.S.C.A. §11151(1) (1995).

31. Joint Commission on Accreditation of Healthcare Organizations, *1998 Comprehensive Accreditation Manual for Hospitals,* MS.5.2.

32. See exception in HCQIA, 42 U.S.C.A. §11112(c)(2) (1995).

33. 486 U.S. 94 (1988) (See Appendix A).

34. 42 U.S.C.A. §11111(a) (1995).

35. *Id.* at §11151(8).

36. *Id.* at §11151(9).

37. *Id.*

38. *Id.* at §11112(a).

39. *Id.* at §11112(b).

40. *Id.* at §11112(a).

41. *Id.* at §11133(1)(B).

42. U.S. Department of Health and Human Services, Public Health Service, Health Resources and Service Administration, *National Practitioner Data Bank Guidebook,* DHHS Pub. no. HRSA-96-255 (Washington, DC: US Government Printing Office, 1996): E-16, E-17.

43. 42 U.S.C.A. §11112(b)(1)(A) (1995).

44. See *Rosenblit v. Fountain Valley Regional Hospital and Medical Center,* 282 Cal. Rptr. 819 (Cal. App. 1991) for excellent discussion of notice issues.

45. See for example, *Huntsville Memorial Hospital v. Honorable Erwin G. Ernst*, 763 S.W.2d 856 (Tex. App. - Houston [14th Dist.] 1998, no writ history).

46. 42 U.S.C.A. §11112(b)(3)(A) (1995).

47. *Id.* at § 11112(b)(3)(C)(i).

48. *Smith v. Ricks,* 31 F.3d 1478 (9th Cir. 1994).

49. 42 U.S.C.A. §11112(b)(3)(D)(i) (1995).

50. *Id.* at §11112(b)(3)(D)(ii) (1995).

51. See *Irving Healthcare System v. Honorable David Brooks,* 927 S.W.2d 12 (Tex. 1995).

52. HCQIA addresses confidentiality, but only as to information provided to the National Practitioner Data Bank. 42 U.S.C.A. § 11137(b) (1995). HCQIA does not afford confidentiality generally to peer review records and proceedings as do most state laws.

53. 42 U.S.C.A. §11111(a)(1) (1995). Keep in mind that HCQIA's immunity only applies to actions involving a "physician," defined as a medical doctor, doctor of osteopathic medicine, or doctor of dental surgery or medical dentistry. *Id.* at §11151(8).

54. *Id.* at §11151(11).

55. *Id.* at §11151(10).
56. *Id.* at §11111(a)(2).
57. *Id.* at §11111(b).
58. *Id.* at §11131.
59. *Id.* at §11132.
60. *Id.* at §11133.
61. *Id.* at §11133(a)(2).
62. Joint Commission on Accreditation of Healthcare Organizations, *1996 Comprehensive Accreditation Manual for Health Care Networks* (Oakbrook Terrace, IL: Joint Commission on Accreditation of Healthcare Organizations, 1996); National Committee on Quality Assurance, *1998 Standards for Managed Care Organizations,* (Washington, DC: National Committee on Quality Assurance, 1998).
63. Joint Commission on Accreditation of Healthcare Organizations, *1997 Accreditation Manual for Preferred Provider Organizations* (Oakbrook Terrace, IL: Joint Commission on Accreditation of Healthcare Organizations, 1996).
64. 1989 WL 153066 (Mo. App.), affirmed, 781 S.W.2d 58 (Mo. 1989) (en banc) (see Appendix A).
65. 604 A.2d 1053 (Pa. Super. Ct. 1992), appeal denied, 616 A.2d 985 (Pa. 1992) (see Appendix A).
66. 42 U.S.C.A. §11133, §11151(4) (1995).
67. Joint Commission on Accreditation of Healthcare Organizations, *1996 Comprehensive Accreditation Manual for Healthcare Networks,* LD.3 (Oakbrook Terrace, IL: Joint Commission on Accreditation of Healthcare Organizations, 1996); National Committee for Quality Assurance, *1998 Guidelines for the Accreditation of Managed Care Organizations,* CR 13 (Washington, DC: National Committee for Quality Assurance, 1998).
68. National Committee for Quality Assurance, *1997 Standards for Certification of Credentials Verification Organizations* (Washington, DC: National Committee for Quality Assurance, 1997): 7.
69. National Committee for Quality Assurance, *1997 Surveyor Guidelines for the Accreditation of Managed Care Organizations* (Washington, DC: National Committee for Quality Assurance, 1997): 172.

Chapter 18

Supporting Fair Hearing Procedures

Cindy A. Gassiot, CMSC, CPCS

As mentioned in an earlier chapter, the medical staff services professional (MSSP) is often the conduit for the medical staff organization to the health care facility's legal counsel. There is no more critical time for the MSSP to contact the medical staff's attorney than when corrective action is contemplated which may trigger the fair hearing process. Medical staff leaders are often unfamiliar with procedures for investigations, corrective actions, and fair hearings, and the legal and time frame requirements that are usually detailed in the medical staff bylaws or a fair hearing plan. It is of critical importance that the MSSP guides medical staff leaders in exact adherence to the bylaws provisions for these activities and ensures that legal advice is obtained early in the process. Should an adversely affected practitioner resort to litigation following exhaustion of due process rights, the courts will carefully scrutinize the process the health care facility used. Good documentation supporting protection of the affected practitioner's rights and evidence that the facility followed its own policies, procedures, and bylaws are obviously the best defenses for any action against the facility.

ROLE OF THE MSSP

The MSSP plays an important role in supporting the corrective action and fair hearing processes that includes planning, adherence to bylaws and legal requirements, documenting the process, and maintaining confidentiality. Making arrangements for a hearing can be very time-consuming and challenging. The MSSP must be prepared to spend many hours conferring with legal counsel, preparing correspondence and evidence notebooks, arranging dates with busy practitioners, arranging for a court reporter and hearing officer, contacting witnesses, and paying careful attention to numerous details.

PLANNING

When an adverse recommendation has been made and the fair hearing procedure has been triggered, meticulous attention must be given to the time frames allowed for each step of the procedure. A checklist (see Table 18-1) outlining each step of the procedure and the time within which the step must be accomplished will be a helpful tool in adhering to the required procedure.

Table 18-1. Sample Checklist for Steps in the Fair Hearing Process.

Procedural Steps	Date Required	Date Accomplished
1. Recommendation for adverse action		
2. Notification to practitioner, including reason for proposed action (30 days to request hearing)		
3. Request for hearing		
4. Hearing panel appointed		
5. Hearing scheduled		
6. Practitioner notified of hearing date, time and place (not less than 30 days from date of notice)		
7. Medical staff representative designated		
8. Court reporter notified		
9. Hearing officer appointed		
10. Hearing panel orientation		
11. Hearing held		
12. Hearing panel report		
13. Notice to practitioner, and others required by Fair Hearing Plan or Bylaws, with basis for recommendation		
14. Appellate Review, if applicable		
15. Final action by governing body		
16. Notice of final decision to affected practitioner with basis for action		
17. NPDB report to State Board of Medical Examiners, if indicated (within 15 days of final action)		

CORRESPONDENCE

When the hearing process has been triggered, the MSSP usually prepares the correspondence to the affected practitioner. Again, careful attention should be given to required time frames when preparing correspondence to the affected practitioner and all correspondence should be reviewed by legal counsel to ensure that legal requirements have been met.

ORIENTATION OF HEARING PANEL

Most practitioners are not familiar with a fair hearing procedure. If a hearing panel or committee is used for the hearing (versus an arbitrator or hearing officer), when the members have been identified, it is helpful to orient them to the procedure. Legal counsel should be engaged to present the orientation, which should describe the manner in which the hearing will be conducted. The facts or details of the matter under consideration are never discussed with the panel prior to the actual hearing; the purpose of the orientation is to prepare panel members for what can be expected to occur in the actual proceeding. A copy of the fair hearing plan or bylaws article should always be provided to panel members and can be used as the basis for the orientation session.

Hearing panel members should be instructed to arrange for practice coverage during the hearing and advised to leave pagers and cell phones turned off.

EVIDENCE NOTEBOOK

Thorough, accurate documentation of all events leading up to a fair hearing procedure is critical. The written results of an investigation will usually be used as evidence in any hearing and plays an important role in the outcome. Many health care facilities use an evidence notebook as a means of supporting the facility's case against the affected practitioner. The MSSP usually prepares this notebook, which must also be made available to the affected practitioner prior to the hearing, as he or she has a right to review all evidence in order to prepare a defense to the allegations made. Again, legal counsel should be consulted to assist in preparation of the evidence notebook and to advise about its release to the affected practitioner and his or her attorney.

ARRANGING THE HEARING ROOM

Since the parties involved in a fair hearing will most likely spend many hours listening to the evidence presented, a comfortable setting is important. Comfortable chairs should be at the top of the list even if chairs have to be brought from other locations in the facility. Food and drink should also be available, as hearings usually go on into the night. The room in which the hearing is held is usually arranged somewhat like a courtroom setting (see Figure 18-1).

Figure 18-1. Room Arrangement for Fair Hearing Procedure.

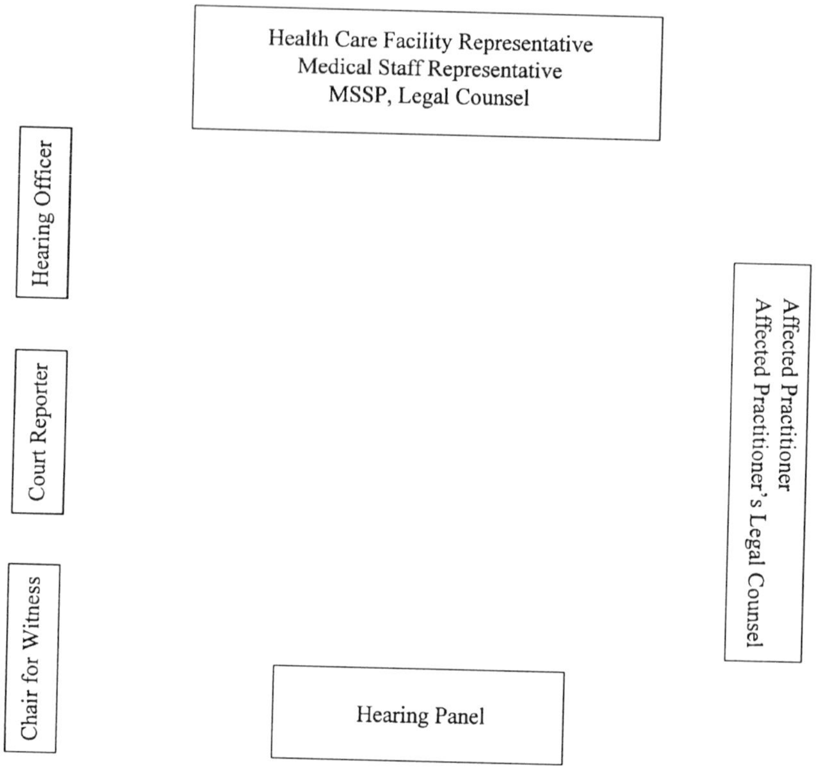

Health Care Facility Representative
Medical Staff Representative
MSSP, Legal Counsel

Hearing Officer

Court Reporter

Chair for Witness

Affected Practitioner
Affected Practitioner's Legal Counsel

Hearing Panel

THE HEARING

The MSSP usually attends the hearing and sits with legal counsel, the medical staff representative, and other health care facility representatives, if present. The MSSP can assist with calling witnesses into the hearing room, referring to the medical staff bylaws, and performing other tasks as needed.

Hearings frequently cannot be completed in one session and the MSSP will be required to schedule subsequent sessions.

FOLLOW-UP

When the hearing panel has reached its decision, the MSSP will assist in preparation of the report and assure that the report is forwarded through channels as outlined in the fair hearing plan or bylaws. Once a final decision is made, the MSSP will prepare the correspondence notifying the affected practitioner. Again, legal counsel should be consulted when preparing any correspondence or other documentation relating to the process.

Fair hearings will test the ability of the MSSP to precisely follow the procedures outlined and to guide medical staff leaders and other participants in doing the same. Assisting with the fair hearing process is one of the most important and interesting functions the MSSP performs.

Index

About the Editors

Cindy A. Gassiot, CMSC, CPCS, began her career in medical staff services and quality management in 1970. She has held the position of director of medical staff services and quality management in several Texas hospitals. She is currently Director of Medical Staff Services at Cook Children's Medical Center in Fort Worth, Texas.

Ms. Gassiot is past president of the National Association Medical Staff Services and was charter president of the Texas Society for Medical Staff Services, which she co-founded. She was the first recipient of the Golden Key Award presented by the National Association Medical Staff Services for contributions to the establishment of the CMSC Certification program. She is an honorary member of the Texas Society for Medical Staff Services and was awarded the Outstanding Medical Staff Services Professional by TSMSS in 1997.

Ms. Gassiot is an adjunct faculty member of the medical staff services program at El Centro College, Dallas, and co-authored the curriculum for the program. She is co-author of *Medical Staff Services Manual* (1981)*, Principles of Medical Staff Services Science* (1987) and the *Handbook of Medical Staff Management* (1990). Ms. Gassiot lives in Grapevine, Texas with her husband John.

Vicki L. Searcy is a Principal of BDO Seidman, LLP, Healthcare Advisory Services. Since 1988, she has been a consultant to health care organizations, primarily in the areas of working with physicians and health care organization leaders on issues related to credentialing, privileging and quality, as well as interpretation and application of accreditation standards and licensing requirements.

Ms. Searcy is a past president of the National Association Medical Staff Services, is a frequent speaker for professional organizations on topics that relate to medical and professional staff organization management and is a surveyor for the National Committee on Quality Assurance's CVO certification program.

Ms. Searcy is a contributing editor to *Health Care Competency & Credentialing Report*, a national monthly publication. She has developed several training manuals for NAMSS that are used to teach seminars, and writes numerous articles which are published in a variety of newsletters and magazines.

Ms. Searcy received the 1998 Woman of Achievement Award in Healthcare from the City of Los Angeles. She serves as a board member on the Juvenile Diabetes Foundation (Los Angeles Chapter).